New Paradigms in Implant Dentistry

New Paradigms in Implant Dentistry

Editor: Victor Martinez

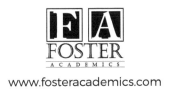

www.fosteracademics.com

www.fosteracademics.com

Cataloging-in-Publication Data

New paradigms in implant dentistry / edited by Victor Martinez.
    p. cm.
Includes bibliographical references and index.
ISBN 978-1-64646-589-7
1. Dental implants. 2. Dental implants--Complications. 3. Mouth--Surgery.
4. Implants, Artificial. 5. Dentures. 6. Dentistry. I. Martinez, Victor.
RK667.I45 N49 2023
617.693--dc23

Foster Academics,
118-35 Queens Blvd., Suite 400,
Forest Hills, NY 11375, USA

ISBN 978-1-64646-589-7 (Hardback)

Contents

Preface

A dental implant is a type of prosthesis, which is introduced in the jaw bone or skull for providing support to dental prosthesis like a denture, facial prosthesis, or crown-bridge. It can also be used as an orthodontic anchor. Success and failure of the dental implants is dependent on the health of the individual undergoing the procedure, as well as the drugs which are administered. The complications and risks related with dental implants that can happen during surgery include nerve injury or excessive bleeding. The long term complications associated with such procedures include mechanical failures and peri-implantitis. Technologies like interactive software applications, cone-beam computed tomography and computed tomography are facilitating the development of significant tools for diagnosis, planning the treatment, and fixing the dental implant along with surgical and restorative procedures. This book explores all the important aspects of implant dentistry in the present day scenario. With state-of-the-art inputs acclaimed by experts in this field, this book targets students and professionals.

This book is the end result of constructive efforts and intensive research done by experts in this field. The aim of this book is to enlighten the readers with recent information in this area of research. The information provided in this profound book would serve as a valuable reference to students and researchers in this field.

At the end, I would like to thank all the authors for devoting their precious time and providing their valuable contribution to this book. I would also like to express my gratitude to my fellow colleagues who encouraged me throughout the process.

Editor

Comparison of 3D-Printed Dental Implants with Threaded Implants for Osseointegration

Ling Li [1,†][iD], Jungwon Lee [2,†][iD], Heithem Ben Amara [1][iD], Jun-Beom Lee [1], Ki-Sun Lee [3][iD], Sang-Wan Shin [4], Yong-Moo Lee [1], Byoungkook Kim [5], Pangyu Kim [5] and Ki-Tae Koo [1,*]

[1] Department of Periodontology and Dental Research Institute, School of Dentistry, Seoul National University, Seoul 03080, Korea; applemint1228@snu.ac.kr (L.L.); benamarahaitham@yahoo.fr (H.B.A.); dentjblee@gmail.com (J.-B.L.); ymlee@snu.ac.kr (Y.-M.L.)

[2] One-Stop Specialty Center, Seoul National University Dental Hospital & Department of Periodontology, School of Dentistry, Seoul National University, Seoul 03080, Korea; jungwonlee.snudh@gmail.com

[3] Department of Prosthodontics, Korea University Ansan Hospital, Ansan 15355, Gyeonggi-do, Korea; kisuns@gmail.com

[4] Department of Advanced Prosthodontics, Graduate School of Clinical Dentistry, Korea University, Seoul 02841, Korea; swshin@korea.ac.kr

[5] 3D Printer R&D Team, Dentium Co., Ltd., Suwon 16229, Gyeonggi-do, Korea; bkkim1@dentium.com (B.K.); pgkim@dentium.com (P.K.)

* Correspondence: periokoo@snu.ac.kr

† These authors contributed equally to this work.

Abstract: This study aimed to compare bone healing and implant stability for three types of dental implants: a threaded implant, a three-dimensional (3D)-printed implant without spikes, and a 3D-printed implant with spikes. In four beagle dogs, left and right mandibular premolars (2nd, 3rd, and 4th) and 1st molars were removed. Twelve weeks later, three types of titanium implants (threaded implant, 3D-printed implant without spikes, and 3D-printed implant with spikes) were randomly inserted into the edentulous ridges of each dog. Implant stability measurements and radiographic recordings were taken every two weeks following implant placement. Twelve weeks after implant surgery, the dogs were sacrificed and bone-to-implant contact (BIC) and bone area fraction occupied (BAFO) were compared between groups. At implant surgery, the primary stability was lower for the 3D-printed implant with spikes (74.05 ± 5.61) than for the threaded implant (83.71 ± 2.90) ($p = 0.005$). Afterwards, no significant difference in implants' stability was observed between groups up to post-surgery week 12. Histomorphometrical analysis did not reveal a significant difference between the three implants for BIC ($p = 0.101$) or BAFO ($p = 0.288$). Within the limits of this study, 3D-printed implants without spikes and threaded implants showed comparable implant stability measurements, BIC, and BAFO.

Keywords: 3D printing; computer-aided design; customized dental implant; patient matched; implant stability

1. Introduction

Various types of dental implants have been developed to replace edentulous areas. Endosseous blade implants and disk implants designed in the 1960s disappeared from the market because of their low survival rate and the extensive bone destruction that would occur around the implant [1,2]. Endosseous dental implants have been considered as the current standard shape, and the surface in contact with the bone is subjected to large shear forces under load [3].

The most widely used implants on the market today are threaded implants. However, such implants are limited in design owing to the need for mass production. Close contact between the recipient site and the implant is essential for proper osseointegration [4]. Therefore, the current implants cannot completely satisfy the requirements of individual patients [5]. Titanium implants with high surface porosity and high core density may allow better load adaptation, while avoiding stress shielding and pressure-induced bone loss [6–8]. However, the manufacturing of personalized implants with this structure is considerably challenging and expensive. In contrast, if a three-dimensional (3D) printing method is used, personalized implants with a complex structure can be manufactured at a lower cost and with more simplicity [9].

Recently, the application of 3D printing technology in dentistry has grown at a rapid pace. The reasons for this rapid development are the possibility of savings on small-scale productions, the ability to manufacture personalized products, the ease of sharing and handling patient imaging data, and the increased number of people who understand and can carry out this process [10]. 3D printing technology is gaining increased attention in the dentistry field thanks to advances in 3D imaging and modeling technologies, such as intraoral scanning and cone-beam computed tomography, and the increasing use of computer-aided design & computer-aided manufacturing (CAD/CAM) technology [11]. 3D printing is also known as additive manufacturing, in which rapid prototyping uses a focused laser beam to create complex shapes layer-by-layer [12]. Implants made using 3D printing technology are custom designed to accommodate the geometry of each individual's anatomic structure, preserving soft and hard tissue and reducing the duration of the healing period [5,13]. The technology makes it easier to create an implant with complex structures. In addition, unlike the cutting or milling process, 3D printing can be conducted without molds or other tools, which is more economical and reduces material loss [14].

Although 3D printing technology is used in many aspects of the dental field, clinical data are still limited regarding the manufacturing of dental implants. The purpose of this study was to compare the sequential implant stability and histologic differences between 3D-printed implants and threaded implants.

2. Materials and Methods

2.1. Animals

The study protocol was approved by the Institutional Animal Care and Use Committee (IACUC), Seoul National University (IACUC No. SNU-190226-4), and the study was conducted in compliance with guidelines of the Institute of Laboratory Animal Resources, Seoul National University. This research regulated by the principle of the 3Rs (replacement, reduction, and refinement). Four male beagle dogs, at 1 year of age and a weight between 10 and 12 kg, were used in the study. At the time of recruitment, all animals were healthy and the dentition was normal. Before the experiment, the beagle dogs were acclimated to the facility for 1 week. The dogs were individually housed in 90 cm × 80 cm × 80 cm (width × depth × height) indoor kennels. They drank freely and were fed a standard pellet dog food diet (HappyRang, Seoulfeed, Korea) or a crushed diet after the implants were placed. The study outline is presented in Figure 1.

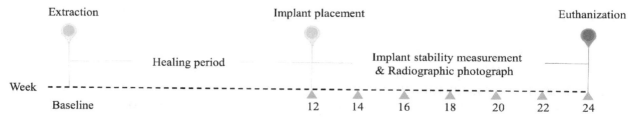

Figure 1. Outline of the experiment. At baseline, the second, third, and fourth premolars and first molars were extracted from the left and right sides of the mandible. After 12 weeks, three different implants were randomly placed in the healing ridges.

2.2. Study Implants

Titanium implants with three different designs, but with similar dimensions, were used in this study (Figure 2): a threaded implant (Superline, Dentium, Seoul, Korea), which was a two-piece bone level implant with 3.7 mm in diameter and 8 mm in length (T; control); a 3D-printed implant without spikes, which was a one-piece tissue level implant with 3.8 mm in diameter and 8 mm in length (3D; test 1); and a 3D-printed implant with spikes, which was a one-piece tissue level implant with 3.8 mm in diameter and 8 mm in length (3DS: test 2).

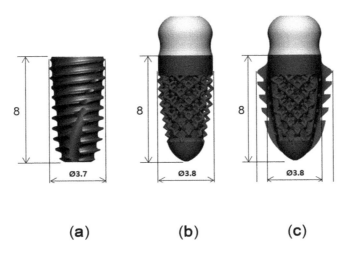

(a)   (b)   (c)

Figure 2. Three implants with different designs. (**a**): SuperLine Fixture (FXS 36 08); (**b**): 3D-printed implant without spikes; (**c**): 3D-printed implant with spikes.

The 3D-printed implant used a dodecahedron lattice structure with a porosity of 70% and a lattice thickness of 250 μm (Figure 3). They were designed with and without spikes to compare the influence of the spikes on implant stability. The spikes' structure was designed in order to provide additional fixation on the extraction site and sidewalls. The 3D-printed implants were printed on a 3D printer Mlab200R (Concept Laser, Lichtenfels, Germany) using Ti-Gr2 (ConceptLaser, Lichtenfels, Germany). The 3D printer uses direct metal laser melting (DMLM) technology to create complex metal 3D geometries. For the surface of the 3D-printed implant, only blasting was performed without any surface treatment. The T implant encompasses sandblasting with large grits and acid etching (SLA) surface and is made of Ti-Gr5.

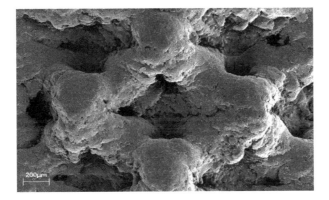

Figure 3. Scanning electron microscopy (SEM) image of the 3D-printed implant without spikes macroporous structure. Both 3D-printed implants feature the same surface.

In order to identify the precision of the 3D-printed products, five rectangular parallelepipedons having a width of 15 mm, a length of 15 mm, and a height of 6 mm were manufactured. When measuring the length of the manufactured rectangular parallelepiped, the maximum error was 9.7 μm (Table 1).

Table 1. Accuracy analysis of 3D-printed products.

Test	x (mm)			y (mm)			z (mm)		
	Reference Values	Measures	Error	Reference Values	Measures	Error	Reference Values	Measures	Error
1		15.0097	0.0097		15.0045	0.0045		6.0034	0.0034
2		15.0081	0.0081		15.0067	0.0067		6.0029	0.0029
3	15.0000	15.0061	0.0061	15.0000	15.0018	0.0018	6.0000	6.0011	0.0011
4		15.0042	0.0042		15.0061	0.0061		6.0005	0.0005
5		15.0084	0.0084		15.0052	0.0052		6.0044	0.0044
Mean		15.0073	0.0073		15.0049	00049		6.0025	0.0025

2.3. Surgical Procedure

All surgical procedures were performed under general anesthesia with an intravenous injection of Zoletil® (5 mg/kg; Virbac, Carros, France), Rompun® (2.3 mg/kg; Bayer Korea, Ansan, Korea), and atropine sulfate (0.05 mg/kg; Jeil Pharm., Daegu, Korea). A complementary local anesthesia was performed at surgical sites with 2% lidocaine HCL with epinephrine (1:1,000,000) (20 mg/kg; Huons, Seongnam, Korea). On the left and right side of the mandible in all dogs, the second, third, and fourth premolars (PM2, PM3, and PM4, respectively) and the first molars (M1) were atraumatically extracted with flap elevation. To reduce damage to the alveolar bone, a hemisection was made in the buccolingual direction of the teeth with diamond fissure burs. The surgical site was closed with a suture (Monosyn 5/0, B Braun Aesculap, Tuttlingen, Germany), and the suture was removed after 1 week.

At 12 weeks after tooth extraction, an incision was made in the crest to place the implants (Figure 4a,b). A full-thickness flap was reflected and drilled for the placement of three different implants. The drilling sequence for the T implant was accomplished following the manufacturer's recommendations. The drilling sequence for the 3D implant started from the initial drill (2.2 mm diameter), a second drill (2.6 mm diameter), two twist drills (2.9 mm and 3.35 mm in diameter), and then ended with the countersink drill (3.6 mm diameter). The drilling sequence for the 3DS implant started from the initial drill (2.2 mm diameter), a second drill (2.6 mm diameter), three twist drills (2.9 mm, 3.35 mm, and 3.85 mm in diameter), and then ended with the countersink drill (4.5 mm diameter). The implants were randomly placed at three positions on each of the left side and the right side of the mandible (six implants per dog). A random sequence was generated using the simple method of the www.random.org website. T implants were placed using a motor-driven handpiece (EXPERTsurg™ LUX, KaVo, Germany) and 3D and 3DS implants heads were directly tapped using a surgical mallet. Subsequently, the T implants were secured with a cover screw. The flap was repositioned and sutured with 5/0 Monosyn® (B Braun Aesculap, Tuttlingen, Germany), and the sutures were removed 1 week later. The surgical procedures were performed by one periodontist.

2.4. Postoperative Management

To mitigate postoperative pain and inflammation, antibiotics (Cefazoline 20 mg/kg; Chongkundang Pharm., Seoul, Korea), analgesics (Toranzin 5 mg/kg; Samsung Pharm., Gyeonggi-do, Korea), and antispasmodics (atropine sulfate 0.05 mg/kg; Jeil Pharm., Daegu, Korea) were intravenously injected after tooth extraction and implant placement. In addition, antibiotics (amoxicillin 500 mg; Chongkundang Pharm., Seoul, Korea) and analgesics (ibuprofen 400 mg, Daewoong Pharm., Seoul, Korea) were mixed with the animals' diet three days after the operations. All dogs were placed under soft diet for one month after surgery to avoid any mechanical interference with the postsurgical healing, and surgical areas were checked twice per week to confirm whether any complications had occurred. Meanwhile, all the surgical sites were rinsed with 0.12% chlorhexidine gluconate solution after feeding (Hexamedine®, Bukwang Pharm., Seoul, Korea).

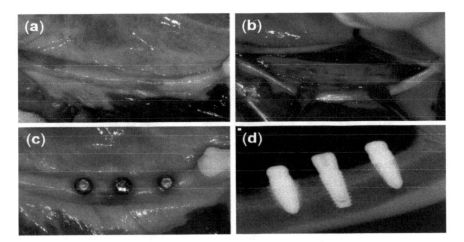

Figure 4. Clinical photographs from the present study. (**a**) Twelve weeks after tooth extraction, (**b**) horizontal incision and flap reflection, (**c**) 8 weeks after implant placement, and (**d**) periapical radiograph of three different types of implants after 8 weeks of healing.

2.5. Implant Stability Measurements

As a result of limitations of resonance frequency analysis in measuring the 3D-printed implants' stability, damping capacity analysis (Anycheck, Neobiotech, Seoul, Korea) was used for implant stability analysis [15]. The implant stability measurements and periapical radiographic recordings were performed every two weeks following implant placement under general anesthesia. Each implant was measured five times on the buccal side. The average value of the measurements from the five times was considered as representative for each implant.

2.6. Histologic Observation and Histomorphometric Analysis

At 12 weeks after implant placement, the beagle dogs were sacrificed by carotid injection with potassium chloride (75 mg/kg; Jeil Pharm., Daegu, Korea). Block biopsies including the extraction sites were collected for histologic observation and histomorphometric analysis. The specimens were placed in a fixative solution containing 10% neutral formalin buffer for 1 week, and subsequently dehydrated in graded ethanol solution. Thereafter, the samples were embedded in resin blocks (Technovit 7200; Heraeus Kulzer, Hanau, Germany) with a UV embedding system (KULZER EXAKT 520, Hanau, Germany) according to the manufacturer's recommendation. The sectioning procedure was performed using a diamond saw. Thereafter, the sections were ground and polished to approximately 80 ± 5 µm, and then stained with Goldner trichrome. On slide scans produced at 20× magnification, histomorphometric analysis was performed using ImageJ 1.51j8 (National Institutes of Health, Bethesda, MD, USA) to measure bone-to-implant contact (BIC) and bone area fraction occupied (BAFO) in a region of interest (ROI) set to the coronal half of each implant (Figure 5).

2.7. Statistical Analyses

The sample size of eight per group was obtained by power analysis under the assumption of a mean difference of 20 among a control group and two experimental groups, with a common sd of 12 (effect size: Cohen's f = 0.786) and 90.0% of power, 0.05 alpha level using GPower version 3.1.9.2.

Statistical analyses were performed using SPSS version 25 (IBM Software, Armonk, NY, USA). Descriptive statistics are expressed as the mean ± standard deviation. The Kruskal–Wallis test was used to compare the effect of different implant designs with the results of implant stability values and histomorphometric data (BIC and BAFO) at an alpha level of 0.05. In the case of statistically significant differences, pairwise post hoc comparisons were performed at $p = 0.017$ significance level using the Mann–Whitney test under the Bonferroni-corrected significance level. The values tested every two weeks were used to observe the correlation of the implant stability values between the three different implants.

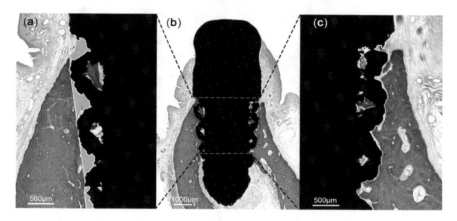

Figure 5. Schematic illustration of histomorphometric analysis in the region of interest (ROI). The ROI was set at the coronal half of each implant (**b**). Areas of the mineralized bone (green) were defined within the implant (**a**). Tissue-to-implant contact within the ROI (**c**) was differentiated into mineralized bone (blue) and void (white).

3. Results

3.1. Clinical and Radiographic Observations

The healing of the implants was uneventful, with no clinical signs of inflammation except at two PM2 sites—a T implant placed on the right side and a 3D implant placed on the left side.

3.2. Implant Stability Measurements

Except for two implants, the stability values for all other implants ranged from 71.18 ± 5.06 to 82.63 ± 4.09 (Table 2). There were significant differences between the three implant types at the time of surgery ($p = 0.007$) and at 2 weeks post-surgery ($p = 0.048$). The pairwise post hoc comparisons showed that the initial fixation force was lower for 3DS implant than for T implant ($p = 0.005$), but no difference was observed after 2 weeks. In addition, no significant differences in mean implant stability were observed from weeks 4 to 12 (Table 2). In 3D and 3DS groups, the implant stability values decreased at the 2-week observation compared with the time of surgery; however, the values gradually increased from week 4 to week 12. In the T group, the implant stability values decreased until 4 weeks post-surgery, but then gradually increased from week 6 to week 12 (Figure 5).

Table 2. Comparison of implant stability measurements among the three different implants.

Time	Threaded Implant (N = 7)	3D-Printed Implant without Spikes (N = 7)	3D-Printed Implant with Spikes (N = 8)	p-Value
Surgery	83.71 ± 2.90 [a]	79.49 ± 3.94 [a),b]	74.05 ± 5.61 [b]	0.007
2 weeks	76.29 ± 2.90	77.06 ± 2.90	71.18 ± 5.06	0.048
4 weeks	75.23 ± 3.22	77.80 ± 2.45	72.28 ± 5.52	0.112
6 weeks	75.86 ± 3.95	78.89 ± 1.37	76.00 ± 4.61	0.221
8 weeks	75.37 ± 5.29	77.89 ± 1.86	76.98 ± 3.57	0.815
10 weeks	76.11 ± 3.79	78.80 ± 1.89	77.75 ± 3.50	0.319
12 weeks	77.00 ± 4.30	80.17 ± 2.97	79.45 ± 2.74	0.349

Values are presented as the mean ± standard deviation. p-values were calculated using the Kruskal–Wallis test to compare implant stability values among the threaded implant, 3D-printed implant without spikes, and 3D-printed implant with spikes ($p < 0.05$). Pairwise post hoc comparisons were performed using the Mann–Whitney test under the Bonferroni-corrected significance level ($p < 0.017$). [a) b)] Significant difference under pairwise post hoc test.

3.3. Histologic Observations

A significant bone loss was found in the implants placed in the PM2 sites (a T implant and a 3D implant). These two implants were not included in the measurements. There was no evidence of inflammatory response in any specimen examined, except for the two implants. The coronal area of the implant showed more bone-to-implant contact, while the apical area showed relatively more contact between bone marrow and the surface of the implants. The region within threads and within lattices were occupied with new bone. Primary bone remodeling had nearly ceased, while secondary remodeling was ongoing around all types of implants (Figure 6).

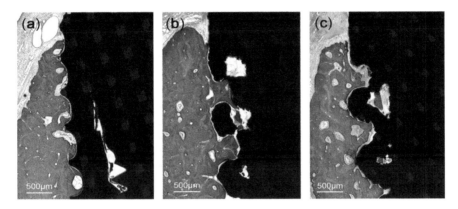

Figure 6. Histologic photograph of threaded implant: (**a**) 3D-printed implant without spikes, (**b**) 3D-printed implant with spikes, and (**c**) at 12 weeks following implant placement. The region within threads and within lattices was occupied with new bone. Primary bone remodeling had nearly ceased, while secondary remodeling was ongoing around all types of implants.

3.4. Histomorphometric Analysis

Mean values (± standard deviation) of BIC and BAFO are presented in Table 3. With regard to BIC, the T implant, the 3D implant, and the 3DS implant averaged $52.27 \pm 13.78\%$, $59.43 \pm 16.98\%$, and $44.28 \pm 15.99\%$, respectively. There were no significant differences in the BICs between the three groups ($p = 0.101$). The mean BAFO was $56.79 \pm 11.25\%$, $56.98 \pm 12.48\%$, and $45.58 \pm 10.77\%$ in T group, in 3D group, and 3DS group, respectively. No significant differences were observed between the three groups ($p = 0.288$).

Table 3. Bone-to-implant contact and bone area fraction occupied in the three implant groups.

Parameter	Thread Implant (N = 7)	3D-Printed Implant without Spikes (N = 7)	3D-Printed Implant with Spikes (N = 8)	p-Value
BIC	52.27 ± 13.78	59.43 ± 16.98	44.28 ± 15.99	0.101
BAFO	56.79 ± 11.25	56.98 ± 12.48	45.58 ± 10.77	0.288

Values are presented as the mean ± standard deviation. BIC: bone-to-implant contact, BAFO: bone area fraction occupied. p-values were calculated using the Kruskal–Wallis test ($p < 0.05$).

4. Discussion

In the present study, 3D-printed implants and conventional threaded implants were compared through stability measurements and histological analysis. Overall, comparable results were found in terms of implant stability, BIC, and BAFO irrespective of the studied implant. However, in this study, the two-dimensional histological assessment of the bone–implant interface was performed. This should be complemented by a 3D evaluation allowing a more accurate comparative analysis.

The lattice structure in the 3D-printed implants (3D and 3DS) did not appear to affect their stability in bone (Table 2). Hence, the 3D implant achieved and preserved primary stability similar to the T implant. A significant difference was found between the primary stability of the 3DS implant and

T implant. This might be explained by the surgical preparation of the 3DS implant bed requiring a larger osteotomy for the spikes. In turn, a gap was created between the bony walls of the surgical bed and the surface of the 3DS implant, translating into lower implant stability measures. These values, however, remain within the favorable range for primary stability [16]. Thereafter, the stability values described a trend toward a decrease followed by an increase over time. This observation is related to the discrepancy that exists between the rate of primary stability decrease and the rise of secondary stability throughout the healing process [17,18], as reported with threaded implants [19–21]. The outcomes from the previous studies, obtained using the resonance frequency analysis, are in line with the results herein, although the latter were produced with the damping capacity analysis [15–22].

Several studies have previously reported the outcomes of 3D-printed titanium implants in pre-clinical and clinical settings. Stubinger et al. [23] used the sheep pelvis model to analyze the in vivo characteristics of implants made by direct metal laser sintering. The implants made by this technology had a porous structure, and when compared with controls with standard machined, sandblasted, and etched surfaces after 2 and 8 weeks, the direct metal laser sintering implant did not show significant differences in BIC as compared with the other implants. Between the two observation time points, the direct metal laser sintering implant showed the highest increase in BIC. Compared with the machined implant and sandblasted and etched implant, the removal torque test of the direct metal laser sintering implant surface showed a significant improvement in the fixed strength after 8 weeks. In the study by Witek et al. [24] comparing a Ti-6Al-4V threaded type implant made by laser sintering to a control group with alumina blast and acid-etched surface after 1, 3, and 6 weeks, the BIC and BAFO values of the laser-sintered implant were higher at 1 week compared with the control group and did not show a significant difference at 3 and 6 weeks. In addition, after 1 and 6 weeks, the laser sintering implant showed a significantly higher removal torque value. Likewise, in a 1-year follow-up of 3D-printed custom-made implants in humans, no impairment of stability or signs of infection were observed simultaneously with a complete function and aesthetic integration [6–25]. Another 3-year follow-up clinical trial reported a survival rate of 94.5% and a crown success rate of 94.3% with 3D-printed implants [26]. Although the direct comparison of the previous studies might be questioned with regard to the different experimental protocols and implants used, the reported results overall indicate that the bone around implants made by 3D-printing displays favorable remodeling features and biomechanical stability. It can also be seen that the 3D printing manufacturing process does not adversely modify the biological or chemical properties of the material.

The microscopic factors and macroscopic factors of the implant are essential factors for implant stability and biological response [27]. To stimulate the growth of new bone into the pores, a materials' porosity superior to 60% is required [28]. This porosity can lead to interconnected porous structures, which facilitates cell ingrowth into porous spaces and facilitates vascularization and metabolite transport [28]. The three-dimensional lattice structure was used to increase the surface area of the 3D-printed implants. Therefore, the lattice structure surface with a porosity of 70% used in this study promotes the growth of new bone into pores to increase bone fixation. To mitigate bacterial colonization around the implant–bone interface, a lattice structure was not used at the top 1.5 mm of the implant texture. The implant with the SLA surface has better cell adhesion and bone neoformation than the machined surface [29]. In this study, 3D-printed implants with untreated surface and threaded implants with SLA surface were compared, and there was no statistically significant difference in histological and biomechanical properties. It is the lack of this research that brings micro and macro factors into the equation. In a follow-up study, SLA surface treatment will be performed on the 3D-printed implant to compensate for the limitation of this pilot study. Several animal models have been used for evaluating the biocompatibility of implants, but the canine model is known to be the most appropriate for implant material testing thanks to its close similarity in bone composition to humans [30,31]. A small amount of research has been conducted thus far on 3D-printed dental implants. In this perspective, the present study provides useful data for the characterization of bone healing at the surface of 3D-printed implants.

5. Conclusions

Within the limits of this study, both types of 3D-printed implants tested in the present study (3D and 3DS) showed comparable implant stability as well as BIC and BAFO values with T implants up to 12 weeks following insertion.

Author Contributions: Conceptualization, J.L. and K.-T.K.; methodology, Y.-M.L., P.K., and B.K.; software, J.L. and L.L.; validation, H.B.A. and K.-S.L.; formal analysis, J.L and L.L.; investigation, L.L.; resources, K.-T.K.; data curation, L.L.; writing—original draft preparation, L.L. and J.L.; writing—review and editing, H.B.A., J.-B.L., K.-S.L., S.-W.S., Y.-M.L., P.K., B.K., and K.-T.K.; visualization, J.-B.L. and L.L.; supervision, J.L. and K.-T.K.; project administration, S.-W.S. and K.-T.K.; funding acquisition, S.-W.S. and K.-T.K. All authors have read and agreed to the published version of the manuscript.

References

1. Smithloff, M.; Fritz, M.E. The Use of Blade Implants in a Selected Population of Partially Edentulous Adults: A Ten-Year Report. *J. Periodontol.* **1982**, *53*, 413–418. [CrossRef] [PubMed]
2. Scortecci, G. Immediate function of cortically anchored disk-design implants without bone augmentation in moderately to severely resorbed completely edentulous maxillae. *J. Oral Implant.* **1999**, *25*, 70–79. [CrossRef]
3. Gaviria, L.; Salcido, J.P.; Guda, T.; Ong, J.L. Current trends in dental implants. *J. Korean Assoc. Oral Maxillofac. Surg.* **2014**, *40*, 50–60. [CrossRef] [PubMed]
4. Harris, W.H.; White, R.E.; McCarthy, J.C.; Walker, P.S.; Weinberg, E.H. Bony Ingrowth Fixation of the Acetabular Component in Canine Hip Joint Arthroplasty. *Clin. Orthop. Relat. Res.* **1983**, *1983*, 7–11. [CrossRef]
5. Chen, J.; Zhang, Z.; Chen, X.; Zhang, C.; Zhang, G.; Xu, Z. Design and manufacture of customized dental implants by using reverse engineering and selective laser melting technology. *J. Prosthet. Dent.* **2014**, *112*, 1088–1095.e1. [CrossRef] [PubMed]
6. Mangano, F.G.; Cirotti, B.; Sammons, R.L.; Mangano, C. Custom-made, root-analogue direct laser metal forming implant: A case report. *Lasers Med. Sci.* **2012**, *27*, 1241–1245. [CrossRef] [PubMed]
7. Mangano, C.; Mangano, F.G.; Shibli, J.A.; Ricci, M.; Perrotti, V.; D'Avila, S.; Piattelli, A. Immediate Loading of Mandibular Overdentures Supported by Unsplinted Direct Laser Metal-Forming Implants: Results From a 1-Year Prospective Study. *J. Periodontol.* **2012**, *83*, 70–78. [CrossRef] [PubMed]
8. Traini, T.; Mangano, C.; Sammons, R.; Macchi, A.; Piattelli, A. Direct laser metal sintering as a new approach to fabrication of an isoelastic functionally graded material for manufacture of porous titanium dental implants. *Dent. Mater.* **2008**, *24*, 1525–1533. [CrossRef]
9. Ciocca, L.; Fantini, M.; De Crescenzio, F.; Corinaldesi, G.; Scotti, R. Direct metal laser sintering (DMLS) of a customized titanium mesh for prosthetically guided bone regeneration of atrophic maxillary arches. *Med. Biol. Eng. Comput.* **2011**, *49*, 1347–1352. [CrossRef]
10. Oberoi, G.; Nitsch, S.; Edelmayer, M.; Janjić, K.; Müller, A.S.; Agis, H. 3D Printing—Encompassing the Facets of Dentistry. *Front. Bioeng. Biotechnol.* **2018**, *6*, 172. [CrossRef]
11. Dawood, A.; Marti, B.M.; Sauret-Jackson, V. 3D printing in dentistry. *Br. Dent. J.* **2015**, *219*, 521–529. [CrossRef] [PubMed]
12. Torabi, K.; Farjood, E.; Hamedani, S. Rapid Prototyping Technologies and their Applications in Prosthodontics, a Review of Literature. *J. Dent. (Shiraz, Iran.)* **2015**, *16*, 1–9.
13. Pirker, W.; Wiedemann, D.; Lidauer, A.; Kocher, A. Immediate, single stage, truly anatomic zirconia implant in lower molar replacement: A case report with 2.5 years follow-up. *Int. J. Oral Maxillofac. Surg.* **2011**, *40*, 212–216. [CrossRef] [PubMed]
14. Wang, X.C.; Laoui, T.; Bonse, J.; Kruth, J.P.; Lauwers, B.; Froyen, L. Direct Selective Laser Sintering of Hard Metal Powders: Experimental Study and Simulation. *Int. J. Adv. Manuf. Technol.* **2002**, *19*, 351–357. [CrossRef]
15. Lee, J.; Pyo, S.-W.; Cho, H.-J.; An, J.-S.; Lee, J.-H.; Koo, K.-T.; Lee, Y.-M. Comparison of implant stability measurements between a resonance frequency analysis device and a modified damping capacity analysis device: An in vitro study. *J. Periodontal Implant. Sci.* **2020**, *50*, 56–66. [CrossRef] [PubMed]
16. Javed, F.; Ahmed, H.B.; Crespi, R.; Romanos, G.E. Role of primary stability for successful osseointegration of dental implants: Factors of influence and evaluation. *Interv. Med. Appl. Sci.* **2013**, *5*, 162–167. [CrossRef]

17.   Suzuki, S.; Kobayashi, H.; Ogawa, T. Implant Stability Change and Osseointegration Speed of Immediately Loaded Photofunctionalized Implants. *Implant. Dent.* **2013**, *22*, 481–490. [CrossRef]

18.   Atsumi, M.; Park, S.-H.; Wang, H.-L. Methods used to assess implant stability: Current status. *Int. J. Oral Maxillofac. Implant.* **2007**, *22*, 743–754.

19.   Kim, S.-J.; Kim, M.-R.; Rim, J.-S.; Chung, S.-M.; Shin, S.-W. Comparison of implant stability after different implant surface treatments in dog bone. *J. Appl. Oral Sci.* **2010**, *18*, 415–420. [CrossRef]

20.   Abrahamsson, L.; Linder, E.; Lang, N.P. Implant stability in relation to osseointegration: An experimental study in the Labrador dog. *Clin. Oral Implant. Res.* **2009**, *20*, 313–318. [CrossRef] [PubMed]

21.   Manresa, C.; Bosch, M.; Echeverría, J.J. The comparison between implant stability quotient and bone-implant contact revisited: An experiment in Beagle dog. *Clin. Oral Implant. Res.* **2013**, *25*, 1213–1221. [CrossRef] [PubMed]

22.   Lee, D.-H.; Shin, Y.-H.; Park, J.-H.; Shim, J.S.; Shin, S.-W.; Lee, J.-Y. The reliability of Anycheck device related to healing abutment diameter. *J. Adv. Prosthodont.* **2020**, *12*, 83–88. [CrossRef] [PubMed]

23.   Stübinger, S.; Mosch, I.; Robotti, P.; Sidler, M.; Klein, K.; Ferguson, S.J.; Von Rechenberg, B. Histological and biomechanical analysis of porous additive manufactured implants made by direct metal laser sintering: A pilot study in sheep. *J. Biomed. Mater. Res. Part B Appl. Biomater.* **2013**, *101*, 1154–1163. [CrossRef] [PubMed]

24.   Witek, L.; Marin, C.; Granato, R.; Bonfante, E.A.; Campos, F.; Bisinotto, J.; Suzuki, M.; Coelho, P.G. Characterization and in vivo evaluation of laser sintered dental endosseous implants in dogs. *J. Biomed. Mater. Res. Part B Appl. Biomater.* **2012**, *100*, 1566–1573. [CrossRef]

25.   Figliuzzi, M.; Mangano, F. A novel root analogue dental implant using CT scan and CAD/CAM: Selective laser melting technology. *Int. J. Oral Maxillofac. Surg.* **2012**, *41*, 858–862. [CrossRef]

26.   Tunchel, S.; Blay, A.; Kolerman, R.; Mijiritsky, E.; Shibli, J.A. 3D Printing/Additive Manufacturing Single Titanium Dental Implants: A Prospective Multicenter Study with 3 Years of Follow-Up. *Int. J. Dent.* **2016**, *2016*, 1–9. [CrossRef]

27.   Albrektsson, T.; Wennerberg, A. Oral implant surfaces: Part 1—Review focusing on topographic and chemical properties of different surfaces and in vivo responses to them. *Int. J. Prosthodont.* **2004**, *17*.

28.   Bram, M.; Schiefer, H.; Bogdanski, D.; Köller, M.; Buchkremer, H.; Stöver, D. Implant surgery: How bone bonds to PM titanium. *Met. Powder Rep.* **2006**, *61*, 26–31. [CrossRef]

29.   Nicolas-Silvente, A.I.; Velasco-Ortega, E.; Ortiz-Garcia, I.; Monsalve-Guil, L.; Gil, F.J.; Jimenez-Guerra, A. Influence of the Titanium Implant Surface Treatment on the Surface Roughness and Chemical Composition. *Materials* **2020**, *13*, 314. [CrossRef]

30.   Aerssens, J.; Boonen, S.; Lowet, G.; Dequeker, J. Interspecies differences in bone composition, density, and quality: Potential implications for in vivo bone research. *Endocrinology* **1998**, *2*, 663–670. [CrossRef]

31.   Pearce, A.; Richards, R.G.; Milz, S.; Schneider, E.; Pearce, S.G. Animal models for implant biomaterial research in bone: A review. *Eur. Cells Mater.* **2007**, *13*, 1–10. [CrossRef] [PubMed]

2

Enhancement of Bone Ingrowth into a Porous Titanium Structure to Improve Osseointegration of Dental Implants: A Pilot Study in the Canine Model

Ji-Youn Hong [1],[†] [iD], Seok-Yeong Ko [2],[†], Wonsik Lee [3], Yun-Young Chang [4], Su-Hwan Kim [5],[6] [iD] and Jeong-Ho Yun [2],[7],[*] [iD]

[1] Department of Periodontology, Periodontal-Implant Clinical Research Institute, School of Dentistry, Kyung Hee University, 26, Kyungheedae-ro, Dongdaemun-gu, Seoul 02447, Korea; jkama7@gmail.com

[2] Department of Periodontology, College of Dentistry and Institute of Oral Bioscience, Jeonbuk National University, 567, Baekje-daero, Deokjin-gu, Jeonju-si, Jeollabuk-do 54896, Korea; dentquartz@naver.com

[3] Advanced Process and Materials R&D Group, Korea Institute of Industrial Technology, 7-47 Songdo-dong, Yeonsu-gu, Incheon 406-840, Korea; wonslee@kitech.re.kr

[4] Department of Dentistry, Inha International Medical Center, 424, Gonghang-ro, 84-gil, Unseo-dong, Jung-gu, Incheon 22382, Korea; bewitme@naver.com

[5] Department of Periodontics, Asan Medical Center, 88, Olympic-ro 43-gil, Songpa-gu, Seoul 05505, Korea; suhwank@gmail.com

[6] Department of Dentistry, University of Ulsan College of Medicine, 88, Olympic-ro 43-gil, Songpa-gu, Seoul 05505, Korea

[7] Research Institute of Clinical Medicine of Jeonbuk National University-Biomedical Research Institute of Jeonbuk National University Hospital, 20, Geonjiro, Deokjin-gu, Jeonju-si, Jeollabuk-do 54907, Korea

[*] Correspondence: grayheron@hanmail.net

[†] These authors contributed equally to this study.

Abstract: A porous titanium structure was suggested to improve implant stability in the early healing period or in poor bone quality. This study investigated the effect of a porous structure on the osseointegration of dental implants. A total of 28 implants (14 implants in each group) were placed in the posterior mandibles of four beagle dogs at 3 months after extraction. The control group included machined surface implants with an external implant–abutment connection, whereas test group implants had a porous titanium structure added to the apical portion. Resonance frequency analysis (RFA); removal torque values (RTV); and surface topographic and histometric parameters including bone-to-implant contact length and ratio, inter-thread bone area and ratio in total, and the coronal and apical parts of the implants were measured after 4 weeks of healing. RTV showed a significant difference between the groups after 4 weeks of healing ($p = 0.032$), whereas no difference was observed in RFA. In the test group, surface topography showed bone tissue integrated into the porous structures. In the apical part of the test group, all the histometric parameters exhibited significant increases compared to the control group. Within the limitations of this study, enhanced bone growth into the porous structure was achieved, which consequently improved osseointegration of the implant.

Keywords: porosity; dental implant; osseointegration; bone formation; titanium

1. Introduction

A dental implant has been accepted as a reliable treatment modality for edentulous ridge with high long-term survival [1], and improvements in implant design, surface treatment, and surgical technique led to a marked increase in implant stability [2,3]. However, the results are mostly based on the selection of subjects with the exclusion of any clinical conditions that might have a negative effect on the healing around the implants. There are several possible risk factors associated with early implant failure or impaired healing, including smoking, head and neck radiation [4,5], bone quality and osteoporosis [6]. Osseointegration was defined as a direct and functional connection between bone and an artificial implant. However, the macroscopic (body structure and thread geometry) and microscopic (chemical composition and surface treatment) characteristics of dental implants could influence the success of the osseointegration [7].

The topographical features in an implant surface can be defined in terms of their scales, which were produced by surface modification treatments such as titanium plasma-spraying, grit-blasting, acid-etching, or combinations [2,8]. Apart from the macro-level that is related to the threaded screw of implant geometry and macroporous surface, mechanical interlocking is maximized by microtopographic roughness [9]. In addition, nanotopography is associated with the biological activities of cells to stimulate bone formation on an implant surface [10]. However, the majority of current surface treatments are unreliable to achieve reproducible nanoscale features as they range randomly from nanometers to millimeters.

Another approach in surface modification was the production of porous bodies of titanium metal and its alloys, and sintering of metal powders onto the surface was commonly used for porous coatings [11,12]. Advantages of porous surface-enhanced implant include the induction of new bone tissue ingrowth and neovascularization into the porous scaffold in three-dimensional (3D) aspects [13], elastic modulus closer to the cancellous bone that allows load distribution [14], and enhanced transport of metabolites and space for new bone through substantial porous interconnectivity [15]. To maximize the potential benefits from the porous structures, precise control of overall porosity and pore size was identified as important, although the optimal ranges were yet to be determined [16]. However, conventional methods had limitations of low volumetric porosity, irregular dimensions of pores, and poor interconnectivity [17]. Furthermore, possible mechanical failures related to a lack of yield strength and separation of coating materials led to soft tissue encapsulation and loosening of implants [18].

Recent approaches have utilized methods such as selective melting with laser or electron beam, 3D printing, casting or vapor deposition to control the internal pore geometry and distribution [12,19]. The porous scaffolds were sometimes combined with threaded implants for additional advantages in terms of primary mechanical stability and removability. One of the products that had been widely studied to adapt the porous structure to the root form implant was the porous tantalum trabecular metal (PTTM) enhanced implant [18,20,21]. PTTM was fabricated by foam-like vitreous carbon scaffold that resulted in the open-cell structure similar to the trabecular bone [18]. The PTTM part was added to the middle portion of the implant by laser welding and was combined with the screw-type design of titanium alloy surface at the cervical and apical portions, which were microtextured by grit-blasting with hydroxyapatite particles. From the animal studies, histomorphometric evaluations have demonstrated more new bone growth at the PTTM occupying the middle portion compared to the conventional surface within the 12-week study periods, and suggested the potential benefits of the porous structures in the compromised bone quality. However, there were limited biomechanical improvements assessed by the resonance frequency analysis in PTTM and the implant stability appeared comparable to the conventional microtextured surface.

In the present study, a novel method of utilizing the powder injection molding technique has been employed to form a porous titanium structure, which was fabricated on the apical portion of the machined screw-type implant. The effect of the newly developed porous structure on osseointegration was compared to the smooth-surfaced implant in the canine model.

2. Materials and Methods

2.1. Design of the Implants

A threaded machined surface implant (c.p. titanium grade 4) with an external-type abutment connection (MegaGen Implant Co., Ltd., Gyeongsan, Korea) was used in the control group. The implant measured 4.1 mm in diameter, 8.1 mm in length, and had a straight configuration of the implant body (core diameter of 3.25 mm) with a homogenous thread height of 0.35 mm (Figure 1a). The test group implant had a porous titanium structure fabricated on the implant core at the apical portion; the core had a reduced diameter of 1.25 mm and a thread height of 1.35 mm to afford the space for the porous scaffold (1 mm in depth and 0.83 mm in width) (Figure 1b). The resulting profile had 3-mm spiral shape threads in the apical part, a regular pitch distance of 1.25 mm and a thread angle of 45°.

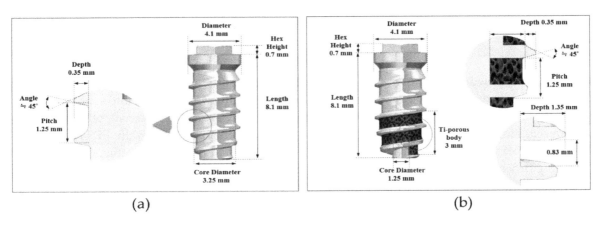

(a)   (b)

Figure 1. Design of the implants: (**a**) overall profiles and dimensions of the implant in the control group; (**b**) overall profiles and dimensions of the implant in the test group.

2.2. Fabrication of Porous Titanium Structure

The porous titanium structure on the implant core was fabricated at the Korea Institute of Industrial Technology (KITECH) using insert powder injection molding technology (Figure 2a). Briefly, a feedstock, which was a mixture of titanium hydride (TiH_2) powder, space holder and some polymeric binders, was prepared as a material for powder injection molding. Expandable polystyrene (EPS) beads with an average diameter of 325 µm were selected as space holders to form open-pore structure made from the contact between the beads during the expansion that occurred above 80 °C. The feedstock was injected into the narrow cavity between the threads at the apical third portion of the implant insert. The molded implants were inserted again into a mold designed for expansion of the EPS beads and kept for 20 min in an oven at 110 °C. The expanded beads were removed in a solvent, resulting in an open-pore structure consisting of TiH_2 powder and binders (Figure 2b). The polymeric binders were removed completely during the thermal debinding process, slowly increasing the temperature up to 700 °C under argon atmosphere. During this process, TiH_2 powder was also transformed to Ti powder by dehydrogenation reaction that occurred in the temperature range of from 350 to 500 °C. Finally, the open-pore scaffold of titanium powder between the threads was sintered for 3 h at 1100 °C in high vacuum (Figure 2c). During sintering, the titanium scaffold and implant core were combined into a single body by interdiffusion of titanium atoms at the interface, and titanium fixtures with open-pore titanium structure between the implant threads were formed. The porous structure had an average porosity of 68.1%, an average strut thickness of 61.4 µm (range: 30 to 100 µm), and an average pore size of 243 µm (range: 200 to 350 µm). The interconnected area between the pores that acts as the path for ingrowth of bone was measured to be 122.0 µm (range: 50 to 235 µm) in mean diameter from 2-dimensional image analysis.

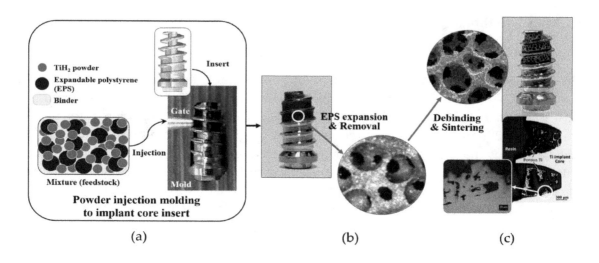

Figure 2. Insert powder injection molding process to fabricate the porous titanium fixture: (**a**) after a titanium implant with a narrow cavity in the deep inter-thread area was inserted into a mold, a mixture of titanium hydride (TiH_2) powder, expandable polystyrene (EPS) beads and some polymeric binders were injected into the narrow cavity between the threads of the implant; (**b**) the EPS beads within the molded area were removed in a solvent after the expansion of EPS; (**c**) subsequently, through the debinding process, binders were removed and after dehydrogenation of TiH_2 to Ti powder and the sintering process, the porous titanium fixtures with an open-pored titanium structure between the implant threads were produced and combined into a single body.

2.3. Animal Experiment

Four 12-month-old male beagle dogs weighing 12.0 to 17.0 kg were used in this study. The dogs were kept in separate cages under standard laboratory conditions. Animal selection, management, surgical procedures, and preparations were performed according to the protocols approved by the Institutional Animal Care and Use Committee at Korea Animal Medical Science Institute, Guri, Korea (Approval No. 16-KE-234). The study was conducted following the Animal Research: Reporting In Vivo Experiments (ARRIVE) guidelines [22].

Surgical procedures were performed under general anesthesia with intravenous injection of a solution (0.1 mL/kg) containing 1:1 ratio of tiletamine/zolazepam (Zoletil 50, Virbac S.A., Virbac Laboratories 06516, Carros, France) and xylazine hydrochloride (Rumpun, Bayer, Seoul, Korea). Infiltration anesthesia with 2% lidocaine HCl with 1:100,000 epinephrine (Huons, Seoul, Korea) was used at the surgical sites. The premolars (P1–P4) and the first molar (M1) in both the mandibles were carefully extracted and a total of 28 implants (14 implants for each group) were placed after 12 weeks. In each quadrant, three or four implants from the control or test group were randomly allocated. After sequential osteotomies, implants were installed under 40 Ncm (newton centimeter) of torque and submerged (Figure 3a–c). Antibiotics and nonsteroidal anti-inflammatory drugs were administered for 5 days. Sutures were removed after one week and animals were sacrificed after 4 weeks of healing by intravenous injection of 1 mL of suxamethonium chloride (50 mg/mL).

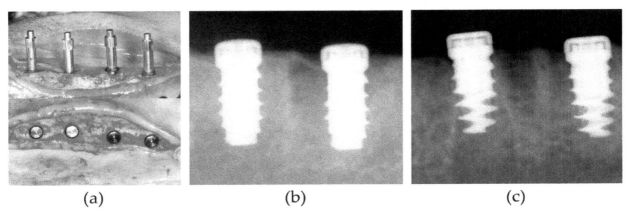

(a)   (b)   (c)

Figure 3. Surgical procedure of implant placement: (**a**) Smartpeg connection to measure implant stability quotient (ISQ) values using the resonance frequency analysis (RFA) device (Osstell Mentor) immediately after the implant placement (upper), and coverscrew connection (lower); (**b**) periapical X-ray images were taken in the control group; (**c**) periapical X-ray images were taken in the test group. Radiolucency near the implant surface was shown at the apical part of the test group compared to the control group.

2.4. Resonance Frequency Analysis (RFA), Removal Torque Test and Topographical Analysis

Implant stability quotient (ISQ) value was measured immediately after the implant placement and at the time of animal sacrifice. A SmartPeg (Type 04, REF 100350, Osstell AB, Gothenburg, Sweden) was connected to each implant and a commercially available RFA equipment (Osstell Mentor, Osstell AB, Gothenburg, Sweden) was adjusted at the mesial and buccal direction of the implant (Figure 3a). The mean ISQ values in the mesial and buccal direction were recorded.

In each group, 7 implants were randomly selected and removal torque values (RTV) were measured using torque meter (MARK-10 torque gauge, MARK-10 Corporation, NY, USA) on the day of sacrifice. Removed implant specimens were dehydrated in graded ethanol series and sputter-coated with platinum (LEICA EM ACE200, sputter current 40 mA, Leica Microsystems, Wetzlar, Germany). Surface topography was examined under a field-emission scanning electron microscope (FE-SEM, SUPRA 40VP, Carl Zeiss, Oberkochen, Germany) and photograph images were taken at the magnifications of 20× and 100× with 5.0 kV.

2.5. Histologic and Histometric Analysis

Among the 14 implants allocated for each group, 7 specimens were processed for histologic and histometric analysis, as the rest of the 7 implants were tested for RTVs described in Section 2.4. Specimens of the implants and surrounding tissues were dissected into blocks and fixed in 10% buffered formalin solution. After sequential ethanol dehydration, nondecalcified specimens were embedded in methylmethacrylate (Technovit 7200, Kulzer GmbH, Hanau, Germany) and sectioned along the implant axis in the bucco-lingual plane using a diamond saw with 30–50 μm thickness. Hematoxylin and eosin (H&E)-stained sections were evaluated under a light microscope fitted with a camera and histometric measurements were completed using an automated image analysis program (Image-Pro Plus, Media Cybernetics, Rockville, MD, USA).

Parameters were measured from two parts (apical and coronal) of the implant, which was transversely divided along its long axis. The apical part included the area between the most apical border of the fixture and 3 mm above and coronal part was from the coronal border of the apical part to the most coronal endpoint thread of the fixture (Figure 4a). The following parameters were measured: (a) the bone-to-implant contact length (BICL, in mm), which was the sum of length of the implant surface in direct contact with surrounding bone; (b) the bone-to-implant contact ratio (BICR, in %), which was the percentage of BICL out of the length measured for the implant surface outline; (c) the inter-thread bone area (BA, in mm^2), which was the sum of bone area observed between the threads;

and (d) the inter-thread bone area ratio (BAR, in %), which was the percentage of BA in the region of interest (ROI). ROI in the control group and coronal part of the test group was determined by outlining the space between the threads (inter-thread space). To determine the corresponding ROI in the apical part of the test group, superimposition of the counterpart in the control implant was performed to outline the virtual boundary of the original shape of the inter-thread area (Figure 4b).

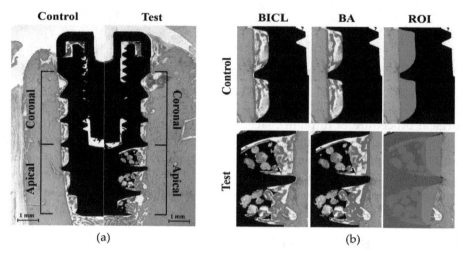

(a)   (b)

Figure 4. Schematic images of the histometric measurements: (**a**) Parameters were measured within the coronal and apical part, which were transversely divided along the long axis of the implant in both the control (left) and test groups (right) (magnification of 20×). (**b**) In each part of the control or test group (magnification of 50×), the bone-to-implant contact length (BICL) was determined by the total length of the implant surface in contact with the surrounding bone (yellow outlines in BICL). The inter-thread bone area (BA) was measured by the total bone area between the threads (red-colored area in BA). The region of interest (ROI) of the control group was outlined for the inter-thread space (blue colored area in ROI at the upper line). The ROI of the apical part in the test group (blue-colored area in ROI at the lower line) was determined by the virtual boundary, which was made from the superimposed counterpart of the control implant (red-colored implant shape in ROI at the lower line). Consequently, the original shape of the inter-thread space was outlined and the BA ratio (BAR) was calculated from the percentage of BA within each ROI.

2.6. Statistical Analysis

Statistical analyses were performed using SPSS Ver. 12.0 (SPSS, Chicago, IL, USA). Normality of data distribution was determined by Shapiro–Wilk test. For ISQ and RTV in both groups, paired t-test was used to compare the differences of the parameters between the two groups at each time period and the differences in ISQ between the baseline and 4 weeks in each group. Regarding histometric parameters, comparisons between the groups in each part and between the two parts (coronal and apical parts) in each group were performed using Student's t-test (in the data of BICL and BICR in the apical part, BA and BAR in the coronal, apical and total area), or Wilcoxon's rank-sum test (in the data of BICL and BICR in apical part and total area). The level of statistical significance was set at $p < 0.05$.

3. Results

3.1. Clinical Findings

The experimental sites in all the animals demonstrated uneventful healing and did not exhibit any adverse reaction throughout the postoperative healing period.

3.2. Resonance Frequency Analysis and Removal Torque Value

No significant differences were observed in ISQ values between the two groups at each time period and between the baseline and 4 weeks in each group. However, RTV in the test group (20.5 ± 6.8) was higher than that of the control group (8.0 ± 3.6) with a significant difference at the 4-week healing period ($p = 0.03$) (Table 1).

Table 1. Implant stability quotient (ISQ) value and removal torque value (RTV) after 4 weeks of healing in the test and control groups (mean ± SD).

		Test Group (n = 14)	Control Group (n = 14)
ISQ Value	Baseline	66.7 ± 4.0	69.5 ± 8.3
	4 weeks	67.5 ± 5.0	68.4 ± 6.3
RTV (Ncm)		Test Group (n = 7)	Control Group (n = 7)
	4 weeks	20.5 ± 6.8 [1]	8.0 ± 3.6

[1] Statistically significant difference between the two groups in the paired t-test ($p < 0.05$).

3.3. Surface Topography from FE-SEM Images

The original surface topography of the test group implant showed a titanium structure with regular distribution of pores in similar size ranging from 200 to 350 μm in the apical part (Figure 5a,b), whereas the control group showed a smooth texture of the machined surface (Figure 5c,d). After the removal torque test, the porous body in the test group exhibited structural destruction with a few integrated bone tissues in close proximity (Figure 5e,f). However, the interface between the porous structure and core of the fixture was maintained. The control group implant did not show any specific destruction, although there were some traces of scrapes on the surface (Figure 5g,h).

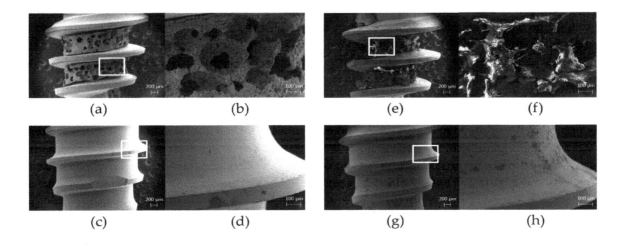

Figure 5. Field-emission scanning electron microscope (FE-SEM) images before the implant placement and after the removal: (**a**) overall image of the test group before the placement (magnification of 20×); (**b**) magnified view of the white box in (**a**) showing a porous titanium structure in the apical part of the test group implant with regularly distributed pores (magnification of 100×); (**c**) overall image of the control group before the placement (magnification of 20×); (**d**) magnified view of the white box in (**c**) showing a smooth machined surface in the control group implant (magnification of 100×); (**e**) overall image of the test group after the removal of implants at 4-week healing periods (magnification of 20×); (**f**) magnified view of the white box in (**e**) showing the destruction of the porous structures and some bone tissues at the porous structure after the removal (magnification of 100×); (**g**) overall image of the control group after the removal of implants at 4-week healing periods (magnification of 20×); (**h**) magnified view of the white box in (**g**) showing no specific destruction in the surface profile except for some scrapes after the removal (magnification of 100×).

3.4. Histologic Analysis

New bone (NB) formation and BIC were observed at entire length of the implants in both the test and control groups (Figure 6a,f). In the coronal part of the test group, newly formed hard tissues projected from the parent bone (PB) surface towards the drilled osteotomy sites along the threads of the implant (Figure 6b,c). Osteoid and NB lined with osteoblast-like cells were found in the space between the threads, which were in direct contact with the implant surface and sometimes bridged PB with the implant surface. Some part of the PB surface underwent a remodeling process with reversal lines parallel to the long axis of the bone wall. These histologic features were also observed at both the coronal (Figure 6g,h) and apical parts (Figure 6i,j) of the control group which had the same surface topography of the coronal part in the test group. In the apical part of the test group, newly formed woven bone with osteoblast-like cells on its surface projected from the PB wall into the drilled space, and ingrowth of NB into the porous structure exhibited direct contact with the implant surface (Figure 6d). NB shown in the porous structure was integrated with the pore entrances and in direct contact with the inner surfaces of regularly distributed porous scaffolds (Figure 6e). NB was bridged between one another or to the PB surface and surrounded by the densely packed connective tissue matrix.

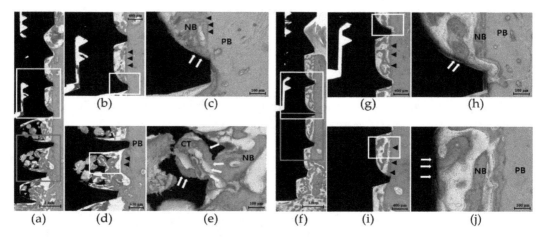

Figure 6. Representative histologic images of the implant in the test group and control group at 4 weeks of healing (H&E staining): (**a**) Overall view of the whole length of the test group implant showing a smooth surface profile in the coronal part (yellow box) and the porous structure in the apical part (red box) (magnification of 20×). (**b**) In the coronal part, new bone (NB) projection from the parent bone (PB) into the drilled osteotomy sites along the implant threads was observed (magnification of 50×). (**c**) Magnified view of the white box in (**b**) showing NB in direct contact with the implant surface (white arrows) (magnification of 200×). (**d**) In the apical part, NB connected with the PB surface and in contact with the surface of the porous structure was shown (magnification of 50×). (**e**) Magnified view of the white box in (**d**) showing NB ingrowth through the pore entrance (yellow arrows) and in direct contact with the surface of the porous scaffold (white arrows) (magnification of 200×). NB was lined with osteoblast-like cells on its surface and surrounded by the densely packed connective tissue matrix (CT). Reversal lines (black arrowheads) at the PB surface were found along the bony wall. (**f**) Overall view of the whole length of the control group implant showing a smooth surface profile in both the coronal (yellow box) and apical parts (red box) (magnification of 20×). (**g**) In the coronal part, new bone (NB) projected from the parent bone (PB) surface and towards the inter-thread space was shown (magnification of 50×). (**h**) Magnified view of the white box in (**g**) showing NB in direct contact with the implant surface (white arrows) and lined with osteoblast-like cells on its surface (magnification of 200×). (**i**) In the apical part, histologic appearance similar to that of the coronal part was shown (magnification of 50×). (**j**) Magnified view of the white box in (**i**) showing NB directly bridged to the implant surface (magnification of 200×). Lamellated reversal lines (black arrowheads) can be seen at the PB surface along the bony wall.

3.5. Histometric Analysis

Significant increases in BICL ($p < 0.007$), BICR ($p = 0.011$), BA ($p = 0.014$) and BAR ($p = 0.028$) of the total area were shown in the test group compared to the control group. The apical part of the test group presented significant increases in BICL ($p < 0.001$), BICR ($p = 0.001$), BA ($p = 0.011$) and BAR ($p = 0.020$) compared to the control group; all the parameters in the coronal part were similar in both the groups. The test group also showed significant differences between the coronal and apical part in BICL ($p = 0.005$), BICR ($p = 0.010$), BA ($p = 0.009$), and BAR ($p = 0.049$), whereas the control group showed no differences between the two parts (Table 2).

Table 2. Histometric parameters after 4 weeks of healing in the test and control groups (mean ± SD).

		Test Group (n = 7)	Control Group (n = 7)
BICL (mm)	Coronal part	1.88 ± 0.98	1.31 ± 0.76
	Apical part	3.43 ± 0.68 [1,2]	1.30 ± 0.78
	Total	5.31 ± 1.28 [1]	2.60 ± 1.21
BICR (%)	Coronal part	17.83 ± 9.53	12.56 ± 7.26
	Apical part	31.70 ± 7.53 [1,2]	12.89 ± 7.57
	Total	24.83 ± 6.44 [1]	12.69 ± 5.74
BA (mm²)	Coronal part	0.28 ± 0.11	0.21 ± 0.08
	Apical part	0.48 ± 0.12 [1,2]	0.25 ± 0.12
	Total	0.77 ± 0.24 [1]	0.45 ± 0.16
BAR (%)	Coronal part	24.9 ± 10.84	20.7 ± 7.74
	Apical part	37.2 ± 10.04 [1,2]	23.0 ± 9.75
	Total	31.5 ± 8.03 [1]	21.8 ± 6.36

BICL, the bone-to-implant contact length; BICR, the bone-to-implant contact ratio; BA, the inter-thread bone area; BAR, the inter-thread bone area ratio. [1] Statistically significant difference from the control group in Wilcoxon's rank-sum test (used for BICL and BICR in total area) and in Student's t-test (used for BICL, BICR, BA, and BAR in apical part, BA and BAR in total area) ($p < 0.05$). [2] Statistically significant difference from the coronal part in Student's t-test ($p < 0.05$).

4. Discussion

In the present study, the porous titanium structure fabricated at the apical portion of the implant resulted in the interconnected open-pore structure, which led to an increase in the implant surface and its osteoconductivity to enhance bone ingrowth into the porous scaffold, thereby improving osseointegration of the implant.

The percentage of porosity on the overall surface and the size of pores are known as the determining factors in bone ingrowth [23]. Conventional methods like the sintering of beads on the titanium alloys have been reported to have limited degree of porosity (around 35%) and exhibit difficulty in controlling the profile of the topography [11]. As per the recent approaches, the PTTM- enhanced titanium implant could exhibit an increased percentage of the porosity (up to 70–80%) owing to the open-cell structure of dodecahedral repeats resembling trabecular bone [17,24]. In animal studies, the porous tantalum implants showed greater bone-to-implant contact with increased osteogenic activity compared to the solid titanium [20,25]. The clinical benefits of porous tantalum implants were also reported in the retrospective studies as there were high survival rates and less peri-implant bone loss [26], and a pilot study of failed implants immediately replaced by using the porous tantalum implants showed successful outcomes in 5 years of follow-up as well although the sample size was limited [27]. However, there still existed difficulty in manipulation of pure tantalum and high costs for purification [28].

The powder injection molding technique was introduced to process the fine ceramics in the past two decades and could offer the reproducible mass production of complicated structures like near-net-shapes, even in hard materials like ceramics [29]. In dental fields, powder injection molding zirconia implants were tested in the animal model, and this technique was suggested to provide an enhanced tissue response to the roughened surface when compared with that of a machined titanium surface [30]. In the present study, porous titanium structure produced by the powder injection molding technique resulted in the formation of interconnected open pores with an average porosity of about 70%. The structure was similar to the alveolar bone of the human mandible with D1 type bone (showing primarily of homogenous dense cortical bone) as evaluated through micro-computed tomography study, thus providing a negative template with a natural trabecular pattern with higher bone density [31]. Potential benefits of rapid vascularization, osteoblastic differentiation, and new bone ingrowth could be expected, as they mimic the natural trabecular bone. As the porosity could be controlled by adjusting the amount of polymers or the temperature of EPS expansion, it might also be possible to alter the characteristics of porous structures to match with the natural bone, or customized as per the need of individual patients.

The multithreaded root-form implant has clinical benefits of simple osteotomy, implant placement, close mechanical proximity to the bone to increase primary stability, and less traumatic retrieval under conditions of failure [3]. When combined with the adequately controlled porous structure, additional effects of enhanced neovascularization and new bone formation inside the porous scaffold termed as osseoincoporation can be expected [32,33]. However, the porous structure in the present study has possible problems, such as a higher risk of bacterial plaque accumulation, mucosal and peri-implant diseases when compared to the machined surface upon exposure to complex oral environments [34]. Hybrid surface implants have been suggested to reduce the prevalence of peri-implantitis by including the machined surface or less roughened texture in the coronal part of the implant together with the rough surface treatments in the apical part, which played important role in healing between the bone and the surface [35]. In correspondence with the rationale of the hybrid implant, the test group implant was expected to have both advantages in terms of accelerated healing and increased bone-to-implant contact by the porous structure at the apical part, and less biological complications related to the inflammation at the coronal smooth surface area. In addition, an external connection was utilized to minimize the risk of fracture from the thinned lateral wall of the body after the decrease in core diameter, while providing space for the porous structure. The crestal bone–implant interface is an important area in stress distribution during load transmission [36], and there exists a lack of data regarding mechanical failure in the porous structure with reference to stress and fatigue when loading, thus stating inappropriateness of this structure in the coronal portion of the implant body.

Implant stability measured using RFA showed ISQ values over 60 in both the groups and at both the observation periods with no significant differences. The ISQ value over 60 was reported to demonstrate clinical stability of the implant despite the differences in implant designs, surgical models, and devices used, and the factors affecting RFA include stiffness of the implant-bone interface, distance to first bone contact, and marginal bone loss [37]. It can be assumed that relatively standardized bone density among the surgical sites, fully engaged implant surface within the surrounding bone, and the same topographic aspects at the coronal portion contribute to the similar outcome of ISQ at baseline and after 4 weeks of healing between the two groups. The presence of a porous titanium structure in the apical portion and its loss of close proximity to the bone wall cut by the twist drill may not have a great influence on the ISQ value. On the other hand, the removal torque test is an indirect method to measure the shear strength that ruptures the bone–implant interface and gives information about the bone growth aspects at the surface [38]. Hence, a significant increase in RTV of the test group implant at 4 weeks might be explained by the increased secondary stability at the porous structure at the apical portion. The fractured bone compartment together with the porous surface in FE-SEM images after the reverse torque rotation also supported the findings of bone ingrowth at the apical portion. However, some of the destructions were observed in the center portion of the porous body, whereas the interface at the attachment to the implant core still remained. The destroyed sites might suggest the weak points in the mechanical properties of the implants, which should further be improved by the development of the manufacturing techniques.

Significant increases in total BICL, BICR, BA, and BAR in the test group implants were attributed to the apical portion, and histologic findings supported the results by showing enhanced NB formation in direct contact with the interconnected open pores with an increased surface area at the apical portion and improved BIC at 4 weeks. Healing in the trabecular compartment relies on the process of osteoconduction and de novo bone formation at the implant surface, resulting in contact osteogenesis [33], and porous configuration could promote osteoconductivity by increasing space for blood clot stabilization and recruitment of various cells involved in biologic cascades of peri-implant healing [39]. A porous structure designed to resemble the trabecular patterns of highest bone quality might permit an adequate osteoconductive scaffold for bone ingrowth, which is in accordance with other studies [40,41]. Apparently, it also might help in providing enhanced micro-mechanical interdigitation with the parent bone and increase primary stability irrespective of the condition of the recipient site, including compromised bone quality such as D4 type bone (showing the fine trabecular bone composing almost the total volume) where the cortical stiffness could not be anticipated and the posterior maxilla that lacks bone height.

In the present study, a porous titanium structure fabricated by the powder injection molding technique was able to provide three-dimensional interconnected porosity on the implant surface and thereby enhanced the new bone ingrowth at the surface. The histometric findings, including the fact that the bone-to-implant contact and new bone formation inside the porous material demonstrated the improvements in osseointegration by the porous structure in the early healing dynamics, were in accordance with some other studies utilizing trabecular-like scaffolds to the dental implants [20,21,25]. However, the test implant used in this study was designed to combine the porous structure with the machined surface implant for a pilot approach to focus on the efficacy of the newly developed structure at the apical portion, and other variables, including overall macrogeometry and topography of the implants, were intended to be controlled. For the clinical applications, various modifications in the microstructures other than the machined surface at the coronal aspect should be considered, and it might also be necessary to develop the macrostructural designs of the implant–abutment connection and the platform that can show more favorable outcomes in the biomechanical aspects. Improvements in the fabrication technologies to standardize porosity and increase the mechanical strength of the porous structures are necessary to obtain reliable clinical outcomes. In addition, the healing events around the porous implants in the long-term period and the tissue dynamics after the loading should further be observed. Finally, the effects of the porous titanium structure on the compromised bone conditions in clinical situations such as osteoporosis, grafted bone or simultaneous sinus floor elevation should be further investigated.

5. Conclusions

The findings of the study suggest that the porous titanium structure might increase apical bone-to-implant contact due to the increased surface area and enhance new bone formation with increased osteoconductivity in the early healing period, thereby leading to improvements in the osseointegration of the implants.

Author Contributions: Conceptualization, S.-Y.K., W.L., and J.-H.Y.; data curation, J.-Y.H., S.-Y.K., and J.-H.Y.; formal analysis, J.-Y.H., S.-Y.K., and J.-H.Y.; funding acquisition, W.L. and J.-H.Y.; methodology, J.-Y.H., S.-Y.K., Y.-Y.C., S.-H.K., and J.-H.Y.; supervision, W.L. and J.-H.Y.; writing—original draft, J.-Y.H. and S.-Y.K.; writing—review and editing, J.-Y.H., W.L., Y.-Y.C., S.-H.K. and J.-H.Y. All authors have read and agreed to the published version of the manuscript.

References

1. Boioli, L.T.; Penaud, J.; Miller, N. A meta-analytic, quantitative assessment of osseointegration establishment and evolution of submerged and non-submerged endosseous titanium oral implants. *Clin. Oral Implants Res.* **2001**, *12*, 579–588. [CrossRef]

2.　Le Guéhennec, L.; Soueidan, A.; Layrolle, P.; Amouriq, Y. Surface treatments of titanium dental implants for rapid osseointegration. *Dent. Mater.* **2007**, *23*, 844–854. [CrossRef]

3.　Javed, F.; Ahmed, H.B.; Crespi, R.; Romanos, G.E. Role of primary stability for successful osseointegration of dental implants: Factors of influence and evaluation. *Interv. Med. Appl. Sci.* **2013**, *5*, 162–167. [CrossRef]

4.　Moy, P.K.; Medina, D.; Shetty, V.; Aghaloo, T.L. Dental implant failure rates and associated risk factors. *Int. J. Oral Maxillofac. Implants* **2005**, *20*, 569–577. [PubMed]

5.　van Steenberghe, D.; Jacobs, R.; Desnyder, M.; Maffei, G.; Quirynen, M. The relative impact of local and endogenous patient-related factors on implant failure up to the abutment stage. *Clin. Oral Implants Res.* **2002**, *13*, 617–622. [CrossRef]

6.　Beikler, T.; Flemmig, T.F. Implants in the medically compromised patient. *Crit. Rev. Oral Biol. Med.* **2003**, *14*, 305–316. [CrossRef] [PubMed]

7.　Giudice, A.; Bennardo, F.; Antonelli, A.; Barone, S.; Wagner, F.; Fortunato, L.; Traxler, H. Influence of clinician's skill on primary implant stability with conventional and piezoelectric preparation techniques: An ex-vivo study. *J. Biol. Regul. Homeost. Agents* **2020**, *34*, 739–745.

8.　Shibata, Y.; Tanimoto, Y. A review of improved fixation methods for dental implants. Part I: Surface optimization for rapid osseointegration. *J. Prosthodont. Res.* **2015**, *59*, 20–33. [CrossRef] [PubMed]

9.　Buser, D.; Schenk, R.K.; Steinemann, S.; Fiorellini, J.P.; Fox, C.H.; Stich, H. Influence of surface characteristics on bone integration of titanium implants. A histomorphometric study in miniature pigs. *J. Biomed. Mater. Res.* **1991**, *25*, 889–902. [CrossRef] [PubMed]

10.　Scopelliti, P.E.; Borgonovo, A.; Indrieri, M.; Giorgetti, L.; Bongiorno, G.; Carbone, R.; Podestà, A.; Milani, P. The effect of surface nanometre-scale morphology on protein adsorption. *PLoS ONE* **2010**, *5*, e11862. [CrossRef]

11.　Pilliar, R.M. Overview of surface variability of metallic endosseous dental implants: Textured and porous surface-structured designs. *Imp. Dent.* **1998**, *7*, 305–314. [CrossRef]

12.　Ryan, G.; Pandit, A.; Apatsidis, D.P. Fabrication methods of porous metals for use in orthopaedic applications. *Biomaterials* **2006**, *27*, 2651–2670. [CrossRef] [PubMed]

13.　Dabrowski, B.; Swieszkowski, W.; Godlinski, D.; Kurzydlowski, K.J. Highly porous titanium scaffolds for orthopaedic applications. *J. Biomed. Mater. Res. B Appl. Biomater.* **2010**, *95*, 53–61. [CrossRef] [PubMed]

14.　Miyazaki, T.; Kim, H.M.; Kokubo, T.; Ohtsuki, C.; Kato, H.; Nakamura, T. Mechanism of bonelike apatite formation on bioactive tantalum metal in a simulated body fluid. *Biomaterials* **2002**, *23*, 827–832. [CrossRef]

15.　Yoo, D. New paradigms in hierarchical porous scaffold design for tissue engineering. *Mater. Sci. Eng. C Mater. Biol. Appl.* **2013**, *33*, 1759–1772. [CrossRef]

16.　Karageorgio, V.; Kaplan, D. Porosity of 3D biomaterial scaffolds and osteogenesis. *Biomaterials* **2005**, *26*, 5474–5491. [CrossRef]

17.　Fujibayashi, S.; Neo, M.; Kim, H.M.; Kokubo, T.; Nakamura, T. Osteoinduction of porous bioactive titanium metal. *Biomaterials* **2004**, *25*, 443–450. [CrossRef]

18.　Bencharit, S.; Byrd, W.C.; Altarawneh, S.; Hosseini, B.; Leong, A.; Reside, G.; Morelli, T.; Offenbacher, S. Development and applications of porous tantalum trabecular metal-enhanced titanium dental implants. *Clin. Implant. Dent. Relat. Res.* **2014**, *16*, 817–826. [CrossRef]

19.　Pattanayak, D.K.; Fukuda, A.; Matsushita, T.; Takemoto, M.; Fujibayashi, S.; Sasaki, K.; Nishida, N.; Nakamura, T.; Kokubo, T. Bioactive Ti metal analogous to human cancellous bone: Fabrication by selective laser melting and chemical treatments. *Acta Biomater.* **2011**, *7*, 1398–1406. [CrossRef]

20.　Lee, J.W.; Wen, H.B.; Gubbi, P.; Romanos, G.E. New bone formation and trabecular bone microarchitecture of highly porous tantalum compared to titanium implant threads: A pilot canine study. *Clin. Oral Implants Res.* **2018**, *29*, 164–174. [CrossRef]

21.　Fraser, D.; Funkenbusch, P.; Ercoli, C.; Meirelles, L. Biomechanical analysis of the osseointegration of porous tantalum implants. *J. Prosthet. Dent.* **2020**, *123*, 811–820. [CrossRef] [PubMed]

22.　Kilkenny, C.; Altman, D.G. Improving bioscience research reporting: ARRIVE-ing at a solution. *Lab. Anim.* **2010**, *44*, 377–378. [CrossRef]

23.　Cornell, C.N.; Lane, J.M. Current understanding of osteoconduction in bone regeneration. *Clin. Orthop. Relat. Res.* **1998**, *355*, S267–S273. [CrossRef]

24. Levine, B.R.; Sporer, S.; Poggie, R.A.; Della Valle, C.J.; Jacobs, J.J. Experimental and clinical performance of porous tantalum in orthopedic surgery. *Biomaterials* **2006**, *27*, 4671–4681. [CrossRef] [PubMed]

25. Fraser, D.; Mendonca, G.; Sartori, E.; Funkenbusch, P.; Ercoli, C.; Meirelles, L. Bone response to porous tantalum implants in a gap-healing model. *Clin. Oral Implants Res.* **2019**, *30*, 156–168. [CrossRef] [PubMed]

26. Edelmann, A.R.; Patel, D.; Allen, R.K.; Gibson, C.J.; Best, A.M.; Bencharit, S. Retrospective analysis of porous tantalum trabecular metal-enhanced titanium dental implants. *J. Prosthet. Dent.* **2019**, *121*, 404–410. [CrossRef]

27. Dimaira, M. Immediate placement of trabecular implants in sites of failed implants. *Int. J. Oral Maxillofac. Implants* **2019**, *34*, e77–e83. [CrossRef] [PubMed]

28. Liu, Y.; Bao, C.; Wismeijer, D.; Wu, G. The physicochemical/biological properties of porous tantalum and the potential surface modification techniques to improve its clinical application in dental implantology. *Mater. Sci. Eng. C Mater. Biol. Appl.* **2015**, *49*, 323–329. [CrossRef]

29. Lin, S.I.E. Near-net-shape forming of zirconia optical sleeves by ceramics injection molding. *Ceram. Int.* **2001**, *27*, 205–214. [CrossRef]

30. Park, Y.S.; Chung, S.H.; Shon, W.J. Peri-implant bone formation and surface characteristics of rough surface zirconia implants manufactured by powder injection molding technique in rabbit tibiae. *Clin. Oral Implants Res.* **2013**, *24*, 586–591. [CrossRef] [PubMed]

31. Lee, J.H.; Kim, H.J.; Yun, J.H. Three-dimensional microstructure of human alveolar trabecular bone: A micro-computed tomography study. *J. Periodontal Implant. Sci.* **2017**, *47*, 20–29. [CrossRef] [PubMed]

32. Bobyn, J.D.; Stackpool, G.J.; Hacking, S.A.; Tanzer, M.; Krygier, J.J. Characteristics of bone ingrowth and interface mechanics of a new porous tantalum biomaterial. *J. Bone Joint Surg. Br.* **1999**, *81*, 907–914. [CrossRef] [PubMed]

33. Davies, J.E. Understanding peri-implant endosseous healing. *J. Dent. Educ.* **2003**, *67*, 932–949. [CrossRef] [PubMed]

34. Hanisch, O.; Cortella, C.A.; Boskovic, M.M.; James, R.A.; Slots, J.; Wikesjö, U.M. Experimental peri-implant tissue breakdown around hydroxyapatite-coated implants. *J. Periodontol.* **1997**, *68*, 59–66. [CrossRef] [PubMed]

35. Lee, C.T.; Tran, D.; Jeng, M.D.; Shen, Y.T. Survival rates of hybrid rough surface implants and their alveolar bone level alteration. *J. Periodontol.* **2018**, *12*, 1390–1399. [CrossRef] [PubMed]

36. Baggi, L.; Cappelloni, I.; Di Girolamo, M.; Maceri, F.; Vairo, G. The influence of implant diameter and length on stress distribution of osseointegrated implants related to crestal bone geometry: A three-dimensional finite element analysis. *J. Prosthet. Dent.* **2008**, *100*, 422–431. [CrossRef]

37. Sennerby, L.; Meredith, N. Implant stability measurements using resonance frequency analysis: Biological and biomechanical aspects and clinical implications. *Periodontology 2000* **2008**, *47*, 51–66. [CrossRef]

38. Klokkevold, P.R.; Johnson, P.; Dadgostari, S.; Caputo, A.; Davies, J.E.; Nishimura, R.D. Early endosseous integration enhanced by dual acid etching of titanium: A torque removal study in the rabbit. *Clin. Oral Implants Res.* **2001**, *12*, 350–357. [CrossRef] [PubMed]

39. Scaglione, S.; Giannoni, P.; Bianchini, P.; Sandri, M.; Marotta, R.; Firpo, G.; Valbusa, U.; Tampieri, A.; Diaspro, A.; Bianco, P.; et al. Order versus disorder: In vivo bone formation within osteoconductive scaffolds. *Sci. Rep.* **2012**, *2*, 274. [CrossRef]

40. Chang, B.S.; Lee, C.K.; Hong, K.S.; Youn, H.J.; Ryu, H.S.; Chung, S.S.; Park, K.W. Osteoconduction at porous hydroxyapatite with various pore configurations. *Biomaterials* **2000**, *21*, 1291–1298. [CrossRef]

41. Götz, H.E.; Müller, M.; Emmel, A.; Holzwarth, U.; Erben, R.G.; Stangl, R. Effect of surface finish on the osseointegration of laser-treated titanium alloy implants. *Biomaterials* **2004**, *25*, 4057–4064. [CrossRef] [PubMed]

3

Radiological Outcomes of Bone-Level and Tissue-Level Dental Implants

Saverio Cosola [1,2,*], Simone Marconcini [2], Michela Boccuzzi [2],
Giovanni Battista Menchini Fabris [2,3], Ugo Covani [2], Miguel Peñarrocha-Diago [1]
and David Peñarrocha-Oltra [1]

[1] Oral Surgery Unit, Department of Stomatology, Faculty of Medicine and Dentistry, University of Valencia, 13, 46010 Valencia, Spain; miguel.penarrocha@uv.es (M.P.-D.); david.penarrocha@uv.es (D.P.-O.)

[2] Tuscan Stomatologic Institute, via Aurelia, 335, 55041 Lido di Camaiore, Italy; simosurg@gmail.com (S.M.); michela.boccuzzi@hotmail.it (M.B.); gbmenchinifabris@yahoo.it (G.B.M.F.); covani@covani.it (U.C.)

[3] Department of Stomatology, University of Studies Guglielmo Marconi, 44, 00193 Roma, Italy

[*] Correspondence: s.cosola@hotmail.it

Abstract: *Background*: to assess the radiological marginal bone loss between bone-level or tissue-level dental implants through a systematic review of literature until September 2019. *Methods*: MEDLINE, Embase and other database were searched by two independent authors including only English articles. *Results*: The search provided 1028 records and, after removing the duplicates through titles and abstracts screening, 45 full-text articles were assessed for eligibility. For qualitative analysis 20 articles were included, 17 articles of them for quantitative analysis counting a total of 1161 patients (mean age 54.4 years) and 2933 implants, 1427 inserted at Tissue-level (TL) and 1506 inserted at Bone-level (BL). The survival rate and the success rate were more than 90%, except for 2 studies with a success rate of 88% and 86.2%. No studies reported any differences between groups in term of success and survival rates. Three studies showed that BL-implants had statistically less marginal bone loss ($p < 0.05$). Only one study reported statistically less marginal bone loss in TL-implants ($p < 0.05$). *Conclusion*: In the most part of the studies, differences between implant types in marginal bone loss were not statistically significant after a variable period of follow-up ranged between 1 and 5 years.

Keywords: tissue-level; bone-level; dental implants; transmucosal; marginal bone loss; systematic review

1. Introduction

Dental implants are the gold standard treatment to restore single edentulous space and partially or completely edentulous jaws because of their long-term success rate, the positive impact on patients' quality of life, and the simplified modern surgical procedures with low morbidity [1,2].

Several factors can influence the preservation of hard and soft tissues around dental implants. Among these factors, the clinician's experience, loading time, surgical protocol, implant neck configuration, implant-abutment connection, the insertion torque, and oral hygiene/maintenance protocols have been shown to influence the different outcomes of the implant therapy [3].

To reach the increasing patients' needs for aesthetic results, low cost and fastest result, several factors must be taken into account before choosing the implant type and the protocol with the goal of a long survival and success rates of the implant-prosthetic rehabilitation. Among these factors, the clinician's experience, the loading time, the type or surgery, the insertion torque, the oral hygiene maintenance protocols, the implant neck configuration and the implant-abutment connection, may influence the preservation of healthy peri-implant hard and soft tissues [4].

Clinical parameters (bleeding score and gingival index) and radiographic parameters (marginal bone loss) are used to evaluate the stability of the peri-implant soft and hard tissues.

The most used and objective clinical and radiological parameters to evaluate the stability of the peri-implant soft and hard tissue, so that the success of the rehabilitations, are respectively bleeding score, gingival index and marginal bone loss (ΔMBL) [5]. Dental implants, after the healing period of 2–5 months, are anchored to the bone because of osseointegration. Traditionally, implants are two-pieces, so they are connected to the prosthetic rehabilitation through a transmucosal component, called abutment [6].

The early bone loss is observed after the connection of the abutment and when the prosthesis is loaded on the implant. It is well-known that there are a lots of factors to explain marginal bone resorption around dental implants such as: the occlusal trauma, biologic width establishment, gingival biotype, insertion torque of the implants, prosthesis loading timing, thickness of the remaining bone, type of surgery, primary stability, lack of bone to implant contact (BIC), bacterial colonization of the implant-abutment junction (IAJ), the macro and micro characteristic of abutment and the coronal portion of the fixture (shoulder/neck of the implant), and the position of the implant [7].

To avoid some of these disadvantages, Schroeder and co-workers introduced a "one-piece" implants to remove the contamination of the implant-abutment junction (IAJ) and to reduce the micromovements in the connection [8].

Nevertheless, one-piece implants have a difficult first surgery due to vertical dimension and due to the orientation of the remaining bone and the final prosthetic rehabilitation. One-piece implants must be inserted according to the final prosthesis position, not only considering hard and soft tissue availability. Moreover, if there are biomechanical complications, it may be more difficult it is not possible to remove to replace the abutment and final prosthesis. the abutment, instead all the implant must be removed.

In modern literature, the term "one-piece implant" has modified its meaning. The new conception of "one-piece implants" regards both endosseous and transmucosal components, but the link with the abutment remains, located at increased distance from the bone, at tissue level [9].

To compare one-piece and two-pieces implants several clinical studies and some systematic review were performed in the last years.

Iglhaut and co-workers stated that the microgrooved surface could be associated with a longer connective tissue attachment and less bone resorption around implants [10].

Even though, considering the literature data, doubts still remain about the question: "What is the difference between one piece (bone-level) and two-piece (transmucosal) dental implants at single or multiple edentulous sites in terms of clinical and radiological outcomes during a long follow-up period?

Focusing on the literature until September 2019, the aim of the present systematic review was to identify whether there are relationships between different implants' position (tissue level or bone level) and radiographic marginal bone loss in single or multiple rehabilitation, after at least 1-year of function. The terminology throughout the manuscript is various to be comprehensive for all synonymous which could be found in literature (e.g., tissue level/transmucosal/one piece versus bone level/two pieces implants).

2. Materials and Methods

The present review has been conducted in accordance with the guidelines for Systematic Reviews and Meta-Analyses (PRISMA) [11].

Before starting the systematic review, a protocol has been developed and registered at PROSPERO, (International prospective register of systematic reviews, National Institute for Health Research, University of York, York, UK) with number: CRD42020157607.

This question follows the PICO (Population, intervention, comparison, outcomes) guidelines. The population (Population) was systemically healthy patients who (Intervention) received at least one implant and those implants that had been in place for at least one year. The Comparison in this type of studies was between two treatment groups according the level of implants: bone level and tissue level implants. The Outcome was the marginal bone loss.

The focused question was: are there any differences in terms of marginal bone loss in single or multiple rehabilitation between bone level implant and transmucosal/tissue level implant?

The rationale is based on the position of implant-abutment connection which could influence the healing process of the peri-implant tissues even after 1 or more years of follow-up, because of inflammation and bacterial infiltration in the micro-gap [12,13].

2.1. Search Strategy

The search was carried out independently by two authors and on four databases (MEDLINE, Embase, Inspec, and Cochrane Central Register of Controlled Trials) using synonyms as [(dental Implant OR abutment) AND (shoulder design OR implant abutment interface OR transmucosal OR bone-level OR scalloped implant OR sloped implant OR flat implant OR one-piece or two-pieces)].

The search was limited to articles in English. No restrictions on date of publication or follow-up period were applied when searching the first electronic databases to be as inclusive as possible. These databases were carried out until September 2019.

The exclusion criteria were applied after the electronic search. The bibliographies of all identified clinical included studies and relevant review articles were checked in order to identify other eligible articles related to the topic.

A complementary manual search that included a complete revision up to September 2019 was made of the following journals: Journal of Clinical Periodontology, Journal of Periodontal Research, Journal of Oral Science & Rehabilitation and Journal of Dental Research.

2.2. Study Selection and Eligibility Criteria

Randomized clinical trials (RCTs), case-control studies, comparative studies, and clinical trials comparing the clinical and/or radiological outcomes of different dental implant shoulder/neck position related to the crestal bone have been searched. The publications with the following inclusion criteria were selected:

- Comparison of different neck/shoulder position (One-piece vs. two-pieces or tissue-level or transmucosal vs. bone-level) of dental implants with at least 1-year follow-up after loading;
- Patients aged between 18 and 70 years old;
- Patients without severe systemic (e.g., recent cardiovascular event or tumoral pathology) or psychiatric disease;
- Clinical and radiological parameters measured were at least respectively bleeding on probing (BoP), and marginal bone loss (ΔMBL);
- Only studies published in English.

The gingival recession was evaluated as a secondary outcome of interest in order to compare the possible association of one type of electric toothbrush with gingival recession prevalence. Reviews, letters, animal model, and vitro studies were excluded. Other exclusion criteria were:

- Studies included orthodontics patients;
- Studies included patients with disabilities;
- Studies included patients who are taking bisphosphonates;
- Studies comparing two or more different types of implant-abutment connections (e.g., switching platform) not focusing on position related to the bone;
- Studies comparing two or more different types of implant surgical technique with similar implant (e.g., one step surgery or two step) not focusing on position related to the bone;
- Studies comparing two or more different types of implant or abutment micro design;

- Studies comparing two or more different types of micro design of the implant neck or of the abutment;
- Final timepoint after less than 1 year after loading;
- Studies evaluating short-implants (in literature defined as implant <8.5 mm) [14];
- Studies analyzing implants and abutments used to retain removable prosthesis;
- Studies published before 1990;
- Duplicated studies or studies with different time points were included only one time with the longest duration.

2.3. Screening and Study Selection

Records identified through database searching were upload on End-Note (ISI Researchsoft 2001, Berkeley, CA, USA, http://www.endnote.com) to exclude the duplicates.

Then, titles and abstracts of all remaining articles were independently scanned by two reviewers following inclusion and exclusion criteria. Disagreements between authors were resolved after discussion by the intervention of a third author.

For studies appearing to meet the inclusion criteria, or for which there were insufficient information in the title and abstract to assess a clear decision, the full-text was obtained. The screening of full-text articles was performed by two reviewers independently to establish whether or not the studies met the inclusion and exclusion criteria. Disagreements were resolved by discussion of two authors. When resolution was not possible, a third reviewer was consulted.

Full-text rejected at this, or subsequent stages, were recorded in the table of excluded studies explaining reasons for exclusion.

All full-text articles meeting the inclusion criteria and assessed for eligibility were evaluated again by three authors to assess the quality of the methodology of each article and to perform data extraction.

2.4. Quality Assessment (Risk of Bias of Included RCTs)

A quality assessment of the included studies was performed according to the Cochrane Handbook for Systematic Reviews of Interventions (version 5.1.0; updated March 2011 by Higgins and Green).

According to handbook guideline five main quality criteria were evaluated:

1. Random sequence generation,
2. Allocation concealment,
3. Blinding of participants, personnel, and outcomes assessors,
4. Incomplete outcome data,
5. Selective outcome reporting.

Depending on the descriptions given for each main article of included studies, these criteria were rated as: low, unclear, or high risk of bias.

2.5. Quantitative Analysis

Mean marginal bone changes values were extracted from each study by one author (S.C.) and compared weighting parameters according to the number of implants for each study using a descriptive statistic. The number of implants was multiplicated by the number of MBL so that a study with a bigger number of implants value more than a study with a lower number of cases. The data were analysed using the T-test with a $p < 0.05$.

3. Results

The purpose of this review was to summarize the available evidences reported in literature of the included studies comparing the marginal bone loss of bone level (BL) versus tissue level implants (TL).

Bone level changes between one-piece (TL) and two-piece (BL) dental implants. The combined search in four databases provided 1028 records (Figure 1).

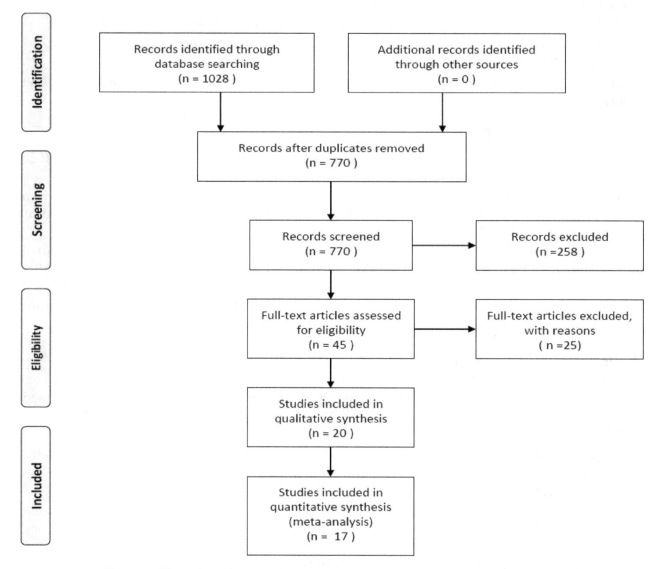

Figure 1. Flow chart diagram (2009) of search strategy adapted from PRISMA.

After removing the duplicates using the software End-Note (ISI Researchsoft 2001) and the screening of title and abstract according to the relevance of the topic 45 articles remained. Following inclusion and exclusion criteria, the full-text of these article was obtained. In Table 1, excluded articles were reported with reasons, three of them (colored in grey) were excluded only from quantitative analysis, but not qualitative [15–42].

Table 1. Excluded articles after full-text screening; the articles marked in grey rows were included for qualitative analysis, but not quantitative one [15–42].

No.	References	Exclusion Motivation
1	Becktor JP, Isaksson S, Billström C. A prospective multicenter study using two different surgical approaches in the mandible with turned Brånemark implants: conventional loading using fixed prostheses [15]	Excluded for the quantitative analysis: The parameter "marginal bone level" was not clearly reported.

Table 1. *Cont.*

No.	References	Exclusion Motivation
2	Bratu EA, Tandlich M, Shapira L. A rough surface implant neck with microthreads reduces the amount of marginal bone loss: a prospective clinical study [16]	Studies comparing 2 or more different types of implant or abutment micro design.
3	de Siqueira RAC, Fontão FNGK, Sartori IAM, Santos PGF, Bernardes SR, Tiossi R. Effect of different implant placement depths on crestal bone levels and soft tissue behavior: a randomized clinical trial [17]	Studies comparing 2 or more different types of implant or abutment micro design.
4	Chappuis V, Bornstein MM, Buser D, Belser U. Influence of implant neck design on facial bone crest dimensions in the esthetic zone analyzed by cone beam CT: a comparative study with a 5-to-9-year follow-up [18]	Excluded for the quantitative analysis: excluded because it reports median, not mean value of MBL.
5	Chien HH, Schroering RL, Prasad HS, Tatakis DN. Effects of a new implant abutment design on peri-implant soft tissues [19]	Studies comparing 2 or more different types of micro design of the implant neck or of the abutment.
6	Cosyn J, Sabzevar MM, De Wilde P, De Rouck T. Two-piece implants with turned versus microtextured collars [20]	Studies comparing 2 or more different types of implant or abutment micro design.
7	Ebler S, Ioannidis A, Jung RE, Hämmerle CH, Thoma DS. Prospective randomized controlled clinical study comparing two types of two-piece dental implants supporting fixed reconstructions—results at 1 year of loading [21]	Studies comparing 2 or more different types of implant surgical technique with similar implant (e.g., one step surgery or two step) not focusing on position related to the bone.
8	Esposito M, Trullenque-Eriksson A, Blasone R, et al. Clinical evaluation of a novel dental implant system as single implants under immediate loading conditions—4-month post-loading results from a multicentre randomised controlled trial [22]	Studies comparing 2 or more different types of implant surgical technique with similar implant (e.g., one step surgery or two step) not focusing on position related to the bone.
9	Hof M, Pommer B, Strbac GD, Vasak C, Agis H, Zechner W. Impact of insertion torque and implant neck design on peri-implant bone level: a randomized split-mouth trial [23]	Studies comparing 2 or more different types of implant or abutment micro design.
10	Herrero-Climent M, Romero Ruiz MM, Díaz-Castro CM, Bullón P, Ríos-Santos JV. Influence of two different machined-collar heights on crestal bone loss [24]	Studies comparing 2 or more different types of implant surgical technique with similar implant (e.g., one step surgery or two step) not focusing on position related to the bone.
11	Judgar R, Giro G, Zenobio E, et al. Biological width around one- and two-piece implants retrieved from human jaws [25]	Studies comparing 2 or more different types of implant surgical technique with similar implant (e.g., one step surgery or two step) not focusing on position related to the bone.
12	Khorsand A, Rasouli-Ghahroudi AA, Naddafpour N, Shayesteh YS, Khojasteh A. Effect of Microthread Design on Marginal Bone Level Around Dental Implants Placed in Fresh Extraction Sockets [26]	Studies comparing 2 or more different types of implant surgical technique with similar implant (e.g., one step surgery or two step) not focusing on position related to the bone.
13	Khraisat A, Zembic A, Jung RE, Hammerle CH. Marginal bone levels and soft tissue conditions around single-tooth implants with a scalloped neck design: results of a prospective 3-year study [27]	Studies comparing 2 or more different types of implant-abutment connections (e.g., Switching platform) not focusing on position related to the bone.
14	Kim JJ, Lee DW, Kim CK, Park KH, Moon IS. Effect of conical configuration of fixture on the maintenance of marginal bone level: preliminary results at 1 year of function [28]	Studies comparing 2 or more different types of implant surgical technique with similar implant (e.g., one step surgery or two step) not focusing on position related to the bone.

Table 1. *Cont.*

No.	References	Exclusion Motivation
15	Kütan E, Bolukbasi N, Yildirim-Ondur E, Ozdemir T. Clinical and Radiographic Evaluation of Marginal Bone Changes around Platform-Switching Implants Placed in Crestal or Subcrestal Positions: A Randomized Controlled Clinical Trial [29]	Studies comparing 2 or more different types of implant surgical technique with similar implant (e.g., one step surgery or two step) not focusing on position related to the bone.
16	Marconcini S, Giammarinaro E, Toti P, Alfonsi F, Covani U, Barone A. Longitudinal analysis on the effect of insertion torque on delayed single implants: A 3-year randomized clinical study [30]	Studies comparing 2 or more different types of micro design of the implant neck or of the abutment.
17	Moberg LE, Köndell PA, Sagulin GB, Bolin A, Heimdahl A, Gynther GW. Brånemark System and ITI Dental Implant System for treatment of mandibular edentulism. A comparative randomized study: 3-year follow-up [31]	Excluded for the quantitative analysis:The parameter "marginal bone level" was not clearly reported.
18	Nóvoa L, Batalla P, Caneiro L, Pico A, Liñares A, Blanco J. Influence of Abutment Height on Maintenance of Peri-implant Crestal Bone at Bone-Level Implants: A 3-Year Follow-up Study [32]	Studies comparing 2 or more different types of micro design of the implant neck or of the abutment.
19	Ormianer Z, Duda M, Block J, Matalon S. One- and Two-Piece Implants Placed in the Same Patients: Clinical Outcomes After 5 Years of Function [33]	It is the topic of the present review but it is a case series.
20	Pellicer-Chover H, Peñarrocha-Diago M, Peñarrocha-Oltra D, Gomar-Vercher S, Agustín-Panadero R, Peñarrocha-Diago M. Impact of crestal and subcrestal implant placement in peri-implant bone: A prospective comparative study [34]	Studies comparing 2 or more different types of implant surgical technique with similar implant (e.g., one step surgery or two step) not focusing on position related to the bone.
21	Peñarrocha-Diago MA, Flichy-Fernández AJ, Alonso-González R, Peñarrocha-Oltra D, Balaguer-Martínez J, Peñarrocha-Diago M. Influence of implant neck design and implant-abutment connection type on peri-implant health. Radiological study [35]	Studies comparing 2 or more different types of implant or abutment micro design.
22	Pozzi A, Agliardi E, Tallarico M, Barlattani A. Clinical and radiological outcomes of two implants with different prosthetic interfaces and neck configurations: randomized, controlled, split-mouth clinical trial [36]	Studies comparing 2 or more different types of implant surgical technique with similar implant (e.g., one step surgery or two step) not focusing on position related to the bone.
23	Pozzi A, Tallarico M, Moy PK. Three-year post-loading results of a randomised, controlled, split-mouth trial comparing implants with different prosthetic interfaces and design in partially posterior edentulous mandibles [37]	Studies comparing 2 or more different types of implant-abutment connections (e.g., Switching platform) not focusing on position related to the bone.
24	Sanz-Martin I, Vignoletti F, Nuñez J, et al. Hard and soft tissue integration of immediate and delayed implants with a modified coronal macrodesign: Histological, micro-CT and volumetric soft tissue changes from a pre-clinical in vivo study [38]	It is a study on animal model (Dog).
25	Shin YK, Han CH, Heo SJ, Kim S, Chun HJ. Radiographic evaluation of marginal bone level around implants with different neck designs after 1 year [39]	Studies comparing 2 or more different types of implant or abutment micro design

Table 1. *Cont.*

No.	References	Exclusion Motivation
26	Tan WC, Lang NP, Schmidlin K, Zwahlen M, Pjetursson BE. The effect of different implant neck configurations on soft and hard tissue healing: a randomized-controlled clinical trial [40]	Studies comparing 2 or more different types of implant surgical technique with similar implant (e.g., one step surgery or two step) not focusing on position related to the bone.
27	Weinländer M, Lekovic V, Spadijer-Gostovic S, Milicic B, Wegscheider WA, Piehslinger E. Soft tissue development around abutments with a circular macro-groove in healed sites of partially edentulous posterior maxillae and mandibles: a clinical pilot study [41]	Studies comparing 2 or more different types of micro design of the implant neck or of the abutment.
28	Wittneben JG, Gavric J, Belser UC, et al. Esthetic and Clinical Performance of Implant-Supported All-Ceramic Crowns Made with Prefabricated or CAD/CAM Zirconia Abutments: A Randomized, Multicenter Clinical Trial [42]	Studies comparing 2 or more different types of micro design of the implant neck or of the abutment.

At the end of the study selection, a last revision was performed again by two authors and 17 articles were included for the final quantitative analysis (20 considering also qualitative analysis as reported in Table 2).

Table 2. All studies included for the qualitative analysis. The 3 studies in grey rowed were excluded from the quantitative analysis as explained in the text [43–59].

	Studies Qualitative Analysis	Study Design	Patients Sample	Number of Implants (BL/TL)	Mean Age Range of the Sample	Type of 6 Implants BL; TL	Type of Prosthetic Restoration	Success Rate BL/TL	Survival Rate BL/TL	Follow-Up
1	Astrand P. [43]	Prospective Randomized Comparative Multicenter Study	28	73/77	61.7 ± SD range: 36–76	BL: Branemark TL:ITI	Fixed Partial Bridges	/	100%	12 Months; 36 Months;
2	Bassi M. [44]	Prospective Clinical Study	133	66/67	60 ± 11 range: 29–75	BL: I-Fiz EVO Conical; TL: Shiner EVO Conical;	52 Single Crown/3 Overdenture/70 Bridges	88%	100%	60 Months;
3	Becktor. [15]	Prospective Multicenter Study	80	206/198	TL: 63.5 ± 9.1 Range: 47–89 BL: 65.5 ± 9.4 Range: 44–84	Branemark System Nobel Biocare AB	Fixed Prosthetic Dentures		97.6%/91.4%	6 Months; 12 Months; 36 Months;
4	Bömicke W. [45]	Randomized Controlled Trial Study	38	19/19	TL: 54.37 ± 14.62 BL: 51.51 ± 13.96	Nobel Biocare AB	Single Zirconia Crown	/	100%/94.7%	12 Months; 36 Months;
5	Cecchinato D. [46]	Multicenter Randomized Controlled Crinical Trial	84	171/153	51.6	Astra Tech	Fixed Prosthetic dentures	/	>98%	12 Months; 24 Months;
6	Cecchinato D. [46]	Multicenter Randomized Controlled Crinical Trial	84	171/153	51.6	Astra Tech	Fixed Prosthetic Dentures	/	>98%	24 Months; 60 Months;
7	Chappuis V. [18]	Comparative Study	61	20/41	TL: 38.8 Range: 24–72 BL: 41.7 Range: 24–60	Straumann	Single Crown	/	/	60 Months;
8	Duda M. [48]	Non Randomized Retrospective Study	33	29/24	TL: 42.5 BL: 53.6	Q Implants Trinon Titanium GmbH		/	100%/91.7%	6, 12, 36 Months; 60 Months;
9	Eliasson A. [49]	prospective clinical study	29	84/84	65	DBA Paragon	Full arch ISFP	86.2%	99.4%	12 Months; 60 Months;
10	Engquist B. [50]	Controlled Prospective Study	82	113/80	TL: 65 BL: 64	Branemark System Noble Blocare AB	Fixed Prosthetic bridges	/	97.5%/93.2%	12 Months;
11	Engquist B. [51]	Controlled Prospective Study	108	110/106	64.9	Branemark System Nobel Biocare AB	Fixed Prosthetic Bridges with Cantilever	/	100%/100%	12 Months; 36 Months;

Table 2. *Cont.*

	Studies Qualitative Analysis	Study Design	Patients Sample	Number of Implants (BL/TL)	Mean Age Range of the Sample	Type of 6 Implants BL; TL	Type of Prosthetic Restoration	Success Rate BL/TL	Survival Rate BL/TL	Follow-Up
12	Ericsson I. [52]	Longitudinal Study	11	33/30	61 Range: 42–72	Branemark System	Fixed Prosthetic Bridges	/	/	12 Months; 18 Months;
13	Gamper F.A. [53]	Randomized Controlled Clinical Trial Study	60	86/65	TL: 47.5 ± 15 BL: 55.8 ± 14	BL: Branemark system Nobel Biocare AB TL: Straumann	Removable Prosthetic Prostheses/Screw Retained prostheses/cemented prostheses	/	98.9%/96.6%	60 Months;
14	Gulati M. [54]	Prospective Randomized Comparative Study	19	10/10	TL: 28.22 ± 3.27 BL: 27.20 ± 2.78 Range: 23–33	Adin Dental Implant System	Screw-Retained Porcelain Fused to Metal Prosthesis	/	/	3 and 6 Months;
15	Hadzik J. [55]	Clinical Study	13	16/16	TL: 46.3 BL: 45.9 Range: 20–63	BL: Osseospeed TX, Astra tech TL: RN SLActive®, Straumann	Cemented Crowns	/	100%	6 Months;
16	Heijdenrijk K. [56]	Prospective Randomized Study	60	38/38	58 ± 11	Unknown	Overdenture with Clip Attachment	/	/	12, 24, 36, 48, and 60 Months;
17	Lago L. [57]	Randomized Clinical Trial	100	102/100	50.5 Range: 25–70	Straumann	Single Crowns		96.1%/98%	12 and 60 Months;
18	Moberg [31]	Randomized Prospective Study	40	103/106	BL: 62.6 ± 7.0 Range: 44.2–75.2 TL: 64.0 ± 6.8 Range: 40.2–77.2	BL: Branemark System Nobel Biocare AB TL: ITI system	Screw Prosthetic Bridges	97.9%/96.8%	/	6 Months; 12 Months; 36 Months;
19	Paolantoni G. [58]	Randomized Controlled Clinical Trial Study	65	29/45	53 ± 4	Thommen Medical AG	Single Crowns		100%	60 Months;
20	Sanz-Martin I. [59]	Prospective Randomized Controlled Clinical Study	33	18/15	Unknown	BL: Branemark System Nobel Biocare AB TL: Straumann	Group 2 Piece: SCs-4FDPs Group 1 Piece: SCs–4FDPs	/	/	12 Months;
	Total		1161	2933						3–60 Months;

3.1. Qualitative Analysis

The data collected from each study were resumed in Table 3 [15,18,31,43–59].

Table 3. The mean values of marginal bone loss (changes) in relation to the number of implants of each study with corresponding *p*-values.

Mean Value Marginal Bone Changes #	Bone Level Implant	Tissue Level	Significance (*p* < 0.05)
3 Months	0.19	0.28	/(Only Gulati 2013)
6 Months	0.33	0.42	0.0169 * (3 studies)
n = 115	*n* = 65	*n* = 50	
12 Months	0.25	0.18	0.0000 * (12 studies)
n = 1850	*n* = 971	*n* = 879	
18 Months	0.05	0.04	/(Only Ericsson 1994)
24 Months	0.18	0.24	0.1907 (2 studies)
36 Months	0.45	0.48	0.5031 (5 studies)
48 Months	1.4	1.6	/(Only Heijdenrijk 2006)
60 Months	0.29	0.38	0.0050 * (7 studies)
n = 1069	*n* = 576	*n* = 493	

The mean values of marginal bone loss (changes) are weighted considering the number of implants of each study.
* The T-test reported significance with $p < 0.05$.

In four studies the implants were positioned in the maxilla [18,43,53,58] in eight studies the implant rehabilitation involved the mandible [45,49–52,54–56] while in the other studies the patients received the implants in both jaws.

In two studis [43,58] the implants were inserted in the anterior region of the maxilla, in one study [53] the implants were positioned in the anterior region of the mandible, whereas in three studies [45,54,55] the implant treatment was performed in the posterior region of the mandible. In the majority of the studies, the patients were treated with the dental implants in both anterior and posterior region of maxillae.

All studies analyzed two types of implant systems: bone level implants and tissue level implants in different groups with different surgery and prosthetic protocols by different clinicians.

The parameter "Marginal Bone Level" was evaluated by the radiographic examination (intraoral radiography) in order to compare the changes in the bone level at the baseline and in the different time of follow-up.

The timing of each follow-up varied considerably through the studies, from a first evaluation at a minimum of 3 months (Gulati 2013) to a maximum of 5 years [31,44,45,49,51,53,56–58], even if the overall follow-up ranged from 1 years to 3 years in the majority of the studies.

The study included 1161 patients (mean age 54.4 years), who needed implants rehabilitation for mandibular and maxilla edentulism by fixed and removable prosthetic prostheses [53].

In total, 2933 implants were placed, 1427 according to the non-submerged protocols and 1506 according to the traditional submerged procedure. In both groups (submerged versus transmucosal group), the most used implants brands were the Branemark implants system Nobel Biocare AB, the ITI systems, the Astra Tech system, and the Straumann systems with exception for some studies as noticed in Table 3.

For both implant systems, the fabrication of fixed prostheses has provided for single crowns and bridges in most cases. Some authors did not specify the prosthetic protocol and no information was given about the design of the framework except for [31,45,53–56].

In the present review, the only parameter used was marginal bone loss changes in the quantitative analysis because of the too wide variability of each studies in other clinical outcomes. The studies analyzed bleeding score did not reported any statically significant differences between groups.

The survival rate and success rate if reported were more than 90%, except for two studies [44,49] that had a success rate of 88% and 86.2% respectively. No studies reported any differences between groups in term of success and survival rates.

Three studies [45,48,57] showed that BL-implants had statistically less marginal bone loss compared with TL-implants ($p < 0.05$). Only one study [53] reported statistically greater peri-implant bone maintenance over time in TL-implants ($p < 0.05$).

In the most part of the studies, differences between implant types in marginal bone loss were not statistical neither clinically significant.

3.2. Quality Assessment

The methodological quality was assessed using the "Downs and Black Scale" and the "New Castle Ottawa Scale Cohort Studies" as suggested by the Cochrane Handbook [60].

The quality scores was graded as high for the studies with a score ≥ 24, medium for the studies with a score between 12 and 24 and low for the studies with a score ≤ 12 [61,62].

Two reviewers investigated the internal validity of the eligible studies and according to the quality assessment tool and the reported results in Figure 2, fourteen studies showed high quality [15,18,31, 45,46,49–51,53–58] meanwhile the other studies showed a moderate quality [18,43,44,47,48,52,58].

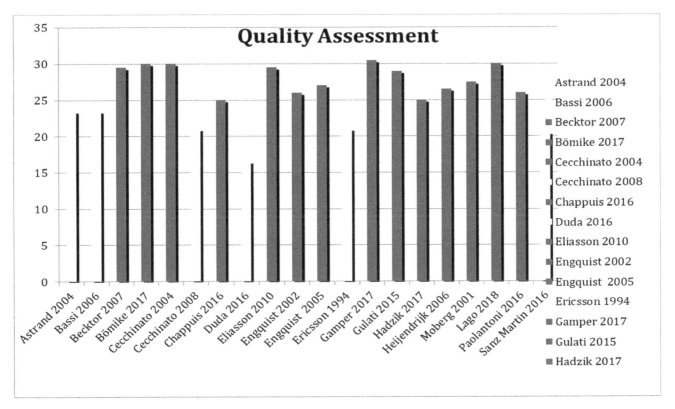

Figure 2. Quality assessment of the studies.

Two authors investigated on the factors that could systematically affect the observations and the conclusions of the studies [63].

The two independent and calibrated authors assessed each single study, according as shown in Figure 3, papers were divided according to risk of bias in three categories: low risk, moderate risk, and high risk [63].

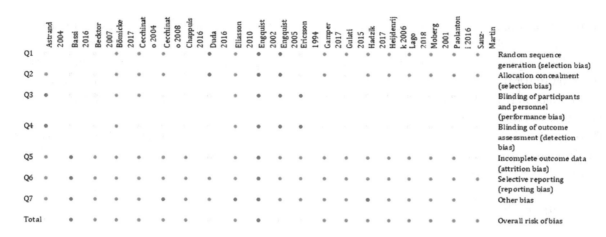

Figure 3. Risk bias word: Risk bias word: red–high risk; yellow–unclear; risk green-low risk.

The tool items were scored as 1 if the item was considered fully fulfilled, as 0 if the item was clearly not fulfilled, and as 0.5 if the item was unclearly or only partially fulfilled.

Studies with a score ≤2.3 were considered high risk of bias, with a score between 2.4 and 4.6 as moderate risk, and with a score ≥4.7 were considered low risk of bias.

The majority of the studies showed a low risk of bias, whereas six studies had a moderate risk of bias: [43,44,48,50–52].

3.3. Quantitative Analysis

Seventeen studies were selected for the quantitative analysis and the marginal bone loss comparison. The radiographic outcome refers to a total of 980 patients and 2260 implants: 1178 implants in BL-groups and 1082 implants in TL-groups.

Three studies reported marginal bone changes at 6 months, twelve studies at 1 year, five studies at 3 year, and seven studies at 5 year, only few studies reported the values at 3 months at 18 months, and finally at 2 year [46].

It had the following follow-up: 6 months, 12 months, 24 months, 36 months, and 60 months reporting better performances of BL-implants in the first time except for 60 months for which there are no radiological values for TL-implants.

The distribution of the mean bone level changes is presented in Table 3. The mean values of marginal bone loss (changes) were weighted considering the number of implants of each study, so that differences between the two intervention groups were calculated with a significance <0.05.

At 3 and 4 months the marginal bone loss was less in BL-groups, but the differences were not significative, plus only one study had such a short follow-up.

At 6 months the marginal bone loss was calculated in a total of 115 implants and it was lower in BL-groups than TL-groups, with a significance <0.05. This statistically significant difference was inverted at 12 months (less in TL than BL) with a sample of 1850 implants ($p < 0.01$). The follow-up at 12 months is the most representative of all included studies. The bone loss reported was again less in TL at 18 months, less in BL at 24 months and 36 months, but these three time-points were not statistically significant.

After 60 months of follow-up the mean marginal bone loss was less in BL-group then in TL-group with a sample of 1069 implants ($p < 0.01$).

4. Discussion

This review gave clinicians an overall view of the topic to improve the knowledge of the marginal bone level changes after several years of follow-up, thus showing if different implant systems (bone level vs. tissue level) could affect bone resorption.

Two recent systematic reviews and meta-analyses conducted by Sanz-Martín and colleagues analyzed all randomized controlled trials (RCTs) until 2016 that investigated macroscopic design, surface topography, and the manipulation of the abutment [64,65]. The authors reported no significant differences between these implants on peri-implant parameters. Only the abutment material had a significant impact on BoP values and ΔMBL.

While Sanz-Martín and colleagues focused on the topic on abutment, other reviews studied the shoulder of the fixture. Starch-Jensen, Christensen, and Lorenzen [66] reported significantly more peri-implant marginal bone loss and higher BoP score in implants with a scalloped implant-abutment connection and not in the flat implant-abutment connection, despite their initial hypothesis, but their review included only three studies.

Also, Tallarico and colleagues, in another systematic review on the topic that also analyzed studies until 2016 (seven RCTs and five comparative studies), highlighted no significant evidence that the implant shoulder position/orientation and design offered improvements in clinical and radiological outcomes [67]. Nevertheless, they also included one-piece implants and they admitted that these results were limited because of the quality of available studies.

In the present analysis, three studies [18,43,59] reported slightly better values in marginal bone loss in BL-groups than TL but with no significance. Also no significant differences were found in the three studies [44,46,47] in which the marginal bone loss was slightly less in TL than in BL; while three studies reported statistically significant bone loss lower for BL than TL and only one study highlighted better radiological outcomes in TL. The other ten studies did not highlight any statistical differences.

Due to the heterogeneity of the included studies according to implant designs, sample sizes, patient parameters, time of evaluation and follow-ups, valid statistical comparisons are not possible, perhaps descriptive statistic for quantitative analysis was used.

The results of this review showed that most parts of the articles reported no differences between BL and TL according to bone loss, survival and success rate, or clinical outcomes. This observation is confirmed by the last review which reported a similar bone loss for both types of implants [68].

Despite the bone level changes being worse in TL-implants than BL-implants at 6 months of follow-up ($p < 0.05$) and 60-months of follow-up ($p < 0.01$), as reported in the results, the time-point the most representative of all quantitative analysis is 12-months because it has the larger sample of implants involving a major number of studies. In fact, 12 studies reported the radiological outcome at 12 months of follow-up, 7 studies at 60 months of follow-up, and only 3 studies at 6 months.

It could be reasonable to assume that the results at 12-months are more important for the number of implants and studies involved, nevertheless there are too many differences for each time-point. Moreover, [48] missed the radiological outcome of TL-implants at 60-months so only the comparison on the other time-point were analyzed.

The results of the present review are limited because of the quality of data, the number of comparable available studies, and the wide variability, all of which could influence the final results, plus, the authors were not calibrated in the screening process.

Also, the different surgical protocols (one-stage or two-stages) may influence the bone changes, especially in the first period of healing and the prosthetic final rehabilitation is not standardized in the included articles, plus some studies did not report the specific information about the kind of prothesis.

Moreover, in the majority of the studies included in this review, the implants were inserted in mandible, but the bone quality and healing are different between upper and lower jaws.

It has been reported that the peri-implant tissues are more susceptible to inflammation than natural teeth [69]. Nevertheless, the definitions of survival rate/success/failure used in the literature do not necessarily reflect the patients' chances of success or the function and aesthetics of the treatment because bleeding on probing (BoP), increasing of pocked probing depth (PPD), and other clinical outcomes are surrogates and the true link with the peri-implant tissues is questionable [70].

It has been reported that the implant type and the surgical protocol (bone level vs. tissue level) is correlated to the soft tissue bleeding response after probing (BoP) because of the presence of a chronic infiltrate at the implant-abutment interface of two-piece implants, attributed to the micro-gap between the implant and the abutment [71].

On the contrary, the peri-implant tissue around transmucosal implants has been reported to be inflammation-free, possibly because of the absence of a micro-gap reporting a lower prevalence of BoP [72,73]. According to the literature, in fact, there is a higher BoP prevalence detected in two-piece implants than in one-piece implants [74].

These studies, plus the biological rationale for the inflammation, have been pushing clinicians and researchers to assess if there are clinical differences in BoP and marginal bone changes in one- and two-piece dental implants. However, in more recent articles, these clinical and radiological differences between types of implants are not statistically significant and are reported probably because of the more efficient platform switching, the surface of the neck, and the type of abutment material [75,76].

Moreover, several authors have reported a lack of correlation between clinical outcomes (PPD and BoP) and crestal bone loss around implants [77,78].

A retrospective study on 4591 implants in 2060 patients with 10-year follow-up reported that, while BoP was very commonly detected on implants (40% of implants in the cohort study), only 3% of these implants had more than 1 mm of marginal bone loss. The study concluded that the minimal bleeding on probing in implants was not correlated with marginal bone loss and therefore probing healthy implants was not recommended [79].

Even if the BoP level is reported to be more frequent in BL implants compared to TL one as a marker of local inflammation in two-pieces implants, the latest systematic review conducted by Paul and Petsch [80] reported no differences between these types of implants, in fact the clinical examination of BoP around dental implants is not completely validated as a clinical outcome to evaluate the bone loss.

In the present review, a statistically less marginal bone loss was reported at one-year follow-up in TL-implants, but after five years of follow-up the BL reported statistically better results. The heterogeneity of the results in the different studies and the oscillation between BL and TL bone loss according to the follow-up are possibly due to other confounding factors such as implant micro surfaces, implant shape, and the implant-abutment connection to prevent bacterial infiltration [81,82].

Implant dentistry needs more prospective studies with more standardized characteristic considering, the bone quality, the site position, the type of loading in order to analyze the bone loss differences associated to one or two-piece implants.

Some patients, especially with chronic disease, may benefit from transmucosal implants because of the lack of bacterial leakage in the implant-abutment connection, but no evidence of long-term effect on bone loss is reported.

Nowadays, the focus should be shifted to the morphology and geometry of the implant neck. This could improve connective and bone stability and guide bone healing, especially in the period immediately after surgery [83].

5. Conclusions

In the present review, no evidence was found for differences in marginal bone loss or implant survival rate between bone-level and transmucosal dental implants after a period of follow-up variable from 12 to 60 months. It could be concluded that many other clinical and surgical variables influence marginal bone level and implant survival. More homogenous clinical trials with larger samples are needed to support these conclusions and to give more precise clinical indications.

Author Contributions: For research articles with several authors, the author individual contributions are provided as follow: Conceptualization, S.C. and U.C.; methodology, D.P.-O.; software, M.B.; validation, S.M., M.P.-D. and D.P.-O.; formal analysis, G.B.M.F.; investigation, S.C.; resources, S.C. and M.B.; data curation, S.C. and M.B.; writing—original draft preparation, S.C. and M.B.; writing—review and editing, S.M. and D.P.-O.; visualization, U.C.; supervision, U.C.; project administration, G.B.M.F.; funding acquisition, U.C. All authors have read and agreed to the published version of the manuscript. Please turn to the CRediT taxonomy for the term explanation. Authorship must be limited to those who have contributed substantially to the work reported.

Abbreviations

BIC — Bone to Implant Contact
BL — Bone-Level (Implants)
BoP — Bleeding on Probing
PPD — Pocked Probing Depth
IAJ — Implant-Abutment Junction
ΔMBL — Marginal Bone Loss
RCTs — Randomized Clinical Trials
TL — Tissue-Level (Implants)

References

1. Buser, D.; Janner, S.F.M.; Wittneben, J.-G.; Bragger, U.; Ramseier, C.A.; Salvi, G. 10-Year Survival and Success Rates of 511 Titanium Implants with a Sandblasted and Acid-Etched Surface: A Retrospective Study in 303 Partially Edentulous Patients. *Clin. Implant. Dent. Relat. Res.* **2012**, *14*, 839–851. [CrossRef] [PubMed]
2. Nagahisa, K.; Arai, K.; Baba, S. Study on Oral Health–Related Quality of Life in Patients after Dental Implant Treatment with Patient-Reported Outcome. *Int. J. Oral Maxillofac. Implant.* **2018**, *33*, 1141–1148. [CrossRef]
3. Barone, A.; Toti, P.; Marconcini, S.; Derchi, G.; Saverio, M.; Covani, U. Esthetic Outcome of Implants Placed in Fresh Extraction Sockets by Clinicians with or without Experience: A Medium-Term Retrospective Evaluation. *Int. J. Oral Maxillofac. Implant.* **2016**, *31*, 1397–1406. [CrossRef] [PubMed]
4. Eckert, S.; Hueler, G.; Sandler, N.; Elkattah, R.; McNeil, D. Immediately Loaded Fixed Full-Arch Implant-Retained Prosthesis: Clinical Analysis When Using a Moderate Insertion Torque. *Int. J. Oral Maxillofac. Implant.* **2019**, *34*, 737–744. [CrossRef]
5. Barone, A.; Covani, U. Maxillary alveolar ridge reconstruction with nonvascularized autogenous block bone: clinical results. *J. Oral Maxillofac. Surg.* **2007**, *65*, 2039–2046. [CrossRef] [PubMed]
6. Grassi, F.R.; Grassi, R.; Vivarelli, L.; Dallari, D.; Nardi, G.M.; Govoni, M.; Kalemaj, Z.; Ballini, A. Design Techniques to Optimize the Scaffold Performance: Freeze-dried Bone Custom-made Allografts for Maxillary Alveolar Horizontal Ridge Augmentation. *Materials* **2020**, *13*, 1393. [CrossRef] [PubMed]
7. Hermann, F.; Lerner, H.; Palti, A. Factors Influencing the Preservation of the Periimplant Marginal Bone. *Implant. Dent.* **2007**, *16*, 165–175. [CrossRef]
8. Schroeder, A.; Van Der Zypen, E.; Stich, H.; Sutter, F. The reactions of bone, connective tissue, and epithelium to endosteal implants with titanium-sprayed surfaces. *J. Maxillofac. Surg.* **1981**, *9*, 15–25. [CrossRef]
9. Hermann, J.S.; Buser, D.; Schenk, R.K.; Higginbottom, F.L.; Cochran, D.L. Biologic width around titanium implants. A physiologically formed and stable dimension over time. *Clin. Oral Implant. Res.* **2000**, *11*, 1–11. [CrossRef]
10. Iglhaut, G.; Schwarz, F.; Winter, R.R.; Mihatovic, I.; Stimmelmayr, M.; Schliephake, H. Epithelial Attachment and Downgrowth on Dental Implant Abutments-A Comprehensive Review. *J. Esthet. Restor. Dent.* **2014**, *26*, 324–331. [CrossRef]
11. Welch, V.; Petticrew, M.; Tugwell, P.; Moher, D.; O'Neill, J.; Waters, E.; White, H. PRISMA-Equity 2012 Extension: Reporting Guidelines for Systematic Reviews with a Focus on Health Equity. *PLoS Med.* **2012**, *9*, e1001333. [CrossRef] [PubMed]
12. Mueller, C.K.; Thorwarth, M.; Schultze-Mosgau, S. Influence of insertion protocol and implant shoulder design on inflammatory infiltration and gene expression in peri-implant soft tissue during nonsubmerged dental implant healing. *Oral Surg. Oral Med. Oral Pathol. Oral Radiol. Endod.* **2010**, *109*, e11–e19. [CrossRef] [PubMed]
13. Merickse-Stern, R.; Aerni, D.; Geering, A.H.; Buser, D. Long-term evaluation of non-submerged hollow cylinder implants. Clinical and radiographic results. *Clin. Oral Implant. Res.* **2001**, *12*, 252–259. [CrossRef] [PubMed]
14. Atieh, M.A.; Zadeh, H.; Stanford, C.M.; Cooper, L.F. Survival of short dental implants for treatment of posterior partial edentulism: A systematic review. *Int. J. Oral Maxillofac. Implant.* **2012**, *27*, 1323–1331.

14. Atieh, M.A.; Zadeh, H.; Stanford, C.M.; Cooper, L.F. Survival of short dental implants for treatment of posterior partial edentulism: A systematic review. *Int. J. Oral Maxillofac. Implant.* **2012**, *27*, 1323–1331.

15. Becktor, J.P.; Isaksson, S.; Billström, C. A Prospective Multicenter Study Using Two Different Surgical Approaches in the Mandible with Turned Brånemark Implants: Conventional Loading Using Fixed Prostheses. *Clin. Implant. Dent. Relat. Res.* **2007**, *9*, 179–185. [CrossRef] [PubMed]

16. Bratu, E.A.; Tandlich, M.; Shapira, L. A rough surface implant neck with microthreads reduces the amount of marginal bone loss: a prospective clinical study [published correction appears in Clin Oral Implants Res. 2009 Oct;20(10):1185]. *Clin. Oral Implants Res.* **2009**, *20*, 827–832. [CrossRef]

17. de Siqueira, R.A.C.; Fontão, F.N.G.K.; Sartori, I.A.M.; Santos, P.G.F.; Bernardes, S.R.; Tiossi, R. Effect of different implant placement depths on crestal bone levels and soft tissue behavior: a randomized clinical trial. *Clin. Oral Implants Res.* **2017**, *28*, 1227–1233. [CrossRef]

18. Chappuis, V.; Bornstein, M.M.; Buser, D.; Belser, U. Influence of implant neck design on facial bone crest dimensions in the esthetic zone analyzed by cone beam CT: A comparative study with a 5-to-9-year follow-up. *Clin. Oral Implant. Res.* **2016**, *27*, 1055–1064. [CrossRef]

19. Chien, H.H.; Schroering, R.L.; Prasad, H.S. Tatakis DN. Effects of a new implant abutment design on peri-implant soft tissues. *J. Oral Implantol.* **2014**, *40*, 581–588. [CrossRef]

20. Cosyn, J.; Sabzevar, M.M.; De Wilde, P.; De Rouck, T. Two-piece implants with turned versus microtextured collars. *J. Periodontol.* **2007**, *78*, 1657–1663. [CrossRef]

21. Ebler, S.; Ioannidis, A.; Jung, R.E.; Hämmerle, C.H.; Thoma, D.S. Prospective randomized controlled clinical study comparing two types of two-piece dental implants supporting fixed reconstructions—Results at 1 year of loading. *Clin. Oral Implants Res.* **2016**, *27*, 1169–1177. [CrossRef] [PubMed]

22. Esposito, M.; Trullenque-Eriksson, A.; Blasone, R.; Blasone, R.; Malaguti, G.; Gaffuri, C.; Caneva, M.; Minciarelli, A.; Luongo, G. Clinical evaluation of a novel dental implant system as single implants under immediate loading conditions—4-month post-loading results from a multicentre randomised controlled trial. *Eur. J. Oral Implantol.* **2016**, *9*, 367–379. [PubMed]

23. Hof, M.; Pommer, B.; Strbac, G.D.; Vasak, C.; Agis, H.; Zechner, W. Impact of insertion torque and implant neck design on peri-implant bone level: a randomized split-mouth trial. *Clin. Implant Dent. Relat. Res.* **2014**, *16*, 668–674. [CrossRef] [PubMed]

24. Herrero-Climent, M.; Romero-Ruiz, M.M.; Díaz-Castro, C.M.; Bullón, P.; Ríos-Santos, J.V. Influence of two different machined-collar heights on crestal bone loss. *Int. J. Oral Maxillofac. Implants* **2014**, *29*, 1374–1379. [CrossRef]

25. Judgar, R.; Giro, G.; Zenobio, E.; Coelho, P.G.; Feres, M.; Rodrigues, J.A.; Mangano, C.; Iezzi, G.; Piattelli, A.; Shibli, J.A. Biological width around one- and two-piece implants retrieved from human jaws. *BioMed Res. Int.* **2014**, *4*, 850120. [CrossRef]

26. Khorsand, A.; Rasouli-Ghahroudi, A.A.; Naddafpour, N.; Shayesteh, Y.S.; Khojasteh, A. Effect of Microthread Design on Marginal Bone Level Around Dental Implants Placed in Fresh Extraction Sockets. *Implant Dent.* **2016**, *25*, 90–96. [CrossRef]

27. Khraisat, A.; Zembic, A.; Jung, R.E.; Hammerle, C.H. Marginal bone levels and soft tissue conditions around single-tooth implants with a scalloped neck design: results of a prospective 3-year study. *Int. J. Oral Maxillofac. Implants* **2013**, *28*, 550–555. [CrossRef]

28. Kim, J.J.; Lee, D.W.; Kim, C.K.; Park, K.H.; Moon, I.S. Effect of conical configuration of fixture on the maintenance of marginal bone level: preliminary results at 1 year of function. *Clin. Oral Implants Res.* **2010**, *21*, 439–444. [CrossRef]

29. Kütan, E.; Bolukbasi, N.; Yildirim-Ondur, E.; Ozdemir, T. Clinical and Radiographic Evaluation of Marginal Bone Changes around Platform-Switching Implants Placed in Crestal or Subcrestal Positions: A Randomized Controlled Clinical Trial. *Clin. Implant Dent. Relat. Res.* **2015**, *17*, e364–e375. [CrossRef]

30. Marconcini, S.; Giammarinaro, E.; Toti, P.; Alfonsi, F.; Covani, U.; Barone, A. Longitudinal analysis on the effect of insertion torque on delayed single implants: A 3-year randomized clinical study. *Clin. Implant Dent. Relat. Res.* **2018**, *20*, 322–332. [CrossRef]

31. Moberg, L.-E.; Sagulin, G.-B.; Köndell, P.-Å.; Heimdahl, A.; Gynther, G.W.; Bolin, A. Branemark System and ITI Dental Implant System for treatment of mandibular edentulism. A comparative randomized study: 3-year follow-up. *Clin. Oral Implant. Res.* **2001**, *12*, 450–461. [CrossRef] [PubMed]

32. Nóvoa, L.; Batalla, P.; Caneiro, L.; Pico, A.; Liñares, A.; Blanco, J. Influence of Abutment Height on Maintenance of Peri-implant Crestal Bone at Bone-Level Implants: A 3-Year Follow-up Study. *Int. J. Periodontics Restorative Dent.* **2017**, *37*, 721–727. [CrossRef] [PubMed]

33. Ormianer, Z.; Duda, M.; Block, J.; Matalon, S. One- and Two-Piece Implants Placed in the Same Patients: Clinical Outcomes After 5 Years of Function. *Int. J. Prosthodont.* **2015**, *29*, 608–610. [CrossRef] [PubMed]

34. Pellicer-Chover, H.; Peñarrocha-Diago, M.; Peñarrocha-Oltra, D.; Gomar-Vercher, S.; Agustín-Panadero, R.; Peñarrocha-Diago, M. Impact of crestal and subcrestal implant placement in peri-implant bone: A prospective comparative study. *Med. Oral Patol. Oral Cir. Bucal.* **2016**, *21*, e103–e110. [CrossRef]

35. Peñarrocha-Diago, M.A.; Flichy-Fernández, A.J.; Alonso-González, R.; Peñarrocha-Oltra, D.; Balaguer-Martínez, J.; Peñarrocha-Diago, M. Influence of implant neck design and implant-abutment connection type on peri-implant health. Radiological study. *Clin. Oral. Implants Res.* **2013**, *24*, 1192–1200. [CrossRef]

36. Pozzi, A.; Agliardi, E.; Tallarico, M.; Barlattani, A. Clinical and radiological outcomes of two implants with different prosthetic interfaces and neck configurations: randomized, controlled, split-mouth clinical trial. *Clin. Implant Dent. Relat. Res.* **2014**, *16*, 96–106. [CrossRef]

37. Pozzi, A.; Tallarico, M.; Moy, P.K. Three-year post-loading results of a randomised, controlled, split-mouth trial comparing implants with different prosthetic interfaces and design in partially posterior edentulous mandibles. *Eur. J. Oral Implantol.* **2014**, *7*, 47–61.

38. Sanz-Martin, I.; Vignoletti, F.; Nuñez, J.; Permuy, M.; Muñoz, F.; Sanz-Esporrín, J.; Fierravanti, L.; Shapira, L.; Sanz, M. Hard and soft tissue integration of immediate and delayed implants with a modified coronal macrodesign: Histological, micro-CT and volumetric soft tissue changes from a pre-clinical in vivo study. *J. Clin. Periodontol.* **2017**, *44*, 842–853. [CrossRef]

39. Shin, Y.K.; Han, C.H.; Heo, S.J.; Kim, S.; Chun, H.J. Radiographic evaluation of marginal bone level around implants with different neck designs after 1 year. *Int. J. Oral Maxillofac. Implants* **2006**, *21*, 789–794.

40. Tan, W.C.; Lang, N.P.; Schmidlin, K.; Zwahlen, M.; Pjetursson, B.E. The effect of different implant neck configurations on soft and hard tissue healing: a randomized-controlled clinical trial. *Clin. Oral Implants Res.* **2011**, *22*, 14–19. [CrossRef]

41. Weinländer, M.; Lekovic, V.; Spadijer-Gostovic, S.; Milicic, B.; Wegscheider, W.A.; Piehslinger, E. Soft tissue development around abutments with a circular macro-groove in healed sites of partially edentulous posterior maxillae and mandibles: a clinical pilot study. *Clin. Oral Implants Res.* **2011**, *22*, 743–752. [CrossRef] [PubMed]

42. Wittneben, J.G.; Gavric, J.; Belser, U.C.; Bornstein, M.M.; Joda, T.; Chappuis, V.; Sailer, I.; Brägger, U. Esthetic and Clinical Performance of Implant-Supported All-Ceramic Crowns Made with Prefabricated or CAD/CAM Zirconia Abutments: A Randomized, Multicenter Clinical Trial. *J. Dent. Res.* **2017**, *96*, 163–170. [CrossRef] [PubMed]

43. Åstrand, P.; Engquist, B.; Anzén, B.; Bergendal, T.; Hallman, M.; Karlsson, U.; Kvint, S.; Lysell, L.; Rundcranz, T. A Three-Year Follow-Up Report of a Comparative Study of ITI Dental Implants® and Brånemark System® Implants in the Treatment of the Partially Edentulous Maxilla. *Clin. Implant Dent. Relat. Res.* **2004**, *6*, 130–141. [CrossRef] [PubMed]

44. Bassi, M.A.; Lopez, M.A.; Confalone, L.; Gaudio, R.M.; Lombardo, L.; Lauritano, D. A prospective evaluation of outcomes of two tapered implant systems. *J. Biol. Regul. Homeost. Agents* **2016**, *30*, 1–6.

45. Bömicke, W.; Gabbert, O.; Koob, A.; Krisam, J.; Rammelsberg, P. Comparison of immediately loaded flapless-placed one-piece implants and flapped-placed conventionally loaded two-piece implants, both fitted with all-ceramic single crowns, in the posterior mandible: 3-year results from a randomised controlled pilot trial. *Eur. J. Oral Implantol.* **2017**, *10*, 179–195.

46. Cecchinato, D.; Olsson, C.; Lindhe, J. Submerged or non-submerged healing of endosseous implants to be used in the rehabilitation of partially dentate patients. *J. Clin. Periodontol.* **2004**, *31*, 299–308. [CrossRef]

47. Cecchinato, D.; Bengazi, F.; Blasi, G.; Botticelli, D.; Cardarelli, I.; Gualini, F. Bone level alterations at implants placed in the posterior segments of the dentition: Outcome of submerged/non-submerged healing. A 5-year multicenter, randomized, controlled clinical trial. *Clin. Oral Implant. Res.* **2008**, *19*, 429–431. [CrossRef]

48. Duda, M.; Matalon, S.; Lewinstein, I.; Harel, N.; Block, J.; Ormianer, Z. One Piece Immediately Loaded Implants Versus 1 Piece or 2 Pieces Delayed: 3 Years Outcome. *Implant Dent.* **2016**, *25*, 109–113. [CrossRef]

49. Eliasson, A.; Narby, B.; Ekstrand, K.; Hirsch, J.; Johansson, A.; Wennerberg, A. A 5-year prospective clinical study of submerged and nonsubmerged Paragon system implants in the edentulous mandible. *Int. J. Prosthodont.* **2010**, *23*, 231–238.

50. Engquist, B.; Astrand, P.; Anzén, B.; Dahlgren, S.; Engquist, E.; Feldmann, H.; Karlsson, U.; Nord, P.G.; Sahlholm, S.; Svärdström, P. Simplified methods of implant treatment in the edentulous lower jaw. A controlled prospective study. Part I: One-stage versus two-stage surgery. *Clin. Implant Dent. Relat. Res.* **2002**, *4*, 93–103. [CrossRef]

51. Engquist, B.; Astrand, P.; Anzén, B.; Dahlgren, S.; Engquist, E.; Feldmann, H.; Karlsson, U.; Nord Dds, P.; Sahlholm, S.; Svärdström, P. Simplified Methods of Implant Treatment in the Edentulous Lower Jaw: A 3-Year Follow-Up Report of a Controlled Prospective Study of One-Stage versus Two-Stage Surgery and Early Loading. *Clin. Implant Dent. Relat. Res.* **2005**, *7*, 95–104. [CrossRef] [PubMed]

52. Ericsson, I.; Randow, K.; Glantz, P.-O.; Lindhe, J.; Nilner, K. Clinical and radiographical features of submerged and nonsubmerged titanium implants. *Clin. Oral Implant. Res.* **1994**, *5*, 185–189. [CrossRef] [PubMed]

53. Gamper, F.B.; Benic, G.I.; Sanz-Martín, I.; Asgeirsson, A.G.; Hämmerle, C.H.F.; Thoma, D.S. Randomized controlled clinical trial comparing one-piece and two-piece dental implants supporting fixed and removable dental prostheses: 4- to 6-year observations. *Clin. Oral Implant. Res.* **2017**, *28*, 1553–1559. [CrossRef]

54. Gulati, M.; Govila, V.; Verma, S.; Rajkumar, B.; Anand, V.; Aggarwal, A.; Jain, N. In Vivo Evaluation of Two-Piece Implants Placed Following One-Stage and Two-Stage Surgical Protocol in Posterior Mandibular Region. Assessment of Alterations in Crestal Bone Level. *Clin. Implant Dent. Relat. Res.* **2015**, *17*, 854–861. [CrossRef] [PubMed]

55. Hadzik, J.; Botzenhart, U.; Krawiec, M.; Gedrange, T.; Heinemann, F.; Vegh, A.; Dominiak, M. Comparative evaluation of the effectiveness of the implantation in the lateral part of the mandible between short tissue level (TE) and bone level (BL) implant systems. *Ann. Anat.* **2017**, *213*, 78–82. [CrossRef] [PubMed]

56. Heijdenrijk, K.; Raghoebar, G.M.; Meijer, H.J.A.; Stegenga, B.; Van Der Reijden, W.A. Feasibility and Influence of the Microgap of Two Implants Placed in a Non-Submerged Procedure: A Five-Year Follow-Up Clinical Trial. *J. Periodontol.* **2006**, *77*, 1051–1060. [CrossRef] [PubMed]

57. Lago, L.; Da Silva, L.; Martínez-Silva, I.; Rilo, B. Crestal Bone Level Around Tissue-Level Implants Restored with Platform Matching and Bone-Level Implants Restored with Platform Switching: A 5-Year Randomized Controlled Trial. *Int. J. Oral Maxillofac. Implant.* **2018**, *33*, 448–456. [CrossRef] [PubMed]

58. Paoloantoni, G.; Marenzi, G.; Blasi, A.; Mignogna, J.; Sammartino, G. Findings of a Four-Year Randomized Controlled Clinical Trial Comparing Two-Piece and One-Piece Zirconia Abutments Supporting Single Prosthetic Restorations in Maxillary Anterior Region. *BioMed Res. Int.* **2016**, *2016*, 1–6. [CrossRef]

59. Sanz-Martín, I.; Benic, G.I.; Hämmerle, C.H.; Thoma, D.S. Prospective randomized controlled clinical study comparing two dental implant types: Volumetric soft tissue changes at 1 year of loading. *Clin. Oral Implant. Res.* **2016**, *27*, 406–411. [CrossRef]

60. Higgins, J.P.; Green, S. *Cochrane Handbook for Systematic Reviews of Interventions*; John Wiley & Sons: Hoboken, NJ, USA, 2011.

61. Downs, S.H.; Black, N. The feasibility of creating a checklist for the assessment of the methodological quality both of randomised and non-randomised studies of health care interventions. *J. Epidemiol. Community Health* **1998**, *52*, 377–384. [CrossRef]

62. Mallen, C.; Peat, G.; Croft, P. Quality assessment of observational studies is not commonplace in systematic reviews. *J. Clin. Epidemiol.* **2006**, *59*, 765–769. [CrossRef] [PubMed]

63. Higgins, J.P.T.; Altman, U.G.; Gøtzsche, P.C.; Jüni, P.; Moher, D.; Oxman, A.D.; Savović, J.; Schulz, K.F.; Weeks, L.; Sterne, J.A.C. The Cochrane Collaboration's tool for assessing risk of bias in randomised trials. *BMJ* **2011**, *343*, d5928. [CrossRef] [PubMed]

64. Sanz-Sánchez, I.; Sanz-Martín, I.; De Albornoz, A.C.; Figuero, E.; Sanz, M. Biological effect of the abutment material on the stability of peri-implant marginal bone levels: A systematic review and meta-analysis. *Clin. Oral Implant. Res.* **2018**, *29*, 124–144. [CrossRef] [PubMed]

65. Sanz-Martín, I.; Sanz-Sánchez, I.; De Albornoz, A.C.; Figuero, E.; Sanz, M. Effects of modified abutment characteristics on peri-implant soft tissue health: A systematic review and meta-analysis. *Clin. Oral Implant. Res.* **2018**, *29*, 118–129. [CrossRef]

66. Starch-Jensen, T.; Christensen, A.-E.; Lorenzen, H. Scalloped Implant-Abutment Connection Compared to Conventional Flat Implant-Abutment Connection: A Systematic Review and Meta-Analysis. *J. Oral Maxillofac. Res.* **2017**, *8*, e2. [CrossRef]

67. Tallarico, M.; Caneva, M.; Meloni, S.M.; Xhanari, E.; Omori, Y.; Canullo, L. Survival and Success Rates of Different Shoulder Designs: A Systematic Review of the Literature. *Int. J. Dent.* **2018**, *2018*, 1–10. [CrossRef]

68. Palacios-Garzón, N.; Velasco-Ortega, E.; López-López, J. Bone Loss in Implants Placed at Subcrestal and Crestal Level: A Systematic Review and Meta-Analysis. *Materials* **2019**, *12*, 154. [CrossRef]

69. Degidi, M.; Artese, L.; Piattelli, A.; Scarano, A.; Shibli, J.A.; Piccirilli, M.; Perrotti, V.; Iezzi, G. Histological and immunohistochemical evaluation of the peri-implant soft tissues around machined and acid-etched titanium healing abutments: A prospective randomised study. *Clin. Oral Investig.* **2012**, *16*, 857–866. [CrossRef]

70. Coli, P.; Sennerby, L. Is Peri-Implant Probing Causing Over-Diagnosis and Over-Treatment of Dental Implants? *J. Clin. Med.* **2019**, *8*, 1123. [CrossRef]

71. Broggini, N.; McManus, L.; Hermann, J.; Medina, R.; Oates, T.; Schenk, R.; Buser, D.; Mellonig, J.; Cochran, D. Persistent acute inflammation at the implant-abutment interface. *J. Dent. Res.* **2003**, *82*, 232–237. [CrossRef]

72. Buser, D.; Weber, H.P.; Donath, K.; Fiorellini, J.P.; Paquette, D.W.; Williams, R.C. Soft Tissue Reactions to Non-Submerged Unloaded Titanium Implants in Beagle Dogs. *J. Periodontol.* **1992**, *63*, 225–235. [CrossRef] [PubMed]

73. Hernández-Marcos, G.; Hernández-Herrera, M.; Anitua, E. Marginal Bone Loss around Short Dental Implants Restored at Implant Level and with Transmucosal Abutment: A Retrospective Study. *Int. J. Oral Maxillofac. Implant.* **2018**, *33*, 1362–1367. [CrossRef] [PubMed]

74. Winitsky, N.; Olgart, K.; Jemt, T.; Smedberg, J.-I. A retro-prospective long-term follow-up of Brånemark single implants in the anterior maxilla in young adults. Part 1: Clinical and radiographic parameters. *Clin. Implant Dent. Relat. Res.* **2018**, *20*, 937–944. [CrossRef] [PubMed]

75. Canullo, L.; Penarrocha-Oltra, D.; Soldini, C.; Mazzocco, F.; Peñarrocha, M.; Covani, U. Microbiological assessment of the implant-abutment interface in different connections: Cross-sectional study after 5 years of functional loading. *Clin. Oral Implant. Res.* **2015**, *26*, 426–434. [CrossRef]

76. Schwarz, F.; Alcoforado, G.; Nelson, K.; Schaer, A.; Taylor, T.; Beuer, F.; Strietzel, F.P. Impact of implant–abutment connection, positioning of the machined collar/microgap, and platform switching on crestal bone level changes. Camlog Foundation Consensus Report. *Clin. Oral Implant. Res.* **2014**, *25*, 1301–1303. [CrossRef]

77. Fransson, C.; Wennström, J.; Berglundh, T. Clinical characteristics and implant with a history of progressive bone loss. *Clin. Oral Implant. Res.* **2008**, *19*, 142–147. [CrossRef]

78. Hashim, D.; Cionca, N.; Combescure, C.; Mombelli, A. The diagnosis of peri-implantitis: A systematic review on the predictive value of bleeding on probing. *Clin. Oral Implant. Res.* **2018**, *29*, 276–293. [CrossRef]

79. French, D.; Cochran, D.L.; Ofec, R. Retrospective Cohort Study of 4591 Straumann Implants Placed in 2060 Patients in Private Practice with up to 10-Year Follow-up: The Relationship between Crestal Bone Level and Soft Tissue Condition. *Int. J. Oral Maxillofac. Implant.* **2016**, *31*, e168–e178. [CrossRef]

80. Paul, S.; Petsch, M.; Held, U. Modeling of Crestal Bone after Submerged vs. Transmucosal Implant Placement: A Systematic Review with Meta-Analysis. *Int. J. Oral Maxillofac. Implant.* **2017**, *32*, 1039–1050. [CrossRef]

81. Agustín-Panadero, R.; Martínez-Martínez, N.; Fernández-Estevan, L.; Faus-López, J.; Solá-Ruíz, M. Influence of Transmucosal Area Morphology on Peri-implant Bone Loss in Tissue-Level Implants. *Int. J. Oral Maxillofac. Implant.* **2019**, *34*, 852–947. [CrossRef]

82. Candotto, V.; Gabrione, F.; Oberti, L.; Lento, D.; Severino, M. The role of implant-abutment connection in preventing bacterial leakage: A review. *J. Biol. Regul. Homeost. Agents* **2019**, *33*, 129–134. [PubMed]

83. Lutz, R.; Sendlbeck, C.; Wahabzada, H.; Tudor, C.; Prechtl, C.; Schlegel, K.A. Periosteal elevation induces supracortical peri-implant bone formation. *J. Cranio-Maxillofac. Surg.* **2017**, *45*, 1170–1178. [CrossRef] [PubMed]

4

Short vs. Standard Length Cone Morse Connection Implants: An In Vitro Pilot Study in Low Density Polyurethane Foam

Luca Comuzzi [1,†]**, Margherita Tumedei** [2,*,†]**, Adriano Piattelli** [2,3,4] **and Giovanna Iezzi** [2]

[1] Private practice, via Raffaello 36/a, 31020 San Vendemiano (TV), Italy; luca.comuzzi@gmail.com

[2] Department of Medical, Oral and Biotechnological Sciences, University "G. D'Annunzio" of Chieti-Pescara, 66100 Chieti, Italy; apiattelli@unich.it (A.P.); g.iezzi@unich.it (G.I.)

[3] Catholic University of San Antonio de Murcia (UCAM), Av. de los Jerónimos, Guadalupe, 135 30107 Murcia, Spain

[4] Villaserena Foundation for Research, 65121 Città Sant'Angelo (Pescara), Italy

* Correspondence: margytumedei@yahoo.it

† These two Authors had an equal contribution to the study. LC for the execution of the experimental portion, MT for data collection, data analysis, statistical evaluation, final editing of the manuscript.

Abstract: The aim of the investigation was to evaluate the insertion torque, pull-out torque and implant stability quotient (ISQ) of short implants (SI) and standard length implants (ST) inserted into linearly elastic and constitutive isotropic symmetry polyurethane foam blocks. Short dental titanium implants with a Cone Morse connection and a conical shape (test implants: Test Implant A—diameter 5.5 mm and length 6 mm) (Test Implant B—diameter 5.5 mm and length 5 mm) were used for the present in vitro investigation. ST implants (4 mm diameter and 10 mm length), with a Cone Morse connection and a conical shape, were used as Control Implant A and as Control Implants B. These two latter implants had a different macro design. A total of 20 implants (5 Test A, 5 Test B, 5 Control A and 5 Control B) were used for the present research. The results were similar when comparing the Test A and Test B implants. The test implants had very good stability in polyurethane 14.88–29.76 kgm^3 density blocks. The insertion torque values were very high for both types of test implant (25–32 Ncm on 14.88 kgm blocks, and up to 45 Ncm in 29.76 kgm^3 blocks). The pull-out test values were very similar to the insertion torque values. The ISQ values were significantly high with 75–80 in 14.88 kgm^3 blocks, and 78–83 in 29.76 kgm^3 blocks. No differences were found in the values of the Control A and Control B implants. In both these implants, the insertion torque was quite low in the 14.88 kgm^3 blocks (16–28 Ncm). Better results were found in the 29.76 kgm^3 blocks. The pull-out values for these control implants were slightly lower than the insertion torque values. High ISQ values were found in both control implants (57–80). When comparing SI and ST implants, the SI had a similar if not better performance in low quality polyurethane foam blocks (14.88–29.76 kgm), corresponding to D3 and D4 bone.

Keywords: bone density; implant stability quotient; insertion torque; polyurethane foam blocks; pull-out torque; resonance frequency analysis; short implants; standard length implants

1. Introduction

Short implants (SI), defined in recent years as implants of less than 10 mm in length [1], seem to have some advantages in certain clinical situations, such as atrophy of the alveolar processes, poor bone quality, and pneumatization of the maxillary sinus [2]. SI are less invasive, simpler to use in the hands of the average clinician, and their surgery is shorter, with a lower morbidity, lower costs and lesser biological complications [1,3–7]. More recently, Ultrashort or Extra-short (<6 mm) implants have been proposed [8–11]. Alternatives to the use of SI are sinus augmentation procedures, the use of zygomatic implants, guided bone regeneration procedures, onlay grafts, inlay grafts, distraction osteogenesis, and lateralization of the inferior alveolar nerve [4,12]. Several recent systematic reviews, some of them with a metanalysis of the data, have shown:

no differences in the in the survival rate between SI and standard length implants (ST);

no differences in marginal bone loss (MBL);

lower biological complications in SI;

good primary stability in SI;

higher mechanical complications in SI [3,4,9,10,13–16].

Primary dental implant stability (PS), i.e., an absence of micromotion of the implant immediately after implant placement, has been reported to have an important role in implant osseointegration [17–19]. PS seemed to be closely correlated to bone quality and quantity, implant macrostructure, implant length and diameter, surgical technique, and the fitting of the implant into the site [17–21]. Bone density has been correlated to the amount of bone-to-implant contact (BIC) [19], and BIC to the PS [17]. Bone density has been measured with the use of different techniques: insertion torque (IT), removal torque (RT), and resonance frequency analysis (RFA), producing a value giving the implant stability quotient (ISQ) [22]. Polyurethane foam has been recognized as a standard material for testing instruments by the American Society for Testing and Materials (ASTM F-1839-08) ("Standard specification for Rigid Polyurethane Foam for Use as a Standard Material for Test Orthopaedic Devices for Instruments"). Polyurethane foam has been widely used as an alternative material in biomechanical tests evaluating, for example, dental implants. It presents consistent mechanical characteristics, has features similar to bone tissue, is very reliable and easy to use, requiring no special handling, and is characterized by linearly elastic and constitutive isotropic symmetry [22–24].

The scope of the present pilot study was to evaluate the insertion torque, pull-out torque and ISQ of SI and ST implants, positioned into polyurethane foam blocks.

2. Materials and Methods

2.1. Dental Implants

The short dental titanium implants with a Cone Morse connection and a conical shape (Implacil De Bortoli, Sao Paulo, Brasil) (Test Implants: Test Implant A—diameter 5.5 mm and length 6 mm) (Test Implant B—diameter 5.5 mm and length 5 mm) were used for the in vitro experimental study. Universal II (UN II) implants (4 mm diameter and 10 mm length), with a Cone Morse connection and a conical shape (Implacil De Bortoli, Sao Paulo, Brasil), were used as Control Implant A, and Universal III (UN III) implants, also with a Cone Morse connection and a conical shape (Implacil De Bortoli, Sao Paulo, Brasil), were used as Control Implants B. These two latter implants differed in their macro design. The UN III macro design differed from the UN II implants regarding its larger thread, the lack of double thread pitch, having a round apex not self-tapping, and in the chambers' patterns between the cutting surface of the threads.

2.2. Study Design

A total of 20 implants (5 Test A, 5 Test B, 5 Control A and 5 Control B) were used in the present investigation. The control implants were inserted following the protocol of the manufacturer: implant lance drill, 2 mm drill (1200 rpm) and 3.5 mm final drill (800 rpm) (Figures 1 and 2). The test implants were inserted following the protocol of the manufacturer: implant lance drill, 2 mm drill (1200 rpm), 3.5 mm conical drill for SI and 4.5 mm final conical drill for SI (800 rpm).

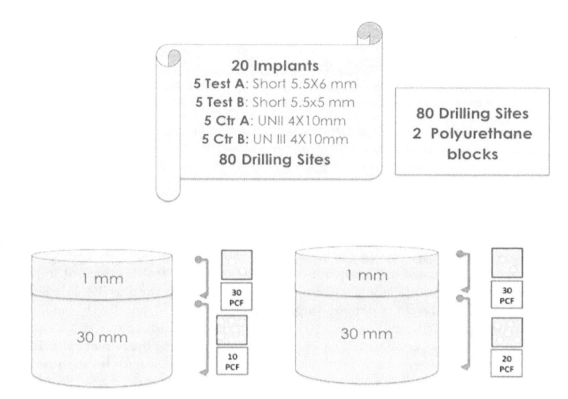

Figure 1. Study design and the experimental groups of the present in vitro investigation. PCF = pound per cubic foot.

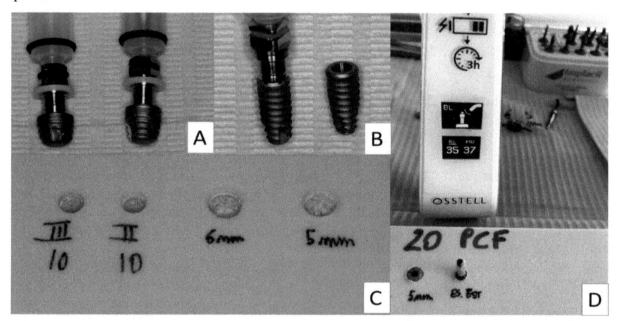

Figure 2. Sequence of the study investigation: (**A**) Test A and Test B; (**B**) Control A and Control B; (**C**) Polyurethane foam block after drilling; (**D**) implant stability quotient (ISQ) measurement device.

The insertion of the implants was made by the handpiece calibrated to 20 rpm speed and a torque of 30 Ncm. The torque peaks were recorded by the software package (ImpDat Plus, East Lansing, Michigan) installed on a digital card. The insertion torque (IT, Ncm) peaks indicated the force of the maximum clockwise movement of the dental fixture positioned into the material. The research was performed by a single operator (LC), recording the fixture insertion and the pull-out torque peaks of the Test A, Test B, Control A and Control B Implants positioned into polyurethane foam blocks in different sizes and densities.

Different types of solid rigid polyurethane foam (SawBones H, Pacific Research Laboratories Inc, Vashon, Washington, USA) with homogeneous densities were selected for the present investigation. The polyurethane foam blocks presented a size of "120 mm × 70 mm × 31 mm".

The block densities of polyurethane samples used in the present investigation were: 16.01 kgm^3 (10 PCF), similar to D3 bone quality, 32.02 kgm^3 (20 PCF), corresponding with and similar to D2 bone; moreover, a 1 mm sheet of polyurethane with a 48.03 kgm^3 (30 PCF) density, similar to D1 bone, was present to simulate a layer of cortical bone. Ten implant site perforations were performed for each type of implant (Test A, Test B, Control A and Control B) for both polyurethane densities (14.88–29.76 kgm^3), for a total of 80 implant site preparations.

2.3. Implant Drill

Test A and Test B implants were inserted following a suggested drill protocol using a lance drill, then a 2 mm bur at 1200 rpm, then a 3.5 mm conical bur, and subsequently a 4.5 mm conical bur (both at 300 rpm) with the implant insertion at 20 Rpm. Control A and Control B Implants were inserted using a surgical lance drill, then a 2 mm bur, and subsequently a conical 3.5 mm bur at 800 Rpm with the implant insertion at 20 rpm.

2.4. Insertion Torque and Pull-Out Torque

The comparative research evaluating the insertion torque and pull-out peaks was conducted using a calibrated torque ratchet (Implacil De Bortoli, Sao Paulo, Brasil) provided by a torque range of 5–80 N/cm. The final 1 mm insertion torque of the implants into the polyurethane blocks was evaluated using a calibrated torque ratchet (Implacil De Bortoli, Sao Paulo, Brasil). In the present investigation, the mechanical torque gauges were used to assess the insertion torque and the pull-out strength values.

2.5. Resonance Frequency Evaluation

After the fixture positioning, the primary stability was evaluated using Resonance Frequency analysis (RFA) values expressed in the implant stability quotient (ISQ) by a hand-screwed Smart-Pegs type 7 for test implants (Osstell Mentor Device, Integration Diagnostic AB, Savadelen, Sweden) (Figure 2). The ISQ values ranged from 0 to 100 (measured by a frequency in the range 3500–85,000 Hz), and was classified into Low (less than 60 ISQ), Medium (in the range 60–70 ISQ), and High stability rate (more than 70 ISQ) [25]. Moreover, RFA evaluation was repeated twice for each sample evaluated. The RFA evaluation was performed following two different orientations separated by a 90-degree angle, and the mean ISQ peaks were calculated.

2.6. Statistical Analysis

The Shapiro–Wilks test was performed to evaluate data normality. Moreover, the differences between the peaks of insertion torque, pull-out strength and the RFA of the study groups were evaluated using a two-way analysis of variance (ANOVA), followed by the Tukey post-hoc test. A p-value < 0.05 was considered statistically significant. The research data and the statistical analysis were performed using the software package Excel (Microsoft Office, Redmond, USA) and GraphPad 6 (Prism, San Diego, USA).

3. Results

The results are similar when comparing the Test A and Test B implants. The test implants had very good stability in polyurethane 14.88–29.76 kgm^3 density blocks (Figures 3 and 4).

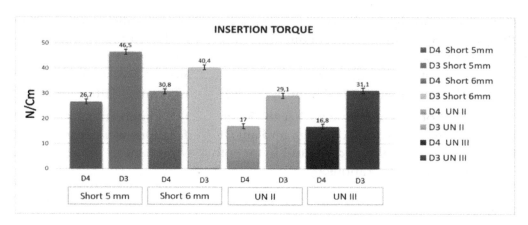

Figure 3. Insertion torque evaluation of the study groups: Test A, Test B. Control A and Control B.

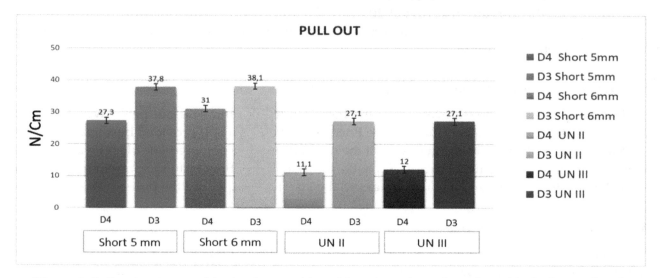

Figure 4. Pull-out outcome of the implant positioned into the polyurethane foam block: Test A, Test B. Control A and Control B.

The insertion torque values were very high for both types of test implant (25–32 Ncm on 14.88 kgm^3 blocks, and up to 45 Ncm in 29.76 kgm^3 blocks) (Figure 3; Tables 1 and 2).

The pull-out test values were very similar to the insertion torque values (Figure 4). The ISQ values were significantly high with 75–80 in 14.88 kgm^3 blocks, and 78–83 in 29.76 kgm^3 blocks (Tables 3 and 4).

Table 1. Summary of the insertion torque value for the implant positioned into polyurethane foam (14.88–29.76 kgm^3); Test A, Test B. Control A and Control B.

Insertion Torque	D4 Density				D3 Density			
	Short 5 mm (A)	Short 6 mm (B)	UN II (C)	UN III (D)	Short 5 mm (E)	Short 6 mm (F)	UN II (G)	UN III (H)
Mean	26.7	30.8	17	16.8	46.5	40.4	29.1	31.1
Std. Deviation	±1.059	±1.033	±0.942	±1.135	±1.269	±1.350	±0.994	±0.994

Table 2. Insertion torque: ANOVA Bonferroni post-hoc comparison test (CI = Confidence Interval; Diff = Difference).

Multiple Comparison Insertion Torque	95.00% CI of Diff,	Adjusted p Value
A-B	−5.577 to −2.623	<0.0001
B-C	12.32 to 15.28	<0.0001
C-D	−1.277 to 1.677	N.S.D.
D-E	−31.18 to −28.22	<0.0001
A-D	8.423 to 11.38	<0.0001
A-C	8.223 to 11.18	<0.0001
B-D	12.52 to 15.48	<0.0001
E-F	4.623 to 7.577	<0.0001
F-G	9.823 to 12.78	<0.0001
G-H	−3.477 to −0.5230	0.0006
E-H	13.92 to 16.88	<0.0001
F-H	7.823 to 10.78	<0.0001
E-G	15.92 to 18.88	<0.0001

N.S.D. (no significant differences).

Table 3. Summary of the pull-out outcome of the implant positioned into polyurethane foam (14.88 D3 Density–29.76 kgm^3 D3 Density); Test A, Test B. Control A and Control B.

Pull Out	D4 Density				D3 Density			
	Short 5 mm (A)	Short 6 mm (B)	UN II (C)	UN III (D)	Short 5 mm (E)	Short 6 mm (F)	UN II (G)	UN III (H)
Mean	27.3	31	11.1	12	37.8	38.1	27.1	27.1
Std. Deviation	±1.059	±1.054	±0.994	±1.247	±0.918	±0.875	±1.101	±1.287

Table 4. Pull-out: ANOVA Bonferroni post-hoc comparison test (CI = Confidence Interval; Diff = Difference).

Multiple Comparison Pull Out	95.00% CI of Diff,	Adjusted p Value
A-B	−5.124 to −2.276	<0.0001
B-C	18.48 to 21.32	<0.0001
C-D	−2.324 to 0.5237	N.S.D.
A-D	13.88 to 16.72	<0.0001
B-D	17.58 to 20.42	<0.0001
A-C	14.78 to 17.62	<0.0001
D-E	−27.24 to −24.36	<0.0001
E-F	−1.724 to 1.124	>0.9999
F-G	9.576 to 12.42	<0.0001
G-H	−1.424 to 1.424	N.S.D.
E-H	9.276 to 12.12	<0.0001
F-H	9.576 to 12.42	<0.0001
E-G	9.276 to 12.12	<0.0001
A-B	−5.124 to −2.276	<0.0001

N.S.D. (no significant differences).

The clinical sensation of the very good stability of the implant was felt at the initial insertion into the polyurethane blocks. No differences were found in the values of the Control A and Control B implants (Tables 1–4). In both these implants, the insertion torque was quite low in the 14.88 kgm^3 blocks (16–28 Ncm) (Tables 1 and 2). Better results were found in the 29.76 kgm^3 blocks, with significantly good stability of the implants. The pull-out values for these control implants were slightly lower than the insertion torque values. High ISQ values were found in both control implants (57–80) (Figure 5; Tables 5 and 6).

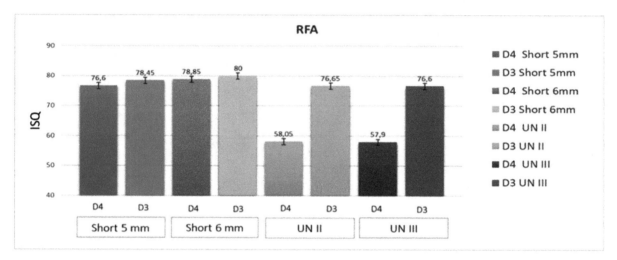

Figure 5. ISQ outcome of the implant positioned into polyurethane foam block: Test A, Test B. Control A and Control B.

Table 5. Summary of the ISQ of the implant positioned into Polyurethane foam (14.88 D4 Density–29.76 kgm^3 D3 Density); Test A, Test B. Control A and Control B.

ISQ	D4 Density				D3 Density			
	Short 5 mm (A)	Short 6 mm (B)	UN II (C)	UN III (D)	Short 5 mm (E)	Short 6 mm (F)	UN II (G)	UN III (H)
Mean	76.6	78.85	58.05	57.9	78.45	80	76.65	76.6
Std. Deviation	±0.966	±0.747	±0.283	±0.809	±0.550	±1.491	±1.001	±0.774

Table 6. ISQ: ANOVA Bonferroni Post-hoc comparison test (CI = Confidence Interval; Diff = Difference).

Multiple Comparison RFA	95.00% CI of Diff,	Adjusted p Value
A-B	−3.430 to −1.070	<0.0001
B-C	19.62 to 21.98	<0.0001
C-D	−1.030 to 1.330	N.S.D.
A-D	17.52 to 19.88	<0.0001
B-D	19.77 to 22.13	<0.0001
A-C	17.37 to 19.73	<0.0001
D-E	−21.74 to −19.36	<0.0001
E-F	−2.730 to −0.3703	0.0027
F-G	2.170 to 4.530	<0.0001
G-H	−1.130 to 1.230	N.S.D.
E-H	0.6703 to 3.030	0.0002
F-H	2.220 to 4.580	<0.0001
E-G	0.6203 to 2.980	0.0003

N.S.D. (no significant differences).

4. Discussion

The atrophy of the posterior regions of the jaws with reduced bone quality and quantity could limit the use of standard length implants (≥10 mm), without doing an invasive sinus grafting procedure. Recently, it has been reported in a few systematic reviews with meta-analysis that, in these cases, short implants could be a suitable alternative [2–8,12,13]. These reviews have reported, for short implants, survival rates similar to those of standard length implants and the capability to osseointegrate and to bear a functional load [8]. In recent years, a reduction in the implant length of short implants has been reported in the literature [1,7,8,12]. Polyurethane foam could be an alternative useful material to provide biomechanical tests substituting, for example, animal bone. ("Standard specification for Rigid Polyurethane Foam for Use as a Standard Material for Test Orthopaedic Devices for Instruments"). Polyurethane presents a cellular structure with constant mechanical characteristics, and similar properties to bone. In the present study, very good stability was obtained for both test and control implants. In the test implants, insertion torque, pull-out torque and ISQ values were all very high, showing the very good stability of both types of SI. Also, all the values for the ST implants were quite high, with better results, and then better stability, in higher density polyurethane blocks. The density of polyurethane blocks is similar to the structure of the bone in the posterior regions in humans. The conical shape of all these implants was probably instrumental in achieving such good levels of stability.

The main reason for measuring the implant primary stability concerns the ability to predict the prognosis of the dental implant procedure. Comuzzi et al., in vitro, reported that in polyurethane foam, ISQ, insertion torque, and pull-out measuring provide the high repeatability and reproducibility that represent suitable indicators for implant stability [26]. In the present investigation, the implant primary stability was evaluated in a controlled reproducible study design and without the variables correlated to the use of animal bone.

The study effectiveness showed that the types of polyurethane used in the present in vitro study were shown to be constituted by a homogenous material.

Moreover, implants with a conical shape have a high stability even in blocks with a low density (D4 Density) and no differences were found between 5 mm and 6 mm long implants, where reasonable values of insertion torque and pull-out tests were found in short implants in both polyurethane densities. Comuzzi et al. reported in vitro that a conical shape, rather than a cylindrical design, provided increased values of insertion torque and pull-out strength [26]. Thus, the ISQ values of both short implants were great, with an increased clinical sensation of the high stability of the implants.

The posterior maxilla is an anatomical region often characterized by poor bone quality and quantity. Thus, the 5 mm short implant could probably be more useful for insertion in this area in cases of reduced bone volume and density.

In fact, the choice of a short implant is clinically indicated as an alternative to more invasive regenerative procedures in cases of bone atrophy of the posterior ridge's regions [3].

The standard length implants had slightly lower values of insertion torque and pull-out torque, and very high ISQ values, where the conometric connection of all the types of implants seemed to also resist quite well to very high torque values (up to 60–80 Ncm).

5. Conclusions

In conclusion, when comparing the SI and ST, the SI had a similar if not better performance in low quality polyurethane foam blocks corresponding to D3 and D4 bone.

Author Contributions: A.P. Conceptualization, L.C. Investigation, A.P., L.C. Methodology; Supervision G.I., Validation A.P., G.I.; M.T. Data Curation, M.T. Formal Analysis; and A.P. and M.T. Writing Original Draft, A.P. and M.T. Writing Review Draft.

References

1. Lombardo, G.; Pighi, J.; Marincola, M.; Corrocher, G.; Simancas-Pallares, M.; Nocini, P.F. Cumulative Success Rate of Short and Ultrashort Implants Supporting Single Crowns in the Posterior Maxilla: A 3-Year Retrospective Study. *Int. J. Dent.* **2017**, *2017*, 8434281. [CrossRef] [PubMed]
2. Nielsen, H.B.; Schou, S.; Isidor, F.; Christensen, A.E.; Starch-Jensen, T. Short implants (≤8 mm) compared to standard length implants (>8 mm) in conjunction with maxillary sinus floor augmentation: A systematic review and meta-analysis. *Int. J. Oral Maxillofac. Surg.* **2019**, *48*, 239–249. [CrossRef] [PubMed]
3. Cruz, R.S.; Lemos, C.A.A.; Batista, V.E.S.; Oliveira, H.F.F.E.; Gomes, J.M.L.; Pellizzer, E.P.; Verri, F.R. Short implants versus longer implants with maxillary sinus lift. A systematic review and meta-analysis. *Braz. Oral Res.* **2018**, *32*, 86. [CrossRef] [PubMed]
4. Tolentino da Rosa de Souza, P.; Binhame Albini Martini, M.; Reis Azevedo-Alanis, L. Do short implants have similar survival rates compared to standard implants in posterior single crown?: A systematic review and meta-analysis. *Clin. Implant. Dent. Relat. Res.* **2018**, *20*, 890–901. [CrossRef] [PubMed]
5. Lemos, C.A.A.; Ferro-Alves, M.L.; Okamoto, R.; Mendonça, M.R.; Pellizzer, E.P. Short dental implants versus standard dental implants placed in the posterior jaws: A systematic review and meta-analysis. *J. Dent.* **2016**, *47*, 8–17. [CrossRef] [PubMed]
6. N Dias, F.J.; Pecorari, V.G.A.; Martins, C.B.; Del Fabbro, M.; Casati, M.Z. Short implants versus bone augmentation in combination with standard-length implants in posterior atrophic partially edentulous mandibles: Systematic review and meta-analysis with the Bayesian approach. *Int. J. Oral Maxillofac. Surg.* **2019**, *48*, 90–96. [CrossRef]
7. Markose, J.; Eshwar, S.; Srinivas, S.; Jain, V. Clinical outcomes of ultrashort sloping shoulder implant design: A survival analysis. *Clin. Implant Dent. Relat. Res.* **2018**, *20*, 646–652. [CrossRef]
8. Urdaneta, R.A.; Daher, S.; Leary, J.; Emanuel, K.M.; Chuang, S.K. The survival of ultrashort locking-taper implants. *Int. J. Oral Maxillofac. Implant* **2012**, *27*, 644–654.
9. Ravidà, A.; Barootchi, S.; Askar, H.; Suárez-López Del Amo, F.; Tavelli, L.; Wang, H.L. Long-Term Effectiveness of Extra-Short (≤6 mm) Dental Implants: A Systematic Review. *Int. J. Oral Maxillofac. Implant.* **2019**, *34*, 68–84. [CrossRef]
10. Bitaraf, T.; Keshtkar, A.; Rokn, A.R.; Monzavi, A.; Geramy, A.; Hashemi, K. Comparing short dental implant and standard dental implant in terms of marginal bone level changes: A systematic review and meta-analysis of randomized controlled trials. *Clin. Implant Dent. Relat. Res.* **2019**, *21*, 796–812. [CrossRef]
11. Deporter, D. *Short and Ultrashort Implants*; Quintessence Publishing: New Malden, UK, 2018; pp. 59–74.
12. Deporter, D.; Ogiso, B.; Sohn, D.S.; Ruljancich, K.; Pharoah, M. Ultrashort sintered porous-surfaced dental implants used to replace posterior teeth. *J. Periodontol.* **2008**, *79*, 1280–1286. [CrossRef] [PubMed]
13. Fan, T.; Li, Y.; Deng, W.W.; Wu, T.; Zhang, W. Short Implants (5 to 8 mm) Versus Longer Implants (>8 mm) with Sinus Lifting in Atrophic Posterior Maxilla: A Meta-Analysis of RCTs. *Clin. Implant Dent. Relat. Res.* **2017**, *19*, 207–215. [CrossRef] [PubMed]
14. Al-Johany, S.S. Survival Rates of Short Dental Implants (≤6.5 mm) Placed in Posterior Edentulous Ridges and Factors Affecting their Survival after a 12-Month Follow-up Period: A Systematic Review. *Int. J. Oral Maxillofac. Implant* **2019**, *34*, 605–621. [CrossRef] [PubMed]
15. Martinolli, M.; Bortolini, S.; Natali, A.; Pereira, L.J.; Castelo, P.M.; Rodrigues Garcia, R.C.M.; Gonçalves, T.M.S.V. Long-term survival analysis of standard-length and short implants with multifunctional abutments. *J. Oral Rehabil.* **2019**, *46*, 640–646. [CrossRef]
16. Felice, P.; Soardi, E.; Pellegrino, G.; Pistilli, R.; Marchetti, C.; Gessaroli, M.; Esposito, M. Treatment of the atrophic edentulous maxilla: Short implants versus bone augmentation for placing longer implants. Five-month post-loading results of a pilot randomised controlled trial. *Eur. J. Oral Implant* **2011**, *4*, 191–202.
17. Gehrke, S.A.; Guirado, J.L.C.; Bettach, R.; Fabbro, M.D.; Martínez, C.P.A.; Shibli, J.A. Evaluation of the insertion torque, implant stability quotient and drilled hole quality for different drill design: An in vitro Investigation. *Clin. Oral Implant Res.* **2018**, *29*, 656–662. [CrossRef]
18. Romanos, G.E.; Delgado-Ruiz, R.A.; Sacks, D.; Calvo-Guirado, J.L. Influence of the implant diameter and bone quality on the primary stability of porous tantalum trabecular metal dental implants: An in vitro biomechanical study. *Clin. Oral Implant Res.* **2018**, *29*, 649–655. [CrossRef]

19. Möhlhenrich, S.C.; Heussen, N.; Elvers, D.; Steiner, T.; Hölzle, F.; Modabber, A. Compensating for poor primary implant stability in different bone densities by varying implant geometry: A laboratory study. *Int. J. Oral. Maxillofac. Surg.* **2015**, *44*, 1514–1520. [CrossRef]

20. Yamaguchi, Y.; Shiota, M.; FuJii, M.; Sekiya, M.; Ozeki, M. Development and application of a direct method to observe the implant/bone interface using simulated bone. *Springerplus* **2016**, *5*, 494. [CrossRef]

21. Falco, A.; Berardini, M.; Trisi, P. Correlation Between Implant Geometry, Implant Surface, Insertion Torque, and Primary Stability: In Vitro Biomechanical Analysis. *Int. J. Oral Maxillofac. Implant* **2018**, *33*, 824–830. [CrossRef]

22. Di Stefano, D.A.; Arosio, P.; Gastaldi, G.; Gherlone, E. The insertion torque-depth curve integral as a measure of implant primary stability: An in vitro study on polyurethane foam blocks. *J. Prosthet. Dent.* **2018**, *120*, 706–714. [CrossRef] [PubMed]

23. Tsolaki, I.N.; Tonsekar, P.P.; Najafi, B.; Drew, H.J.; Sullivan, A.J.; Petrov, S.D. Comparison of Osteotome and Conventional Drilling Techniques for Primary Implant Stability: An In Vitro Study. *J. Oral Implant* **2016**, *42*, 321–325. [CrossRef] [PubMed]

24. Oliveira, P.S.; Rodrigues, J.A.; Shibli, J.A.; Piattelli, A.; Iezzi, G.; Perrotti, V. Influence of osteoporosis on the osteocyte density of human mandibular bone samples: A controlled histological human study. *Clin. Oral Implant Res.* **2016**, *27*, 325–328. [CrossRef] [PubMed]

25. Sennerby, L.; Meredith, N. Implant stability measurements using resonance frequency analysis: Biological and biomechanical aspects and clinical implications. *Periodontology* **2008**, *47*, 51–66. [CrossRef]

26. Comuzzi, L.; Iezzi, G.; Piattelli, A.; Tumedei, M. An In Vitro Evaluation, on Polyurethane Foam Sheets, of the Insertion Torque (IT) Values, Pull-Out Torque Values, and Resonance Frequency Analysis (RFA) of NanoShort Dental Implants. *Polymer* **2019**, *11*, 1020. [CrossRef]

5

Intraosteal Behavior of Porous Scaffolds: The mCT Raw-Data Analysis as a Tool for Better Understanding

Andrés Parrilla-Almansa [1], Carlos Alberto González-Bermúdez [2], Silvia Sánchez-Sánchez [1],
Luis Meseguer-Olmo [3], Carlos Manuel Martínez-Cáceres [4], Francisco Martínez-Martínez [5],
José Luis Calvo-Guirado [6], Juan José Piñero de Armas [7], Juan Manuel Aragoneses [8],
Nuria García-Carrillo [9] and Piedad N. De Aza [10],*

[1] Image Diagnostic Service, Virgen de la Arrixaca University Hospital, El Palmar, 30120 Murcia, Spain;
    aparrilla10@gmail.com (A.P.-A.); silviasanchez@gmail.com (S.S.-S.)
[2] Faculty of Medicine, Universidad de Murcia, Instituto Murciano de Investigación Biosanitaria Virgen de la
    Arrixaca (IMIB-Arrixaca), 30.100 Murcia, Spain; cagb1@um.es
[3] Department of Orthopaedic Surgery and Trauma, School of Medicine, Lab of Regeneration and Tissue
    Repair, UCAM-Universidad Catolica San Antonio de Murcia, Guadalupe, 30107 Murcia, Spain;
    lmeseguer.doc@gmail.com
[4] Pathology Unit, Biomedical Research Institute of Murcia (IMIB-Arrixaca-UMU), El Palmar, 30120 Murcia,
    Spain; cmmarti@um.es
[5] Orthopaedic and Trauma Service, Virgen de la Arrixaca University Hospital, El Palmar, 30120 Murcia, Spain;
    fmtnez@gmail.com
[6] Department of Oral Surgery and Implant Dentistry, Faculty of Health Sciences, UCAM- Universidad
    Católica San Antonio de Murcia, Guadalupe, 30107 Murcia, Spain; jlcalvo@ucam.edu
[7] Cátedra Internacional de Análisis Estadístico y Big Data, Universidad Católica de Murcia, 30107 Murcia,
    Spain; jjpinero@ucam.edu
[8] Department of Dental Research in Universidad Federico Henriquez y Carvajal (UFHEC),
    Santo Domingo 10107, Dominican Republic; jaragoneses@ufhec.edu.do
[9] Department of Medicina Oral, Facultad de Medicina, Universidad de Murcia, Instituto Murciano de
    Investigación Biosanitaria Virgen de la Arrixaca (IMIB-Arrixaca), 30.100 Murcia, Spain; ngc2@um.es
[10] Instituto de Bioingenieria, Universidad Miguel Hernandez, 03202 Elche, Spain
*   Correspondence: piedad@umh.es

Abstract: The aim of the study is to determine the existing correlation between high-resolution 3D imaging technique obtained through Micro Computed Tomography (mCT) and histological-histomorphometric images to determine in vivo bone osteogenic behavior of bioceramic scaffolds. A Ca-Si-P scaffold ceramic doped and non-doped (control) with a natural demineralized bone matrix (DBM) were implanted in rabbit tibias for 1, 3, and 5 months. A progressive disorganization and disintegration of scaffolds and bone neoformation occurs, from the periphery to the center of the implants, without any differences between histomorphometric and radiological analysis. However, significant differences ($p < 0.05$) between DMB-doped and non-doped materials where only detected through mathematical analysis of mCT. In this way, average attenuation coefficient for DMB-doped decreased from 0.99 ± 0.23 Hounsfield Unit (HU) (3 months) to 0.86 ± 0.32 HU (5 months). Average values for non-doped decreased from 0.86 ± 0.25 HU (3 months) to 0.66 ± 0.33 HU. Combination of radiological analysis and mathematical mCT seems to provide an adequate in vivo analysis of bone-implanted biomaterials after surgery, obtaining similar results to the one provided by histomorphometric analysis. Mathematical analysis of Computed Tomography (CT) would allow the conducting of long-term duration in vivo studies, without the need for animal sacrifice, and the subsequent reduction in variability.

Keywords: ceramic scaffolds; demineralized bone matrix; bone regeneration; micro-CT; histomorphometry

1. Introduction

Imaging techniques have contributed to some of the most significant advances in biomedicine, and this trend is accelerating [1]. Development of image-capture techniques has required parallel advances in image processing and characterization, being consolidated as a specific research discipline in biomedicine. Digital image processing and analysis are aimed to develop methods of information extraction from images generated by different capture techniques, as well as to integrate the information obtained [2].

Compare to others, Computed Tomography (CT) offers the best radiographic method for morphological and qualitative analysis of bone and solid structures [3]. The images obtained through CT are the result of a volumetric decomposition of the body in units or voxels. From each voxel, a data set of attenuation coefficients is extracted, being known as "raw data". This volumetric set of raw data is mathematically reconstructed (iterative reconstruction, filtered retro projection algorithms) to obtain a pixelated image [4,5].

Strongly related to the size/number of voxels, and to the resolution of the acquisition system, the reconstruction from a volumetric object in a pixelated and multiplanar image is associated with the loss of data, as well as to the introduction of errors. In this way, despite presenting different attenuation coefficient, data contained in a voxel would contribute to the final pixel conformation [5]. Apart from the previously explained sources of miss information, the interpretation of radiological images is associated with other problems. At this respect, Garland (1949) [6] warned the scientific community about the error inherent in the radiological interpretation. Among the frequent mistakes identified during imaging analysis, perceptual errors or miss evaluation of images with a limited interpretive value are included [7]. Alternatively, cognitive errors of interpretation have been also described as frequent [8]. Work overload and environment factors are also decisive in radiological interpretation as, among others, they determine staff fatigue or eyestrain [9]. To reduce errors and false negative rates of image interpretation, a computer-assisted detection (CAD) program has been developed. CAD is software to analyze digital data set of the images, and estimate the probability of a specific disease based on algorithms developed to identify structural distortions. So far it has been used on mammographic studies but with limited results [10,11].

New strategies in the management of bone lesions include the implantation of porous biomaterial scaffolds. These biomaterials can enhance bone healing capacity and favor new bone formation when it is comprised (for instance: lack of vascularization, infections, lack of mechanical stability, or tissue loss) [12]. Histomorphometry and Micro Computed Tomography (mCT) proved to be dominant imaging techniques in the preclinical evaluation of cortical and medullary bone structure. These techniques enable the measurement and the assessment of in vivo bone formation and resorption. By using the mCT, either the anatomic correlation in 2D or the spatial bone microstructure in 3D can be analyzed [13,14]. Algorithmic studies have been conducted to ensure the greatest correspondence in the correlation between the image obtained by mCT and the one obtained by histology [12,15]. The development of a standardized method based on raw-data analysis would contribute to non-destructively quantify the formation of new bone tissue at the periphery and within the implanted biomaterial, reducing the variability associated with CT image processing and its interpretation.

The aim of the study is to determine the possible role of a global imaging analysis, which includes imaging descriptive analysis, mCT raw-data mathematical analysis, and histomorphometric analysis in order to objectively elucidate the osteogenic behavior observed after implant porous biomaterial scaffolds in tibias from New Zealand rabbits as preclinical model.

2. Materials and Methods

2.1. Porous Scaffold Implants Composition and Fabrication

Porous scaffolds were produced by partial sintering method [16–19]. Laboratory previously synthesized tricalcium phosphate ($Ca_3(PO_4)_2$) [TCP] and dicalcium silicate (Ca_2SiO_4) [C2S] were used as raw materials [20,21]. C2S (45% wt.) and TCP (55% wt.) were attrition-milled in isopropyl media, dried (60°C overnight), isostatically pressed (200 MPa) and heated inside platinum crucibles for 2 h to 1000 °C. Homogeneous bars were obtained after being grounded, pressed and reheated (1300 °C, 24 h). One part of the material was grounded to obtain a coarse fraction powder of ~1–2 mm particle size, whereas the other part was milled to ~2 μm. Scaffold implants were obtained after mixing 90% of 1–2 mm coarse fraction powder with 10% of 2 μm particles, using polyvinyl acetate (10%) as binder. Mixture was then heated to 1170° for 2 h, allowing cooling to room temperature inside furnace for 24 h. Finally, cylinders (height = 6 mm; diameter = 4.5 mm) were cut and sterilized by means of hydrogen peroxide gas-plasma (Sterrad® 100S, Germany) at low temperature (Figure 1A).

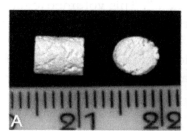 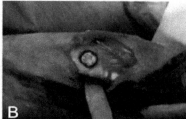 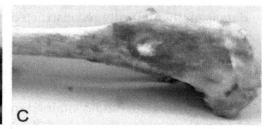

Figure 1. (**A**) Non-doped porous scaffold implants (before being implanted); (**B**) Intrasurgical image (proximal anteromedial metaphysis of right tibia) showing the implanted material; (**C**) Sample collection after tibia removal.

After sterilization, 60% of scaffolds were immersed in 231.3 ± 1.35 mg of Demineralized Bone Matrix Gel (DBM-gel, labeled as DMB-doped)) Activagen® (Bioteck, Arcugnano, Italy) for 3 minutes. Each scaffold was weighed to ensure an impregnated amount of DBM of 79.06 ± 0.47 mg. DBM is being defined as osteogenic inductor, promoting a rapid vascularization and osteoblast differentiation [22]. The remaining 40% of pellets were untreated (labeled as non-doped).

2.2. Animal Selection and Conditioning

Fifteen New Zealand white rabbits were included in this study. Inclusion criteria were: pathogen-free male, with an initial weight of 3.500–4.000 g and aged 26–28 weeks to ensure skeletal maturity and physical closure [23,24]. Ethical approval for the experiment was obtained from the Ethics Committee in Animal Research of the University of Murcia (A13150102). Before the experimental stage, each animal was housed individually for 5 days, under the optimal vivarium conditions for the detailed specie (temperature, light/darkness cycle, maximum noise, and relative humidity). These conditions are legally established by the EU Directive/63/2010 and by the Spanish Royal Decree 53/2013. During the entire study, animals received ad libitum food and water.

After conditioning, animals were randomly allocated into three groups ($n = 5$ each) in correspondence to three defined study periods (1, 3 and 5 months) respectively.

2.3. Scaffold Implantation: Anesthetic and Surgical Method

All surgical procedures were performed under rigorous aseptic conditions. Animal anesthesia and post-operative analgesia was performed following the previously established and approved protocol described by Ros-Tarraga et al. (2016) [25,26]. Premedication and anesthesia was achieved with atropine sulfate (0.3 mg k^{-1}, im), chlorpromazine hydrochloride (10 mg k^{-1}, im), xylacine (0,25 mg k^{-1}, im) and ketamine hydrochloride (50 mg k^{-1}, im). Animals were treated with a prophylactic single dose of enrofloxacin (mg k^{-1}, im) (Virbac, Barcelona, Spain) to reduce the risk of surgical site infections.

Surgical surface was shaved, washed and sterilized with clorhexidine® (Bohm SA, Madrid, Spain) and povidone iodine 10% (Betadine™; Meda Pharma, Madrid, Spain). Sterile fenestrates adhesive drapes were used for delimitation of surgical area. A 1.5–2 mm long and deep skin incision was made at the proximal anteromedial metaphysis, in parallel to the right tibial shaft axis. Anterior tibial tuberosity was landmarked as surgical reference to minimize incisional variability. After dissection of fascia and periostium, a unicortical ~4.5 mm diameter bone defect was created with a surgical bone drill, coupled to a micromotor at low revolutions and continuous irrigation with saline solution. Bone medullar cavity was not invaded. Surgical defects were debrided and washed with physiological saline solution before being grafted with porous cylindrical implants as it has been shown in Figure 1B. Within each previously defined animal group, the DBM-doped: non-doped scaffold ratio implanted was 3:2. Surgical wound was sutured in anatomical layers with 3-0 Coated Vicryl® and 3-0 Vicryl rapide® (Johnson & Johnson Medical Devices & Diagnostics, New Brunswick, NJ, USA and covered by the application of a thin layer of NovecutanTM plastic dressing spray (Inibsa, Barcelona, Spain). Post-operative analgesia was assessed by the application of subcutaneous mepivacaine (1%) around the surgical wound and buprenorphine (0.3 mg k^{-1}, im, every 12 h for 4 days). After 4 days, individual analgesia was provided in case of pain symptoms, local swelling, or stress. After surgery, limb free movements were permitted. All animals used during the study survived and appeared to be in good health status.

2.4. Euthanasia and Samples Collection

Three different sampling times were considering across the study (1, 3 and 5 months after surgery). For each sampling time, a group of animals ($n = 5$) was deeply sedated with a single dose of ketamine hydrochloride (50 mg k^{-1}, im) and euthanized by an intracardiac overdose of pentobarbital (Dolethal®, Lab Vetoquinal, Cedex, France). For each animal, right limb tibia was removed, cleaned of soft tissue and fixed in neutral buffered formalin (10%) (Figure 1C). Samples were stored at 4 °C until analyses.

2.5. mCT Imaging Protocol and Descriptive Analysis

The imaging study was performed using the Albira tri-modal preclinical-scanner (Bruker®, Billerica, MA, USA). Fixed scanning parameters were 45 Kv, 0.2 mA, 0.05 mm voxels. From each sample, a set of 1000 axial projections of 0.05 mm thickness was obtained using a digital flat panel detector with 2400 × 2400 pixels and a 70 × 70 mm field of view (FoV). Tibial images were spatially reconstructed by the filtered back projection (FBP) algorithm, and Bone Mineral Density (BMD) in the implanted area was quantified in Hounsfield Unit (HU). With this purpose, a medical image data examiner (AMIDE, UCLA University, LA, USA) and online 3D image analysis software (Volview, mm^3, Inc) were used. Images were pre-described by two experienced radiologists (A and B), based on a double-blind visual analysis, evaluating evolution of implanted material along the study (pre-implanted material and 1, 3 and 5 months after surgery). Final report was concluded by consensus among A and B. To homogenize image description, the visual analysis was centered on the following items: (1) loss of homogeneity of implanted material with respect to the pre-implanted one; (2) loss of implant contour sharpness in relation to the peripheric tissue; (3) presence of neoformed bone trabeculations inside the implanted biomaterial; (4) dispersion of biomaterial in the peripheric tissue; (5) neoformed trabeculations between implant surface and adjacent cortical bone. Figure 2 shows the mCT and 3D mCT images evaluated by radiologists.

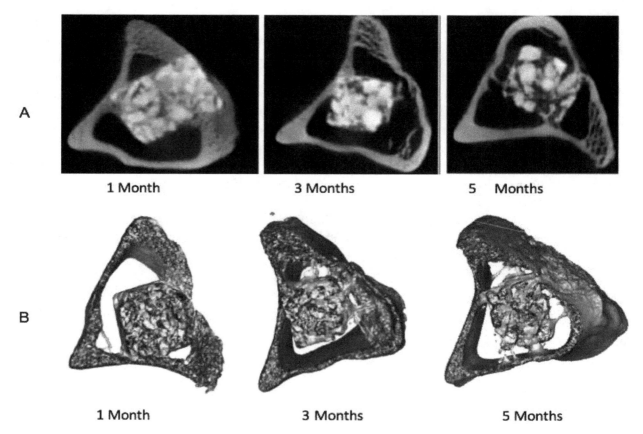

Figure 2. (**A**) Transverse mCT images of implanted area, obtained at different times of study (1, 3 and 5 months); (**B**) 3D mCT image reconstruction of samples obtained at 1, 3 and 5 months of study. Figure show the non-doped scaffold as a representative of both materials.

2.6. Mathematical Processing of mCT Raw Data

Selection and mathematical study of raw data was conducted at the Biostatistics Department of San Antonio Catholic University (Murcia, Spain). With this purpose, three regions of interest (ROIs) were selected by consensus (Figure 3), according to the following criteria: (A) implanted biomaterial (4×4 mm^3 cylindrical ROI) to evaluate implant resorption, degradation or integration by bone tissue; (B) implanted biomaterial and peripheral corticomedullar bone ($10 \times 10 \times 10$ mm cubical ROI) to assess the dispersion undergone by biomaterial fragments within the peripheral host bone; (C) surgically unaltered cortical bone distanced from the implanted area (3×3 mm cylindrical ROI) to determine the spontaneous evolution of unaltered cortical bone, as control measurement and yardstick of analysis. In parallel, two unimplanted porous scaffolds cylinders were analyzed as basal values, being represented as time 0 in the study.

From each ROI and sample, raw data were obtained after voxel selection. According to the basal values obtained, and with the aim of analyzing the interactions between porous scaffold implants and bone tissue, voxels with average values $> +1.10$ HU were preselected as implanted material from cubical ROI ($10 \times 10 \times 10$). In the same way, outranged voxels representing medullar/cortical bone or soft tissue were suppressed. Based on this selection, material dispersion was estimated as follows: A "center of mass" of the whole piece was calculated, determining the mean distance from each preselected voxel to this center. This mathematical study makes it possible to analyze the time evolution of variability in voxel standardized attenuation coefficients (HU), as well as to quantify how much biomaterial had dispersed within the peripheral host bone.

To visually clarify the effect of time on scaffold resorption and dispersion values per each group of implants (DBM-doped and non-doped), trend lines have been added. It must be taken into account that pre-implanted scaffolds were excluded for trend-line adjustment, as resorption and dispersion were not possible.

ROIs selection and raw data were obtained with Albira CT software (Bruker®, Billerica, MA, USA), in conjunction with Volview software (Kitware Inc), and Medical Image Data Analysis software (AMIDE, UCLA University, Los Angeles, CA, USA).

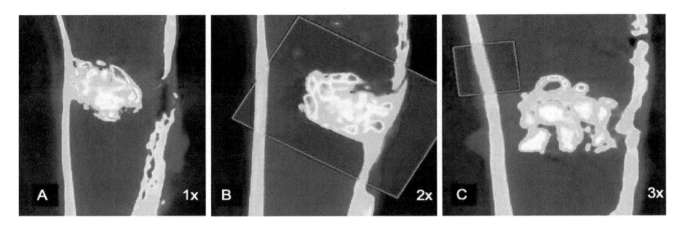

Figure 3. mCT images processed with AMIDE software. Defined Regions of interest (ROIs): (**A**) Implanted biomaterial (Cylindrical 4 × 4 mm), (1×); (**B**) implanted biomaterial and peripheral corticomedullar bone (10 × 10 × 10 mm cubical ROI) (2×). Red squares describe the ROI of cortical area; (**C**) surgically unaltered cortical bone (3 × 3 mm cylindrical ROI) (3×). Red squares describe the cortical area. Different color values correspond to different Hounsfield Unit (HU) ranges: HU > + 1100 (yellow-orange) correspond to different states of the implanted biomaterial. + 0.50–+ 1.00 HU (green) correspond to cortical bone and reabsorbed biomaterial. HU + 0.20–+ 0.40 HU (blue) correspond to connective and medullary bone tissue.

2.7. Histological and Histomorphometric Study

Samples were cross-sectioned perpendicular to the longitudinal axis of tibia with an electric circular saw (Figure 4A). Pieces of 3–4 mm thickness were fixed in neutral buffered formalin (10% formalin in 0.08 M sodium phosphate, pH 7.4) for 48 h and decalcified by the addition of hydrochloride acid (Osteomoll®, Merck Chemical, Darmstadt, Germany). Samples were subsequently dehydrated in alcohol and embedded in paraffin. Histologic and histomorphometric analysis was performed in hematoxylin-eosin stained sections of 4 µm thicknesses. A panoramic histological image (low magnification, ×5.4) of implanted area in each section was obtained (Figure 4B) using a Leica Z6 Apo macroscope (Leica Microsystems, Barcelona, Spain), connected to a Leica CDC500 digital camera and image-capture software (Leica Application Suite). Equipment was provided by the Image Analysis Service of the University of Murcia, Spain (SAI-UMU).

Total implanted area surface (TIS) was calculated, and consecutives microscopic fields were captured under ×50 magnification (Figure 4C). Magnified images were obtained by a bright-field Zeiss Axio Scope A.1 optical microscope (Carl Zeiss, Jenna, Germany), connected to a digital camera (AxioCam IcC3, Carl Zeiss). Equipment was supplied by Pathology Platform of "Instituto Murciano de Investigación Biosanitaria Virgen de la Arrixaca" (IMIB-Arrixaca), Murcia, Spain. As it can be seen in Figure 5, from each 50x field, 4 identifiable components were analyzed: (1) Floury and acidophilic material, identified as "non-absorbed implanted material"; (2) "neoformed bone tissue"; (3) "connective tissue"; (4) floury and basophilic material, located between components 1 and 2, named "unidentifiable material". For components 2, 3 and 4, the surface area was outlined manually using AxioVision rel. 4.8 (Zeiss, Canada) software. To calculate "non-absorbed-implanted material" surface area, the following formula was used:

$$Surface\ area\ (1) = TIS - (2 + 3 + 4) \tag{1}$$

With the aim of an accurate quantification of each component surface extension, the morphometric analysis was repeated on three different levels per sample (inter-level distance 300 μm).

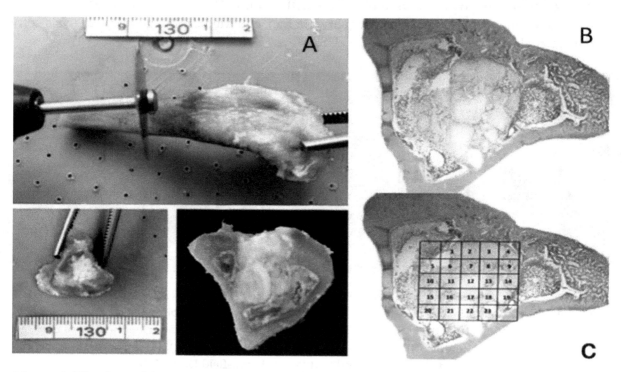

Figure 4. Histological-Histomorphometric procedure. (**A**) Samples including implanted area were obtained perpendicularly to the long axis of tibia, using an electric circular saw; (**B**) Panoramic histological view (×5.4) containing porous material; (**C**) ×50 magnified and consecutives images on a panoramic histological view.

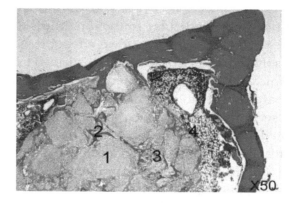

Figure 5. 50× magnified image obtained from the panoramic histological view of the non-doped scaffold as a representative of both materials. Four different components can be identified in the study: (1) non-absorbed implanted material; (2) neoformed bone tissue; (3) connective tissue; (4) special material.

2.8. Statistical Analysis

Statistical analysis was performed using R software v.3.2.3. A previous statistical descriptive analysis was performed to data characterization. Raw data were mathematically processed using a linear regression analysis, which simultaneously included 14,153 points from all the pieces. Linear regression was aimed to detect significant relations ($p < 0.05$) between the average HU of each ROI. As variables, the analysis included: Area location (ROIs), implant composition (DBM-doped or non-doped) and sampling time (non-implanted materials (0), 1, 3 and 5 months). In addition, biomaterial dispersion was analyzed with a to interpretative mathematical study of the biomaterial's

HU values respect the center of mass, establishing its evolution across the study (1, 3 and 5 months) regardless if it is DBM-doped or non-doped

Regarding Histological and Histomorphometric study, a Mann–Whitney non-parametric test was performed. Statistically significant differences (* $p < 0.05$, ** $p < 0.05$) between each previously defined component (1, 2, 3 and 4) in relation to time of sampling (non-implanted material (0), 1, 3 and 5 months) were analyzed.

3. Results

3.1. Descriptive Analysis of mCT Images

mCT images were pre-evaluated by a double-blind interpretation. Final report was issued by consensus based on the previously described procedure. As can be seen on Figure 2A, when mCT images where visually analyzed, both radiologist A and B, concluded that during the 5-month study period, implanted material underwent progressive dispersion into the host bone medulla after matrix disaggregation and disintegration.

According to the final report, when 1-, 3-, and 5-months 3D mCT images (Figure 2B) were visually compared, a progressive disintegration and disorganization of initial implant morphology (from a compact cylindrical block to a fragmented and porous mass) as well as a neoformation of bone tissue were descripted. These findings were more noticeable and earlier detected at the periphery than at the central portion of implanted material. Consensuated descriptional analysis of mCT and 3D mCT images was not able to distinguish differences between the behavior of DMB-doped and no-doped implants across the study period.

Previously, explained findings in descriptive analysis of mCT and 3D mCT (Figure 2) were related to an increment in biomaterial porosity, as well as to the dispersion of implant fragments. This fragmentation seems to be more evident at the scaffold periphery, allowing neoformation of trabecular bone both inside the implanted material and around its surface.

3.2. mCT Raw-Data Analysis

The evolution of scaffold during the study period (pre-implanted material, 1, 3 and 5 months after surgery) was analyzed in the defined cylindrical 4x4mm ROIs, which contained the implanted material (> + 1.10 HU). As can be seen in Figure 6A, a significant relation ($p < 0.05$) was defined in each selected ROI between the average standardized attenuation coefficient (average HU value) and time, accompanied by an increment in voxels HU variability. This relation has been represented by the adjusted trend lines per each group of implants (DBM-doped and non-doped), which suggest a time-dependent decrease of average HU values. To be concrete, pre-implanted scaffolds showed an average attenuation coefficient of 1.13 ± 0.18 HU. Three months after surgery, the attenuation coefficient decreased to average values of 0.99 ± 0.23 HU (DBM-doped scaffolds) and 0.86 ± 0.25 HU (non-doped scaffolds). Five-month attenuation coefficients reached minimum values of 0.86 ± 0.32 HU (DBM-doped scaffolds) and 0.66 ± 0.33 HU (non-doped scaffolds). As can be deduced from these results, DBM-doped scaffolds showed a more gradual decrease of average HU values than non-doped implants, resulting in significant differences ($p < 0.05$) between both groups average values.

Biomaterial dispersion in peripheral tissue was analyzed selecting cubical ROIs ($10 \times 10 \times 10$ mm^3) and a > + 1.10 HU window. As can be seen in Figure 6B, the variation of global distance (mm) of selected voxels with respect to the center of mass of implanted material, increased at a rate of ~ 0.16 mm per month, from the beginning (1 month) to the end (5 months) of post-surgical period analyzed. The dispersion value increment between different stages of study were statistically significant ($p < 0.05$); however, no differences were found between DBM-doped and no-doped implants.

As control measurement, the average standardized attenuation coefficient in surgically unaltered cortical bone (0.50–1.00 HU window) was analyzed in cylindrical ROI (3×3 mm^3). According to the results obtained, average unaltered cortical HU values remained stable across the study (0.83 ± 0.12 HU), with no significant differences between different sampling times (1, 3 and 5 months after surgery).

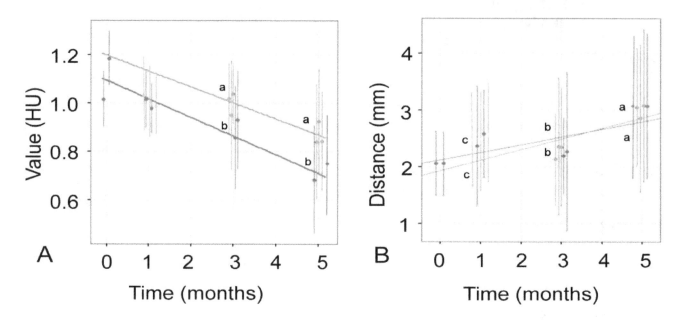

Figure 6. Evolution of implanted material after 1, 3, and 5 months post-implantation in each animal group ($n = 5$). Pre-implanted material results are considered as time 0. Doped (Activagen®-treated) and no-doped material have been represented as blue and red dots, respectively. (**A**) For evaluation of implant resorption, results have been presented as the average HU ± S.D. in each preselected cylindrical ROI (4×4 mm^3). Different letters a, b denote significant differences between type of material for each time of study. (**B**) Per each cubical ROI ($10 \times 10 \times 10$ mm^3), implanted material dispersion in the peripheral tissue has been presented as the center of mass per each implant (dot) and the global variation of distance (mm) of the preselected voxels (>1.10 HU) from this center of mass (bars). A > 1.10 HU window was set to identify voxels corresponding to biomaterial. Different letters a, b, c denote significant differences between time).

3.3. Histological and Histomorphometrical Results

According to Figure 7A, there was a good visual correspondence between mCT images and histological preparations. Implanted scaffolds were degraded and resorbed during the time of study, being transformed into fragments which were smaller at the periphery and larger at the central portion of the implant. When the sites between remaining scaffold fragments were histologically analyzed (Figure 7B,C), it consisted of osteogenic tissue (fibroblasts, osteoclasts and osteoblast, surrounded by extracellular matrix) with signs of active angiogenesis.

Histological image of implant was divided in consecutives ×50 microscopic fields for histomorphometric analysis (Figure 4C). The surface area of each histologic component considered in the study [(A) non-absorbed implanted material; (B) neoformed bone tissue; (C) connective tissue; (D) unidentifiable material] was calculated. In Figure 8, the evolution of these components surfaces with time of study (1, 3 and 5 months) have been shown. A progressive and significant increase in bone tissue (Figure 8B) was observed from 1 to 5 month after surgery. In this way, bone tissue significantly increased ($p < 0.05$) from 1.27 ± 0.30 mm^2 (non-doped) and 1.09 ± 0.32 mm^2 (DBM-doped), to 2.12 ± 0.21 mm^2 (non-doped) and 2.15 ± 0.35 mm^2 (DBM-doped) 3 months post-surgery. This increment become more evident 5 months post-surgery ($p < 0.005$), reaching final values of 3.91 ± 0.39 mm^2 (non-doped) and 3.43 ± 0.27 mm^2 (DBM-doped).

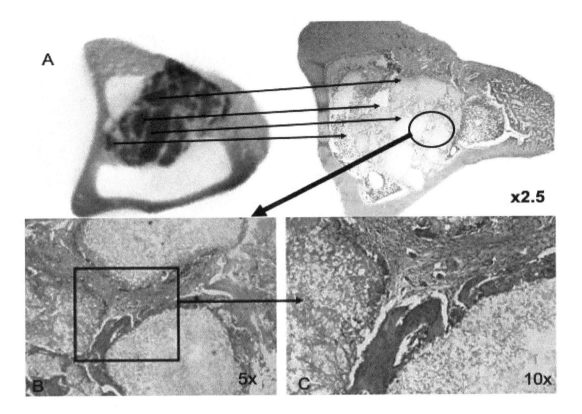

Figure 7. (**A**) Visual correlation between histological (hematoxylin and eosin stain) and axial mCT images. (**B,C**) Detailed view (×5 and ×10 magnification) of area contained between scaffolds fragments. Corresponding to the non-doped scaffold as a representative of both materials.

In parallel to bone tissue increment, a significant progressive reduction in surface of implanted material (Figure 8A) and basophilic component surrounding neoformed bone tissue (unidentifiable material) (Figure 8D) can be described. Regarding implanted material, its surface decreased from 27.21 ± 5.28 mm^2 (non-doped) and 26.92 ± 4.19 mm^2 (DBM-doped), to 15.88 ± 5.01 mm^2 (non-doped) and 16.52 ± 3.28 mm^2 (DBM-doped) 5 months post-surgery. Similar behavior was described for unidentifiable material surface, decreasing from 1.75 ± 0.90 mm^2 (non-doped) and 1.64 ± 0.46 mm^2 DBM-doped) at 1 month, to a final value of 0.30 ± 0.29 mm^2 (non-doped) and 0.36 ± 0.23 mm^2 (DBM-doped) 5 months post-surgery.

When the post-surgery evolution of surface occupied by connective tissue was analyzed (Figure 8C), significant differences were found between 1 month (1.10 ± 0.75 and 1.22 ± 0.41 mm^2, non-doped and DBM-doped respectively) and 3 months (1.63 ± 0.92 and 1.78 ± 0.71 mm^2, non-doped and DBM-doped material respectively). However, at 5 months after surgery, connective tissue decreased to 0.43 ± 0.29 mm^2 (non-doped) and 0.68 ± 0.26 mm^2 (DBM-doped). Five-month results, were statistically significant ($p < 0.005$) only when compared to DBM-doped implanted materials at 1 and 3 months after surgery.

After the analysis of the effect of scaffold composition (non-doped and DBM-doped material), no statistical differences were found for each time considered in the study (1, 3 and 5 months after surgery). Despite this fact, when average values for each material after 5 months were compared, DBM-doped scaffolds resulted in an average lower reduction of connective tissue (Figure 8C) and a lower bone tissue formation (Figure 8B), than the average values obtained for non-doped implant. Differences in average values between DBM-doped and non-doped materials, were less noticeable for the evolution of surface area of residual implanted material (Figure 8A) and unidentifiable material (Figure 8D), than for the evolution of connective tissue and bone tissue formation.

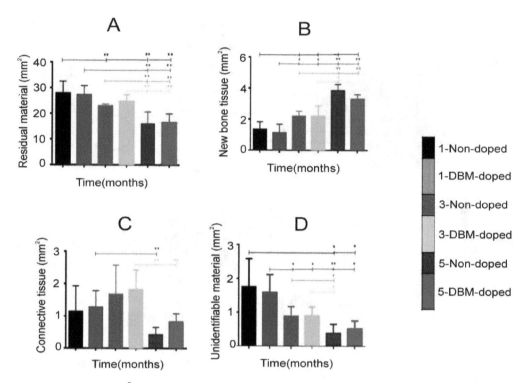

Figure 8. Surface area (mm^2) evolution of different histological components. (**A**) residual biomaterial, (**B**) new bone tissue, (**C**) connective tissue and (**D**) unidentifiable material in sliced histological samples]. Results have been presented as means ± S.D. Horizontals bars represent the Mann–Whitney–Wilcoxon test for two samples comparison (* $p < 0.05$ and ** $p < 0.005$).

4. Discussion

As has been widely described, bone repair process consists of (1) the recruitment of mesenchymal cells, which differentiates into fibroblast and osteogenic cells, (2) extracellular chondroid matrix formation, and (3) mineralization/chondroid matrix resorption [27]. Current bone tissue engineering includes the implantation of porous calcium phosphate and silicate scaffolds. Their presence induces a response similar to the one described for bone remodeling [28–32]. It has been described that when porous scaffolds are implanted, they are progressively resorbed and substituted by neoformed bone tissue. These process follows a concentric evolution, from the periphery to the center of the implanted material [33–35]. The results of this work agree with this process. After implantation, scaffolds were progressively degraded from 1 to 5 months after surgery. This degradation commenced at the periphery of the implanted material and advanced to its nucleus. Consensuated descriptive analysis of 3D mCT was able to describe this process as a progressive disintegration and disorganization of scaffold initial morphology, accompanied by the neoformation of bone tissue. However, descriptive analysis was not able neither, to detect the evolution of the connective matrix, nor quantify the time evolution of scaffold degradation and dispersion/bone neoformation. To clarify these issues, it was necessary to resort to histomorphometric and mCT raw-data analysis. The need to compliment the mCT results with other techniques for in vivo time scaffold evolution can be noticed in the previously published bibliography [30,36] including mathematical image analysis, histological macro and microscopic analysis, or design of specific algorithm for mCT data analysis.

As it has been explained, raw-data analysis showed that scaffold dispersion took place at a rate of ~ 0.16 mm per month. This material dispersion reflects the implanted material degradation. Considering a total scaffold surface area of 116.63 mm^2, and according to histomorphometric results, implant surface showed an approximate time-dependent degradation of 12-24% after 5 months post-implantation. These results can be partially compared to those showed by Sweedy et al. (2017) [22], who defined a scaffold resorption ratio of 22.16 ± 3.3%–31.66 ± 6.8% for a 6 weeks study period using Swiss Alpine sheep. However, it must be taken into account that this resorption ratio not only depends on animal species, but also is affected by scaffold porous size, implant composition or scaffold total size [37–39]. Furthermore, Bohner et al. (2017) [21] described that scaffold resorption and bone/mineralized tissue formation is not a uniform process, with a rapid increase in the first 4–10 weeks followed by a slow decrease after 10–12 weeks post-implantation. Based in the previously exposed results, scaffold degradation was uniform during the 5-month post-surgery period. By contrast, bone tissue formation and extracellular matrix resorption of the physical characteristics of scaffolds (e.g., micro- and macropore diameter) were not set during this study, and the differences between both scaffolds in resorption/bone repair process evolution cannot be really discussed. Bohner et al. (2017) [21] concluded in their work that mineralized matrix and ulterior bone formation needed an interconnected porous net, with a pore size larger than 1–10 μm. This would mean that a previous scaffold degradation process is needed to provide a suitable structure for bone repair, explaining the progressive scaffold degradation and the initial slow extracellular matrix resorption and bone formation previously described.

Regarding scaffold composition, the treatment with DBM-doped did not result in significant differences between doped and non-doped implants. Only raw-data mathematical analysis was able to detect significant differences in scaffold HU average values across the study between both types of materials. In fact, doped materials resulted in a more gradual decrease of average HU than no-doped implants. These results could be due to a higher phagocytic and osteoclastic resorption when non-doped scaffolds were implanted. However, no significant differences were described when implant dispersion, extracellular matrix resorption and bone tissue formation were analyzed. DBM-doped is composed of lyophilized granules of collagen type I [12]. After implantation to bone defects, biomaterial is degraded by osteoclasts, leading to the release of protein factors which induces mesenchymal cells differentiation into osteoblasts [30,31,38,40]. Shalash et al. (2013) [33], published a 6-month study based on the comparison between the use of TCP alone, and TCP plus DBM, for maxillary alveolar ridges deficiencies regeneration before implants placement. According to this study, after 6 months, TCP plus DBM resulted in a higher bone formation and TCP resorption than TCP alone. As it has been previously exposed, implantation of non-doped biomaterial, resulted in a higher resorption of scaffolds with no differences in new bone formation. Although the reason for these results remains unclear, a possible explanation could be the early stimulation of osteoblasts differentiation when DBM is added, controlling resorptive activity of osteoclasts [41]. It must be taken into account that the study was performed over 5 months, and synthesis of new bone tissue seemed to be more active at the end of this period. To obtain significant differences in new bone formation between both materials (doped and non-doped), a longer study would be needed.

Beyond these results, it is important to point out that medical invasive techniques are being substituted by minimally or non-invasive alternatives. Recent advances in CT technology are contributing to this purpose. Clear examples can be found in CT angiography, which is a non-invasive alternative to classical coronary angiography [35,36]. Applied to biomedical experimentation on animal models, improvement of imaging analysis techniques can replace invasive histological studies. This would lead to the refinement of experiments, due to the reduction of the number of animals needed, and to the continuous data collection without the need for animal sacrifice at intermediate experimental points [37]. Regarding in vivo assessment of bone quality and regeneration, preclinical research requires the combination of image and histomorphometric analysis [37–40]. Against visual image analysis and volumetric estimation of average standardized X-ray attenuation coefficients, histology provides a direct method to assess the bone regeneration process at a macroscopic and microscopic level, without resolution or standardization limitations. However, histomorphometric analysis requires to foreseeing the sacrifice of different groups of animals during the experiment, preventing from a continuous study and increasing both intragroup variability and number of animals needed [40–42]. Mathematical analysis of CT raw data could help to refine preclinical assays in bone regeneration studies. Their mathematical analysis could improve research based on image analysis. Budán et al. (2018) [43] performed an experiment with rats to develop a new method for evaluation of bone regeneration. With this purpose, CT and single photon emission computed tomography (SPECT) with marked methyl diphosphonate (MDP) as tracer were combined. Based on the cubic voxel reconstruction and calculation of summarized absorbance of VOI after normalization of bone total X-ray attenuation, quantification of bone regeneration was performed through the bone opacity changes, as well as marked MDP activity. Despite normalization, authors declared that as raw data were visually compared, not enough information was provided for proper quantitative evaluation and significant statistical analysis, especially during the early period of the experiment. The mathematical analysis of raw data could help to could help avoid these limitations in the methodology.

5. Conclusions

Mathematical analysis of CT raw data is often used separately by researchers, with no connection to radiological studies. Nevertheless, an adequate exploration of raw data seems to provide an objective analysis of radiological image. The present study shows the necessity of combining both radiological imaging studies and mathematical analysis of CT raw data to perform an adequate in vivo analysis of implanted bone scaffold and its evolution after surgery. Furthermore, as the results obtained seem to be similar to the anatomopathological ones, mathematical analysis of CT raw data would allow the conducting of long-term duration in vivo studies, without the need for animal sacrifice and the subsequent reduction in variability.

The combination of imaging and mathematical analysis could be extended to other areas in radiology practice, allowing clinicians to obtain a more accurate and objective image description, as well as to quantify the evolution of lesions or implants, without having to resort to aggressive techniques such as biopsy. In this way, future studies would be needed to assess these applications, and standardize the mathematical analysis of raw data applied to the radiological practice.

Author Contributions: Conceptualization: A.P.-A., C.A.G.-B.; methodology, S.S.-S., L.M.-O., C.M.M.-C., F.M.-M.; software, J.L.C.-G., J.J.P.d.A., N.G.-C. and J.M.A.; validation, J.J.P.d.A., N.G.-C., P.N.D.A.; formal analysis, J.J.P.d.A., C.A.G.-B.; investigation, A.P.-A., C.A.G.-B., S.S.-S.; resources, C.M.M.-C., F.M.-M., data curation, N.G.-C., P.N.D.A., A.P.-A.; writing—original draft preparation, A.P.-A., J.J.P.d.A., N.G.-C., P.N.D.A.; writing—review and editing, F.M.-M., J.L.C.-G., L.M.O.; visualization, F.M.-M., J.L.C.-G., N.G.-C., P.N.D.A.; supervision, J.L.C.-G., P.N.D.A. and J.M.A.; project administration, P.N.D.A., A.P.-A., C.A.G.-B., S.S.-S.; funding acquisition, P.N.D.A.

Acknowledgments: We want to thank to the department of Biostatistical of UCAM for its invaluable support in this work.

References

1. Lehmann, T.M.; Meinzer, H.P.; Tolxdorff, T. Advances in biomedical image analysis ast present and future challenges. *Methods Inf. Med.* **2004**, *43*, 308–314.
2. Lehmann, T.M.; Handels, H.; Maier-Hein ne Fritzsche, K.H.; Mersmann, S.; Palm, C.; Tolxdorff, T.; Wagenknecht, G.; Wittenberg, T. Viewpoints on medical image processing: From science to application. *Curr. Med. Imaging Rev.* **2013**, *9*, 79–88. [CrossRef]
3. Bouxsein, M.L.; Boyd, S.K.; Christiansen, B.A.; Guldberg, R.E.; Jepsen, K.J.; Müller, R. Guidelines for assessment of bone microstructure in rodents using microcomputed tomography. *J. Bone Miner. Res.* **2010**, *25*, 1468–1486. [CrossRef]
4. Höhne, K.H.; Bomans, M.; Pommert, A.; Riemer, M.; Schiers, C.; Tiede, U. 3D visualization of tomographic volume data using the generalized voxel model. *Vis. Comput.* **1990**, *6*, 28–36. [CrossRef]
5. Beister, M.; Kolditz, D.; Kalender, W.A. Iterative reconstruction methods in X-ray CT. *Phys. Med.* **2012**, *28*, 94–108. [CrossRef]
6. Garland, L.H. On the scientific evaluation of diagnostic procedures: Presidential address thirty-fourth annual meeting of the Radiological Society of North America. *Radiology* **1949**, *52*, 309–328. [CrossRef]
7. Berlin, L. Radiologic errors, past, present and future. *Diagnosis* **2014**, *1*, 79–84. [CrossRef]
8. Bruno, M.A.; Walker, E.A.; Abujudeh, H.H. Understanding and confronting our mistakes: The epidemiology of error in radiology and strategies for error reduction. *RadioGraphics* **2015**, *35*, 1668–1676. [CrossRef]

8.   Bruno, M.A.; Walker, E.A.; Abujudeh, H.H. Understanding and confronting our mistakes: The epidemiology of error in radiology and strategies for error reduction. *RadioGraphics* **2015**, *35*, 1668–1676. [CrossRef]

9.   Waite, S.; Scott, J.; Gale, B.; Fuchs, T.; Kolla, S.; Reede, D. Interpretive error in radiology. *Am. J. Roentgenol.* **2017**, *208*, 739–749. [CrossRef]

10.   Castellino, R.A. Computer aided detection (CAD): An overview. *Cancer Imaging* **2005**, *5*, 17–19. [CrossRef]

11.   Doi, K. Computer-aided diagnosis in medical imaging: Historical review, current status and future potential. *Comput. Med. Imaging Graph.* **2007**, *31*, 198–211. [CrossRef]

12.   Parrilla-Almansa, A.; García-Carrillo, N.; Ros-Tárraga, P.; Martínez, C.M.; Martínez-Martínez, F.; Meseguer-Olmo, L.; de Aza, P.N. Demineralized bone matrix coating Si-Ca-P ceramic does not improve the osseointegration of the scaffold. *Materials* **2018**, *11*, 1580. [CrossRef]

13.   Martinez, I.M.; Velasquez, P.A.; de Aza, P.N. Synthesis and stability of α-tricalcium phosphate doped with dicalcium silicate in the system $Ca_3(PO_4)_2$–Ca_2SiO_4. *Mater. Charact.* **2010**, *61*, 761–767. [CrossRef]

14.   Kim, S.Y.; Kim, Y.K.; Park, Y.H.; Park, J.C.; Ku, J.K.; Um, I.W.; Kim, J.Y. Evaluation of the healing potential of demineralized dentin matrix fixed with recombinant human bone. Morphogenetic protein-2 in bone grafts. *Materials* **2017**, *10*, 1049. [CrossRef]

15.   Schmidt, R.; Muller, L.; Kress, A.; Hirschfelder, H.; Aplas, A.; Pitto, R.P. A computed tomography assessment of femoral and acetabular bone changes after total hip arthroplasty. *Int. Orthop.* **2002**, *26*, 299–302. [CrossRef]

16.   Mate-Sanchez de Val, J.E.; Calvo-Guirado, J.L.; Delgado-Ruiz, R.A.; Ramirez-Fernandez, M.P.; Negri, B.; Abboud, M.; Martinez, I.M.; de Aza, P.N. Physical properties, mechanical behavior, and electron microscopy study of a new α-TCP block graft with silicon in an animal model. *J. Biomed. Mater. Res. A* **2012**, *100*, 3446–3454. [CrossRef]

17.   Calvo-Guirado, J.L.; Ramirez-Fernandez, M.P.; Delgado-Ruiz, R.A.; Mate-Sanchez de Val, J.E.; Velasquez, P.; de Aza, P.N. Influence of biphasic β-TCP with and without the use of collagen membranes on bone healing of surgically critical size defects. A radiological, histological and histomorphometric study. *Clin. Oral Implant Res.* **2014**, *25*, 1228–1238. [CrossRef]

18.   Ros-Tarraga, P.; Mazon, P.; Rodriguez, M.A.; Meseguer-Olmo, L.; de Aza, P.N. Novel resorbable and osteoconductive calcium silicophosphate scaffold induced bone formation. *Materials* **2016**, *9*, 785. [CrossRef]

19.   Marsell, R.; Einhorn, T.A. The biology of fracture healing. *Injury* **2011**, *42*, 551–555. [CrossRef]

20.   Ramirez-Fernandez, M.P.; Mazon, P.; Gehrke, S.A.; Calvo-Guirado, J.L.; de Aza, P.N. Comparison of two xenograft materials used in sinus lift procedures: Material characterization and in vivo behavior. *Materials* **2017**, *10*, 623. [CrossRef]

21.   Bohner, M.; Baroud, G.; Bernstein, A.; Dobelin, N.; Galea, L.; Hesse, B.; Heuberger, R.; Meille, S.; Miche, P.; von Rechenberg, B.; et al. Characterization and distribution of mechanically competent mineralized tissue in micropores of β-tricalcium phosphate bone substitutes. *Mater. Today* **2017**, *20*, 106–115. [CrossRef]

22.   Sweedy, A.; Bohner, M.; Baroud, G. Multimodal analysis of in vivo resorbable CaP bone substitutes by combining histology, SEM, and microcomputed tomography data. *J. Biomed. Mater. Res. Part B Appl. Biomater.* **2017**, *106*, 1567–1577. [CrossRef]

23.   Mate-Sanchez de Val, J.E.; Mazón, P.; Piattelli, A.; Calvo-Guirado, J.L.; Bueno, J.M.; de Aza, P.N. Comparison among the physical properties of calcium phosphate-based bone substitutes of natural or synthetic origin. *Int. J. Appl. Ceram. Technol.* **2018**, *15*, 930–937. [CrossRef]

24.   Calvo-Guirado, J.L.; Ballester-Montilla, A.M.; de Aza, P.N.; Fernández-Domínguez, M.; Gehrke, S.A.; Cegarra-Del Pino, P.; Mahesh, L.; Pelegrine, A.A.; Aragoneses, J.M.; Maté-Sánchez de Val, J.E. Particulate extracted human teeth characterization by SEM-EDX evaluation as a biomaterial for socket preservatio: An in vitro study. *Materials* **2019**, *12*, 380. [CrossRef]

25.   Mate Sanchez de Val, J.E.; Calvo Guirado, J.L.; Delgado Ruiz, R.A.; Gomez Moreno, G.; Ramírez Fernández, M.P.; Romanos, G.E. Bone neo-formation and mineral degradation of 4Bone.®Part I: Material characterization and SEM study in critical size defects in rabbits. *Clin. Oral. Implants Res.* **2015**, *26*, 116–1169.

26.   Barone, A.; Toti, P.; Quaranta, A.; Alfonsi, F.; Cucchi, A.; Calvo-Guirado, J.L.; Negri, B.; Di Felice, R.; Covani, U. Volumetric analysis of remodelling pattern after ridge preservation comparing use of two types of xenografts. A multicentre randomized clinical trial. *Clin Oral Implants Res.* **2016**, *27*, e105–e115. [CrossRef]

27. Dozza, B.; Lesci, I.G.; Duchi, S.; Della Bella, E.; Martini, L.; Salamanna, F.; Falconi, M.; Cinotti, S.; Fini, M.; Lucarelli, E.; et al. When size matters: Differences in demineralized bone matrix particles affect collagen structure, mesenchymal stem cell behavior, and osteogenic potential. *J. Biomed. Mater. Res. Part A* **2017**, *105*, 1019–1033. [CrossRef]

28. de Aza, P.N.; Rodríguez, M.A.; Gehrke, S.A.; Mate-Sanchez de Val, J.E.; Calvo-Guirado, J.L. A Si-αTCP scaffold for biomedical applications: An experimental study using the rabbit tibia model. *Appl. Sci.* **2017**, *7*, 706. [CrossRef]

29. Velasquez, P.; Luklinska, Z.B.; Meseguer-Olmo, L.; Mate-Sanchez de Val, J.E.; Delgado-Ruiz, R.A.; Calvo-Guirado, J.L.; Ramirez-Fernandez, M.P.; de Aza, P.N. αTCP ceramic doped with dicalcium silicate for bone regeneration applications prepared by powder metallurgy method: In vitro and in vivo studies. *J. Biomed. Mater. Res. Part A* **2013**, *101*, 1943–1954. [CrossRef]

30. Lugo, G.J.; Mazón, P.; de Aza, P.N. Phase transitions in single phase Si-Ca-P-based ceramic under thermal treatment. *J. Eur. Ceram. Soc.* **2015**, *35*, 3693–3700. [CrossRef]

31. Lugo, G.J.; Mazón, P.; de Aza, P.N. Material processing of a new calcium silicophosphate ceramic. *Ceram. Int.* **2016**, *42*, 673–680. [CrossRef]

32. Rubio, V.; de la Casa-Lillo, M.A.; de Aza, S.; de Aza, P.N. The system $Ca_3(PO_4)_2$–Ca_2SiO_4: The sub-system Ca_2SiO_4-$7CaOP_2O_52SiO_2$. *J. Am. Ceram. Soc.* **2011**, *94*, 4459–4462. [CrossRef]

33. Shalash, M.A.; Rahman, H.A.; Azim, A.A.; Neemat, A.H.; Hawary, H.E.; Nasry, S.A. Evaluation of horizontal ridge augmentation using beta tricalcium phosphate and demineralized bone matrix: A comparative study. *J. Clin. Exp. Dent.* **2013**, *5*, e253–e259. [CrossRef]

34. Andersen, T.L.; Del Carmen Ovejero, M.; Kirkegaard, T.; Lenhard, T.; Foged, N.T.; Delaissé, J.M. A scrutiny of matrix metalloproteinases in osteoclasts: Evidence for heterogeneity and for the presence of MMPs synthesized by other cells. *Bone* **2004**, *35*, 1107–1119. [CrossRef]

35. Benedek, I.; Chitu, M.; Kovacs, I.; Balazs, B.; Benedek, T. Incremental value of preprocedural coronary computed tomographic angiography to classical coronary angiography for prediction of PCI complexity in left main stenosis. *World J. Cardiovasc. Dis.* **2013**, *3*, 573–580. [CrossRef]

36. Chow, B.J.; Hoffmann, U.; Nieman, K. Computed tomographic coronary angiography: An alternative to invasive coronary angiography. *Can. J. Cardiol.* **2005**, *21*, 933–940.

37. Beckmann, N.; Ledermann, B. Noninvasive small rodent imaging: Significance for the 3R principles. In *Small Animal Imaging*; Kiessling, F., Pichler, B., Hauff, P., Eds.; Springer: Berlin, Germany, 2017.

38. Oryan, A.; Eslaminejad, M.B.; Kamali, A.; Hosseini, S.; Moshiri, A.; Baharvand, H. Mesenchymal stem cells seeded onto tissue-engineered osteoinductive scaffolds enhance the healing process of critical-sized radial bone defects in rat. *Cell Tissue Res.* **2018**, *374*, 63–81. [CrossRef]

39. González-Gil, A.B.; Lamo-Espinosa, J.M.; Muiños-López, E.; Ripalda-Cemboráin, P.; Abizanda, G.; Valdés-Fernández, J.; López-Martínez, T.; Flandes-Iparraguirre, M.; Andreu, I.; Elizalde, M.R.; et al. Periosteum-derived mesenchymal progenitor cells in engineered implants promote fracture healing in a critical-size defect rat model. *J. Tissue Eng. Regen. Med.* **2019**. [CrossRef]

40. Develos Godoy, D.J.; Banlunara, W.; Jaroenporn, S.; Sangvanich, P.; Thunyakitpisal, P. Collagen and mPCL-TCP scaffolds induced differential bone regeneration in ovary-intact and ovariectomized rats. *Bio-Med. Mater. Eng.* **2018**, *29*, 389–399. [CrossRef]

41. Francois, E.L.; Yaszemski, M.J. Preclinical bone repair models in regenerative medicine. *Princ. Regen. Med.* **2019**, *43*, 761–767.

42. Ruehe, B.; Niehues, S.; Heberer, S.; Nelson, K. Miniature pigs as an animal model for implant research: Bone regeneration in critical-size defects. *Oral Surg. Oral Med. Oral Pathol. Oral Radiol. Endod.* **2009**, *108*, 699–706. [CrossRef]

43. Budán, F.; Szigeti, K.; Weszl, M.; Horváth, I.; Balogh, E.; Kanaan, R.; Berényi, K.; Lacza, Z.; Máthé, D.; Gyöngyi, Z. Novel radiomics evaluation of bone formation utilizing multimodal (SPECT/X-ray CT) in vivo imaging. *PLoS ONE* **2018**, *13*, e0204423. [CrossRef]

6

A Clue to the Existence of Bonding between Bone and Implant Surface: An In Vivo Study

Taek-Ka Kwon [1,†], Jung-Yoo Choi [2,†], Jae-Il Park [3] and In-Sung Luke Yeo [4,*]

[1] Division of Prosthodontics, Department of Dentistry, St. Catholic Hospital, Catholic University of Korea, Suwon 16247, Korea; tega95@naver.com
[2] Dental Research Institute, Seoul National University, Seoul 03080, Korea; jychoi55@snu.ac.kr
[3] Animal Facility of Aging Science, Korea Basic Science Institute, Gwangju 61186, Korea; jaeil74@kbsi.re.kr
[4] Department of Prosthodontics, School of Dentistry and Dental Research Institute, Seoul National University, 101 Daehak-ro, Jongro-gu, Seoul 03080, Korea
* Correspondence: pros53@snu.ac.kr
† These authors contributed equally to this work.

Abstract: We evaluated the shear bond strength of bone–implant contact, or osseointegration, in the rabbit tibia model, and compared the strength between grades 2 and 4 of commercially pure titanium (cp-Ti). A total of 13 grades 2 and 4 cp-Ti implants were used, which had an identical cylinder shape and surface topography. Field emission scanning electron microscopy, X-ray photoelectron spectroscopy, and confocal laser microscopy were used for surface analysis. Four grades 2 and 4 cp-Ti implants were inserted into the rabbit tibiae with complete randomization. After six weeks of healing, the experimental animals were sacrificed and the implants were removed en bloc with the surrounding bone. The bone–implant interfaces were three-dimensionally imaged with micro-computed tomography. Using these images, the bone–implant contact area was measured. Counterclockwise rotation force was applied to the implants for the measurement of removal torque values. Shear bond strength was calculated from the measured bone–implant contact and removal torque data. The t-tests were used to compare the outcome measures between the groups, and statistical significance was evaluated at the 0.05 level. Surface analysis showed that grades 2 and 4 cp-Ti implants have similar topographic features. We found no significant difference in the three-dimensional bone–implant contact area between these two implants. However, grade 2 cp-Ti implants had a higher shear bond strength than grade 4 cp-Ti implants ($p = 0.032$). The surfaces of the grade 2 cp-Ti implants were similar to those of the grade 4 implants in terms of physical characteristics and the quantitative amount of attachment to the bone, whereas the grade 2 surfaces were stronger than the grade 4 surfaces in the bone–surface interaction, indicating osseointegration quality.

Keywords: osseointegration; titanium; bone–implant interface; shear strength; torque

1. Introduction

Modern endosseous dental implants have been used widely in dental practice since the Toronto conference in 1982 [1,2]. Modern implants have demonstrated reliable longevity and success, and have become a routine dental therapeutic protocol in edentulous patients. However, the bonding mechanism between the bone and the dental implant is still unclear.

Bone-to-implant contact (BIC) in dental implantology is defined as the direct attachment of bone to an implant observed on an undecalcified histologic slide under a light microscopic view without intervening soft tissue. The nature of BIC, whether a real bond exists between the bone and implant or only simple contact, remains unknown [3]. BIC has been suggested to be hard tissue encapsulation, or the bony isolation of the osseointegrated dental implant [4–6]. If such a foreign body reaction is the case, it is highly possible that BIC should be a simple physical attachment between the bone and implant. Therefore, if the implants have identical physical features, such as surface topography and implant design, the shear bond strength or removal torque per unit area of implant would be similar, regardless of the material compositions on implant surfaces. Conversely, different bond strengths imply osseointegration quality at the interface, which suggests the bone has biologic affinity depending on materials, rather than the bony isolation. To the best of our knowledge, no calculation of the interfacial binding per unit area has been published to test whether BIC is only frictional or has its own quality.

This study was designed to test the hypothesis that no significant difference would be found in the removal torque per unit of bone contact area, calculated by micro computed tomography (CT), in a comparison of interfacial bindings composed of grades 2 and 4 commercially pure titanium (cp-Ti), if BIC is a simple contact between the bone and implant. The grades 2 and 4 cp-Ti implants used had an identical geometry and microstructure.

2. Materials and Methods

2.1. Implant Preparation

Twenty-six experimental implants (Deep Implant System, Seongnam, Korea) were prepared, composed of a different grade of cp-Ti: Grade 2 and 4 ($n = 13$ for each grade). All the implants were conventional external hex designed, 3.0 mm in diameter, and 4.0 mm in length. The implants were formed without thread and surface modification: Solid rod or cylindrical design and turned surface (Figure 1A).

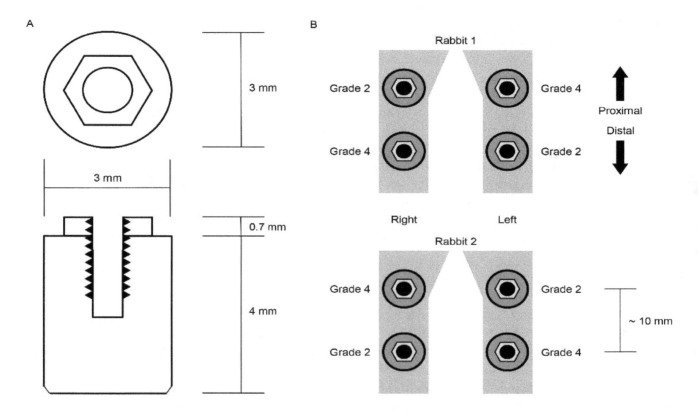

Figure 1. *Cont.*

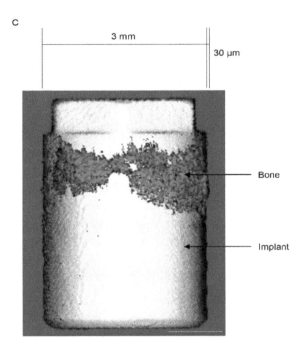

Figure 1. Schematic diagram of the specimens used in this study and the arrangement of the specimens. (**A**) The implant specimens had a simple geometric form: a cylinder that facilitates biomechanical calculations. (**B**) The grades 2 and 4 commercially pure titanium implants were installed into rabbit tibiae according to the Latin Square randomization technique. The distance between the centers of the proximal and distal implants was approximately 10 mm. (**C**) The three-dimensional (3D) bone–implant interfaces were reconstructed via digital image processing. A bone–implant contact surface is shown here. Note that the image of the bone is cut and processed in 30-μm thicknesses.

2.2. Surface Characteristics Analysis

Nine cp-Ti grades 2 and 4 implants were used in the surface character analysis test. Three surface analysis tests were performed for implants of each cp-Ti grade: Field emission scanning electron microscopy (FE-SEM), X-ray photoelectron spectroscopy (XPS), and confocal laser microscopy (CLSM). The FE-SEM (model S-4700, Hitachi, Tokyo, Japan) was used to capture several scaled images of each implant surface ($n = 3$). XPS (Sigma Probe, Thermo Fisher Scientific, Waltham, MA, USA) was used to identify the elemental content and quantify the atomic concentration of the tested surfaces; measurements were repeated three times for each specimen ($n = 3$). CLSM (LSM 800, Carl Zeiss AG, Oberkochen, Germany) was used to measure the surface topographical features of implant sides on three different areas (measurement area: 150 μm × 150 μm on a 200 × optically- and 3 × digitally-magnified image) for each specimen ($n = 3$). The images were filtered using a Gaussian low-pass filter with a cut-off wavelength of 80 μm. The average surface deviation (Sa) and developed surface area ratio (Sdr) were measured.

2.3. In Vivo Implant Surgery and Euthanasia

The animal study was approved by the Ethics Committee of the Animal Experimentation of the Institutional Animal Care and Use Committee (CRONEX-IACUC 201702001; Cronex, Hwasung, Korea). All the animal study procedures, including animal selection, management, preparation, and surgical protocols, were performed according to the guidelines of Animal Research: Reporting In Vivo Experiments (ARRIVE) [7]. We installed grades 2 and 4 cp-Ti implants in two male New Zealand white rabbits, each weighing 2.5 to 3.0 kg and aged about six months. They showed no sign of disease or illness before the experiment. Two implants were installed in each rabbit tibia using a standard Latin Square design (Figure 1B). Prior to surgery, the rabbits were anesthetized with an intramuscular injection of tiletamine/zolazepam (15 mg/kg; Zoletil 50, Virbac Korea, Seoul, Korea) and xylazine

(33 mg/kg; Rompun, Bayer Korea Ltd., Seoul, Korea). The animals received an intramuscular injection of 33 mg/kg Cefazolin (Yuhan, Seoul, Korea), a preoperative prophylactic antibiotic. The skin of each rabbit's proximal tibia area was shaved with an electric shaving machine and sterilized with povidone iodine solution, and local anesthetic, lidocaine (1:100,000 epinephrine; Yuhan, Seoul, Korea), was injected into each surgical site. The skin was incised with a surgical blade, and full-thickness periosteal flap reflection was performed to expose each tibia. The implant preparation drilling was conducted on the flat surface of the tibia using a 3-mm-diameter final dental implant drill under simultaneous sterile saline irrigation. The implant was inserted into the drill hole so that the top of the implant was 0.5 mm above the upper cortex of the rabbit tibia without contacting the lower cortex using a silicone ring. Four implants were installed into each rabbit—two grade 2 cp-Ti implants and two grade 4 cp-Ti implants—in a Latin Square design (2 × 2 Latin Square, $n = 4$). After the insertion of the implants, the surgical sites were sutured layer by layer. We allowed a relatively long healing period to present similar bone–implant contacts for the two different types of implants. Rabbits were sacrificed after six weeks of bone healing by intravenous administration of potassium chloride following anesthetization. The implants were exposed by full thickness periosteal elevation and retrieved en bloc with the adjacent bone collar.

2.4. Measurement of Three-Dimensional Bone–Implant Contact Area

CT imaging of the harvested implants and bone was performed using a Quantum GX μCT imaging system (PerkinElmer, Hopkinton, MA, USA), located at the Korea Basic Science Institute (Gwangju, Korea). The X-ray source was set to 90 kV and 88 μA with a 10 mm field of view (voxel size = 20 μm; scanning time = 57 min). The CT data were visualized using the Quantum GX's three-dimensional (3D) viewing software. 3D images of the implant specimens and bone growth were constructed. Image processing for the calculation of the bone–implant contact area was described in a previous study [8]. Briefly, following scanning, the images were segmented using Analyze software version 12.0 (AnalyzeDirect, Overland Park, KS, USA) and filtered to reduce imaging noise. Then, the dataset was manually reoriented using Analyze software to visualize standard coronal, sagittal, and horizontal planes through the implants. The images were reformatted to cubic volume (3D) with a resliced 30-μm image thickness of the surface area on the implant outer surface for the cross-sectional and longitudinal axes. The segmentations of implant and bone-growth images were also performed on Analyze software. As such, 3D rendering of the implants and bone growth was completed. To determine the bone volume on the implant surface in 30-μm thicknesses, the original scanned images were rotated by 10 degrees and the segmentations and 3D rendering were repeated. These 18 repetitions produced the overall 3D bone growth image on the implant surface in 30-μm thicknesses (Figure 1C). The 3D BIC area was the bone formation area on the cylindrical surface of the implant. Assuming that the volume in 30-μm thicknesses was homogeneously filled with bone, the 3D BIC area was determined by dividing the bone volume by the thickness (30 μm).

2.5. Measurement of Shear Bond Strength of Bone and Implant

After CT scanning, implant removal torque values were measured within 24 h. The experimental implants had no thread and no fixation via screw action. The constant-speed counter-clockwise rotation of the implant or collar bone results in the disintegration of the BIC or shear bond failure. This continuous removal torque test produces accurate and uniform results [9,10]. Implant removal torque was measured with a motorized torque test stand (TSTM, Mark-10 Co., Long Island, NY, USA). The rotation speed was 0.3 rpm for the lowest angular speed to ensure peak implant removal torque was not skipped between sampling intervals (65 samples/s). The peak implant removal torque was selected from the time–torque curve data. The shear bond strength (MPa) between the bone and osseointegrated dental implant, or binding force per unit area in this study, was calculated by dividing the peak implant removal torque (Ncm) by the determined 3D BIC area (mm^2) and the implant radius (1.5 mm). The units were adjusted before calculation.

2.6. Statistics

The independent t-test was used to determine the statistical significance of the surface roughness parameters, Sa and Sdr, between the grade 2 and 4 cp-Ti implants. The paired t-test was used to compare the 3D BIC area and the shear bond strength between the groups. All data were evaluated at the significance level of 0.05.

3. Results

3.1. Surface Characteristics Analysis

The FE-SEM image of each surface area is shown in Figure 2. The grades 2 and 4 cp-Ti surfaces show similar surface characteristics, which resulted from the computer numerical control machining manufacturing process. The results of the CLSM analysis showed that the means of Sa were 0.49 ± 0.082 µm for grade 2 cp-Ti implants and 0.45 ± 0.088 µm for grade 4 cp-Ti implants. No significant difference was found for Sa between the Ti grades ($p = 0.63$). The means of Sdr were $16.9\% \pm 1.5\%$ for the grade 2 implant group and $14.4\% \pm 2.1\%$ for the grade 4 implant group, and no significant difference was found between the groups ($p = 0.18$). These results indicate that the grades 2 and 4 cp-Ti implants used in this study had similar surface topographical features. However, surface chemistry depended on the Ti grades. The XPS showed that the atomic composition of the grade 2 cp-Ti surface was significantly different from that of the grade 4 surface (Table 1).

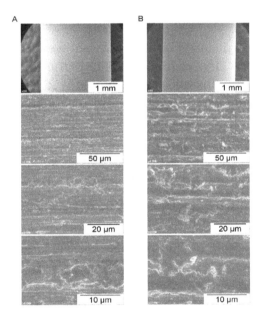

Figure 2. Field emission scanning electron microscopy (FE-SEM) images of commercially pure titanium of (**A**) grade 2 and (**B**) grade 4. Many machining grooves were observed. Similar surface characteristics were found for both grades, which implies that the influence of topographical features on the biological response should not be different between the commercially pure titanium grades used in this study.

Table 1. The atomic composition of surfaces of grades 2 and 4 commercially pure titanium (cp-Ti) obtained by X-ray photoelectron spectroscopy (XPS).

Element	Cp-Ti Grade 2	Cp-Ti Grade 4	p-Value
Carbon (C)	$3.66\% \pm 0.21\%$	$4.03\% \pm 0.39\%$	2.3×10^{-1}
Oxygen (O)	$1.15\% \pm 0.10\%$	$3.21\% \pm 0.29\%$	3.0×10^{-4} *
Iron (Fe)	$0.26\% \pm 0.02\%$	$0.39\% \pm 0.05\%$	2.0×10^{-2} *
Titanium (Ti)	$94.93\% \pm 0.32\%$	$92.38\% \pm 0.13\%$	2.1×10^{-4} *

* Statistically significant.

3.2. Three-Dimensional Bone–Implant Contact Area and Shear Bond Strength

The bone–implant contact surface area and three-dimensional bone–implant contact ratio are summarized in Table 2. The means and standard deviations of the contacted surface area for grades 2 and 4 cp-Ti implants were 12.7 ± 1.2 mm^2 and 11.5 ± 1.6 mm^2, respectively. The 3D bone–implant contact percentages of grades 2 and 4 cp-Ti implants were $33.6\% \pm 3.2\%$ and $30.5\% \pm 4.3\%$, respectively. Neither the contacted surface area nor the 3D bone–implant contact showed any statistical difference between the two grades. The peak implant removal torques of grades 2 and 4 cp-Ti implants were 2.9 ± 0.4 Ncm and 1.9 ± 0.3 Ncm, respectively. The shear bond strength of grade 2 cp-Ti implants was 1.5 ± 0.2 MPa, which was statistically significantly higher than that of the grade 4 cp-Ti implants, which was 1.1 ± 0.1 MPa ($p = 0.032$) (Table 2).

Table 2. Three-dimensional bone-to-implant contact (BIC) area and shear bond strength.

	Grade 2 cp-Ti	Grade 4 cp-Ti	p-Value
3D BIC area (mm^2)	12.7 ± 1.2	11.5 ± 1.6	0.35
3D BIC ratio (%)	33.6 ± 3.2	30.5 ± 4.3	0.35
Implant removal torque (Ncm)	2.9 ± 0.4	1.9 ± 0.3	0.052
Torque per unit (Ncm/cm^2)	23.2 ± 3.5	16.5 ± 1.0	0.032 *
Shear bond strength (MPa)	1.5 ± 0.2	1.1 ± 0.1	0.032 *

* Statistically significant.

4. Discussion

The grades 2 and 4 cp-Ti implants used in this study showed similar surface topographic features in SEM images and CLSM analysis. The grade 2 cp-Ti implants showed higher shear bond strength than the grade 4 implants despite the similar 3D bone–implant contact ratios between these two grades. Considering the significant differences in the compositions between the grades 2 and 4 cp-Ti surfaces, the bone response was evaluated to be stronger to grade 2 than to grade 4. The results of this study suggest that the bone would have its own affinity, depending on the materials, and that an actual bond would exist in addition to the physical contact and friction between bone and an implant surface [3]. Although further verification studies are required, the osseointegration phenomenon of a Ti dental implant appears to be a bioaffinitive response to the Ti surface beyond the bony isolation.

The pull-out test of integrated implants has been widely adopted to test osseointegration strength [11–15]. However, we used rotating force instead of pull-out force because the removal direction for the pull-out test could be nonparallel to the long axis of the implant, imposing unintentional lateral force on the implant, which can introduce measurement error. This adverse effect was minimized in this study by using rotational force for implant removal and a motorized torque test stand to simplify adjustment to the long axis [10].

This study compared the grades 2 and 4 implants using the rabbit tibia model. Sample size determination and randomization are important to reduce the number of sacrificed animals [7]. Following the guidelines of the 3Rs (replacement, reduction, and refinement) of ARRIVE, this study used the 2×2 Latin Square design, which minimized the sample size and accomplished complete randomization in the arrangement of the implant groups [7]. Considering the standard deviation of the 3D BIC area and ratio measures, the number of sacrificed animals (two) was estimated to be adequate although sample size calculation was not performed in this study, which would require more animals than two.

Many studies reported significant differences in the amount of bone–implant contact when implant surfaces were topographically changed [16]. Further studies are needed to evaluate the effects of surface topography on the quality of osseointegration. A roughened surface increases the bone–implant area, increasing the physical interlocking between bone and the surface, which would result in the same shear bond strength or removal torque per unit area when the implant surfaces, topographically changed or not, have the same chemical composition. Conversely, the topographical change could have a qualitative influence on the bone–implant contact, which remains to be verified. In addition, further studies are required to evaluate osseointegration qualities by comparing the bone–implant contact and shear bond strength at the different phases of bone healing after implant placement.

5. Conclusions

Grades 2 and 4 cp-Ti surfaces with similar topographical features showed different bond strengths in the bone–implant contact. Considering the results of this study, an actual bond may occur between bone and a Ti dental implant surface beyond the physical attachment of bone to the surface.

Author Contributions: T.-K.K. and I.-S.L.Y. designed the experiments; T.-K.K., J.-Y.C., and I.-S.L.Y. performed the experiments; T.-K.K. and J.-I.P. obtained the data; J.-Y.C. and I.-S.L.Y. analyzed the data; T.-K.K., J.-Y.C., J.-I.P., and I.-S.L.Y. wrote the manuscript. T.-K.K. and J.-Y.C. equally contributed to this study and I.-S.L.Y. had correspondence.

References

1. Block, M.S. Dental Implants: The Last 100 Years. *J. Oral Maxillofac. Surg.* **2018**, *76*, 11–26. [CrossRef] [PubMed]

2. Brånemark, P.I.; Zarb, G.A.; Albrektsson, T. *Tissue-Integrated Prostheses: Osseointegration in Clinical Dentistry*; Quintessence Publishing: Chicago, IL, USA, 1985.

3. Brunski, J. On Implant Prosthodontics: One Narrative, Twelve Voices-2. *Int. J. Prosthodont.* **2018**, *31*, s15–s22. [PubMed]

4. Albrektsson, T. On Implant Prosthodontics: One Narrative, Twelve Voices-1. *Int. J. Prosthodont.* **2018**, *31*, s11–s14. [PubMed]

5. Jemt, T. On Implant Prosthodontics: One Narrative, Twelve Voices-4. *Int. J. Prosthodont.* **2018**, *31*, s31–s34. [PubMed]

6. Trindade, R.; Albrektsson, T.; Galli, S.; Prgomet, Z.; Tengvall, P.; Wennerberg, A. Osseointegration and foreign body reaction: Titanium implants activate the immune system and suppress bone resorption during the first 4 weeks after implantation. *Clin. Implant. Dent. Relat. Res.* **2018**, *20*, 82–91. [CrossRef] [PubMed]

7. Kilkenny, C.; Browne, W.J.; Cuthill, I.C.; Emerson, M.; Altman, D.G. Improving bioscience research reporting: The ARRIVE guidelines for reporting animal research. *Osteoarthr. Cartil.* **2012**, *20*, 256–260. [CrossRef] [PubMed]

8. Choi, J.Y.; Park, J.I.; Chae, J.S.; Yeo, I.L. Comparison of micro-computed tomography and histomorphometry in the measurement of bone–implant contact ratios. *Oral Surg. Oral Med. Oral Pathol. Oral Radiol.* **2019**, in press. [CrossRef] [PubMed]

9. Kwon, T.K.; Lee, H.J.; Min, S.K.; Yeo, I.S. Evaluation of early bone response to fluoride-modified and anodically oxidized titanium implants through continuous removal torque analysis. *Implant. Dent.* **2012**, *21*, 427–432. [CrossRef] [PubMed]

10. Lee, H.J.; Yeo, I.S.; Kwon, T.K. Removal Torque Analysis of Chemically Modified Hydrophilic and Anodically Oxidized Titanium Implants with Constant Angular Velocity for Early Bone Response in Rabbit Tibia. *Tissue Eng. Regen. Med.* **2013**, *10*, 252–259. [CrossRef]

11. Gracco, A.; Giagnorio, C.; Incerti Parenti, S.; Alessandri Bonetti, G.; Siciliani, G. Effects of thread shape on the pullout strength of miniscrews. *Am. J. Orthod. Dentofac. Orthop.* **2012**, *142*, 186–190. [CrossRef] [PubMed]

12. Nonhoff, J.; Moest, T.; Schmitt, C.M.; Weisel, T.; Bauer, S.; Schlegel, K.A. Establishment of a new pull-out strength testing method to quantify early osseointegration-An experimental pilot study. *J. Cranio-Maxillofac. Surg.* **2015**, *43*, 1966–1973. [CrossRef] [PubMed]

13. Velasco, E.; Monsalve-Guil, L.; Jimenez, A.; Ortiz, I.; Moreno-Munoz, J.; Nunez-Marquez, E.; Pegueroles, M.; Perez, R.A.; Gil, F.J. Importance of the Roughness and Residual Stresses of Dental Implants on Fatigue and Osseointegration Behavior. In Vivo Study in Rabbits. *J. Oral Implantol.* **2016**, *42*, 469–476. [CrossRef] [PubMed]

14. Watanabe, T.; Nakada, H.; Takahashi, T.; Fujita, K.; Tanimoto, Y.; Sakae, T.; Kimoto, S.; Kawai, Y. Potential for acceleration of bone formation after implant surgery by using a dietary supplement: An animal study. *J. Oral Rehabil.* **2015**, *42*, 447–453. [CrossRef] [PubMed]

15. Yashwant, A.V.; Dilip, S.; Krishnaraj, R.; Ravi, K. Does Change in Thread Shape Influence the Pull Out Strength of Mini Implants? An In vitro Study. *J. Clin. Diagn. Res.* **2017**, *11*, ZC17–ZC20. [CrossRef] [PubMed]

16. Yeo, I.S. Reality of dental implant surface modification: A short literature review. *Open Biomed. Eng. J.* **2014**, *8*, 114–119. [CrossRef] [PubMed]

7

Effects of Liner-Bonding of Implant-Supported Glass–Ceramic Crown to Zirconia Abutment on Bond Strength and Fracture Resistance

Yong-Seok Jang [1], Sang-Hoon Oh [2], Won-Suck Oh [3], Min-Ho Lee [1], Jung-Jin Lee [4] and Tae-Sung Bae [1,*]

[1] Department of Dental Biomaterials, Institute of Biodegradable Materials, BK21 plus Program, School of Dentistry, Chonbuk National University, Jeonju 54896, Korea

[2] Haruan Dental Clinic, Department of Dental Biomaterials, Institute of Biodegradable Materials, BK21 plus Program, School of Dentistry, Chonbuk National University, Jeonju 54896, Korea

[3] Department of Biologic and Materials Sciences Division of Prosthodontics, School of Dentistry, University of Michigan, Ann Arbor, MI 48109, USA

[4] Department of Prosthodontics, Institute of Oral Bio-Science, School of Dentistry, Chonbuk National University and Research Institute of Clinical Medicine of Chonbuk National University-Biomedical Research Institute of Chonbuk National University Hospital, Jeonju 54907, Korea

* Correspondence: bts@jbnu.ac.kr

Abstract: This study was conducted to test the hypothesis that heat-bonding with a liner positively affects the bond strength and fracture resistance of an implant-supported glass–ceramic crown bonded to a zirconia abutment produced by a computer-aided design/computer-aided milling (CAD/CAM) procedure. Lithium disilicate-reinforced Amber Mill-Q glass ceramic blocks were bonded to 3 mol% yttria stabilized tetragonal zirconia polycrystal (3Y-TZP) blocks by heat-bonding with a liner or cementation with a dual-cure self-adhesive resin cement for a microtensile bond strength test. CAD/CAM implant-supported glass ceramic crowns were produced using Amber Mill-Q blocks and bonded to a milled 3Y-TZP zirconia abutments by heat-bonding or cementation for a fracture test. A statistical analysis was conducted to investigate the significant differences between the experimental results. The mode of failure was analyzed using high-resolution field emission scanning electron microscopy. Chemical bonding was identified at the interface between the zirconia ceramic and liner. The mean tensile bond strength of the liner-bonded group was significantly higher than that of the cement-bonded group. The initial chipping strength of the liner-bonded group was significantly higher than that of the cement-bonded group, although no statistically significant difference was found for the fracture strength. The mode of failure was mixed with cohesive fracture through the liner, whereas the cement-bonded group demonstrated adhesive failure at the interface of bonding.

Keywords: CAD/CAM all-ceramic restoration; fracture strength; liner treatment; resin cement; tensile bond strength; zirconia abutment

1. Introduction

Implant-supported crowns restore oral functions and aesthetics without affecting the integrity of adjacent teeth. These crowns are usually connected to the implants by means of titanium abutments. However, the use of a metallic abutment may compromise the gingival aesthetics of implant crowns, particularly in patients presenting with a thin biotype gingival architecture. The grayish metallic color can be pronounced with a light reflected from the metallic surface of the abutment [1,2]. In addition, the submucosal placement of a crown margin can restrict the cement removal procedure and lead to develop peri-implantitis [3].

Ceramic abutments are biocompatible and aesthetic by mimicking the color of natural teeth [4,5]. In addition, the use of ceramic abutments is versatile with the development of CAD (computer-aided design)/CAM (computer-aided milling) technology, which allows for the design and milling of zirconia ceramics. Though concerns regarding the mechanical properties of zirconia abutments (i.e., brittleness, stress corrosion cracking, and low temperature degradation) have been addressed, their clinical application has been expanded for the anterior and premolar regions [6–9]. Furthermore, all abutments made of zirconia or titanium can be customized to produce a desired size, shape, angle, and location of a crown margin for better aesthetics [10–12].

Zirconia abutments are commonly designed as one-piece system to support implant crowns and establish the implant–abutment interface with a zirconia ceramic. This system eliminates the negative effects of titanium abutments related to aesthetics. However, the implant–abutment interface may experience an excessive wear under occlusal loading due to dissimilarities between the zirconia ceramic and the titanium implant [13,14]. Complications may include a discoloration of the peri-implant mucosa associated with the embedment of titanium particles dislodged from implants, abutment screw loosening, and the fracture of ceramic abutments and crowns [14,15]. This type of abutments have also shown very low fracture resistance when compared to zirconia abutments using a titanium base [16,17].

The two-piece system of zirconia abutments was designed to avoid the possible consequences related to the use of the one-piece system. This system consists of a ceramic core and a titanium link to establish the implant–abutment interface with titanium-to-titanium without compromising the aesthetics of the ceramic abutment. The ceramic core is customized using CAD/CAM technology and is bonded to the titanium base with adhesive resin cement [18]. This two-piece system was found to demonstrate a higher flexural resistance than one-piece system [1,19] without compromising the emergence profile, crown orientation, and coronal contour matching the prosthesis and anatomical shape of the mucosa [20].

However, problems may occur when bonding a final prosthesis to a zirconia ceramic abutment [18,21,22]. The resin cement may not adhere to the zirconia ceramic abutment because of the lack of undercut features commonly created by blasting with air-borne particle abrasion technology and/or etching with hydrofluoric acid. The final prosthesis can be at a risk of chipping or cracking due to the relatively weak bond strength of the resin cementing the abutment. In addition, the luting procedure of the final prosthesis to the abutment is inconvenient and can be problematic when combined with the submucosal margin.

A lithium disilicate-reinforced liner has recently been developed to overcome the weak linkage of the final prosthesis of a glass–ceramic to a zirconia abutment designed to replace single anterior and posterior teeth. However, no scientific research has been conducted to elucidate the bond characteristics of the liner. The objective of this in vitro study was to investigate the effect of heat-bonding with the liner on the bond strength and fracture resistance of an implant-supported glass–ceramic crown bonded to a two-piece system zirconia abutment produced by a CAD/CAM procedure. The null hypothesis was set to test no significant difference between the liner-bonding and the cement-bonding of the implant-supported ceramic crown to the zirconia abutment on the initial chipping and fracture strengths of crowns, as well as the microtensile bond strength.

2. Materials and Methods

2.1. Bond Strength Test

2.1.1. Preparation of Specimen

Three CAD/CAM 3Y-TZP zirconia ceramic blocks (Zirtooth, O98FGJ1701, Hass, Gangneung, Korea) were machined to fabricate 6 zirconia ceramic specimens with dimensions of 10 × 10 × 5 mm, and they were sintered in an electric furnace (Programat EP3000/G2, Ivoclar Vivadent, Schaan, Liechtenstein) at 1450 °C. In addition, lithium disilicate-reinforced Amber Mill-Q glass ceramic blocks (Hass, Gangneung, Korea) were machined to fabricate 6 glass ceramic specimens matching the zirconia ceramic specimens (10 mm × 10 mm × 5 mm).

For bonding with the liner, the liner (Hass, Gangneung, Korea), consisting of 5–15 wt.% Li_2O, 55–65 wt.% SiO_2, and 5–25 wt.% other trace elements of oxides and colorants was applied on the surfaces of 3 zirconia ceramic specimens. Then, heat-bonding with 3 lithium disilicate-reinforced glass ceramic specimens was conducted at 800 °C.

For bonding with a resin cement, 3 lithium disilicate-reinforced glass ceramic specimens were acid-etched with 9.5% hydrofluoric acid gel (Bisco, IL, USA) for 30 s, washed with distilled water, dried, and silane primer (Espe[TM] Sil, 3M/ESPE, Seefeld, Germany) coated. The surfaces of 3 zirconia ceramic specimens were roughened using an air-borne particle abrasion technology with 50 μm alumina particles (Hi-aluminas, Shofu, Japan) under the pressure of 3 atm at a distance of 10 mm [23]. After placing the specimens in an electric furnace (Programat EP3000/G2), the temperature was raised to 1000 °C at a rate of 50 °C/min, held for 10 min, and then cooled to 25 °C in the furnace to restore the phase transformations occurred during the blasting procedure. Then, a 10-methacryloyloxydecyl dihydrogen phosphate (MDP)-containing primer (Z-PRIME[TM] plus, BISCO, Schaumburg, IL, USA) was coated on the surface of zirconia ceramic specimens [24]. The cement bonding between the lithium disilicate-reinforced glass and zirconia ceramics was performed using a self-adhesive dual-cure resin cement (Rely-X[TM] U200, 3M/ESPE, Neuss, Germany) with an equal amount of base and catalyst pastes mixed for 20 s. The cement was applied to the prepared ceramic surface and a pressure of 49 N was applied to the ceramic specimens under a constant-load device. After the removal of excess cement, the resin cement was photopolymerized using an light emitting diode (LED) curing unit (G-Light, GC Corporation, Tokyo, Japan) for 20 s from each of the four directions for a total of 80 sec under a light intensity of 550 mW/cm^2 at a distance of 2 mm. The specimens were kept under pressure for additional 10 min, relieved from the constant-load device and immersed in distilled water for 24 h.

The bonded ceramic blocks were serially sectioned perpendicular to the bonded surface. The first cut was made through each specimen using a high-speed diamond cutting machine (Accutom-50, Struers Inc, Cleveland, OH, USA) to produce a 1 mm thick plate, and the sliced plate was cut using a low-speed diamond cutting machine (Metsaw-LS, Topmet, Daejeon, Korea) after rotating 90° for second set of cuts. Twelve specimens (1.0 mm × 1.0 mm × 10 mm) were prepared with 3 ceramic blocks per each group by selecting 4 specimens from the middle of a bonded ceramic block (10 mm × 10 mm × 10 mm). Thus, a total of 24 specimens (12 × 2 groups) were used for the bond strength test. Figure 1 schematically shows the preparation process of specimens for the microtensile bond test.

2.1.2. Microtensile Bond Strength Test

The prepared ceramic specimens were attached to the grip of metal holders, mounted, and subjected to tensile force in a universal testing machine (Instron, Model 5569, Instron Co., Norwood, MA, USA) at a crosshead speed of 0.5 mm/min [25,26]. The microtensile bond strength was calculated in MPa with the failure load (N) divided by the cross-sectional area (mm^2) of each test specimen.

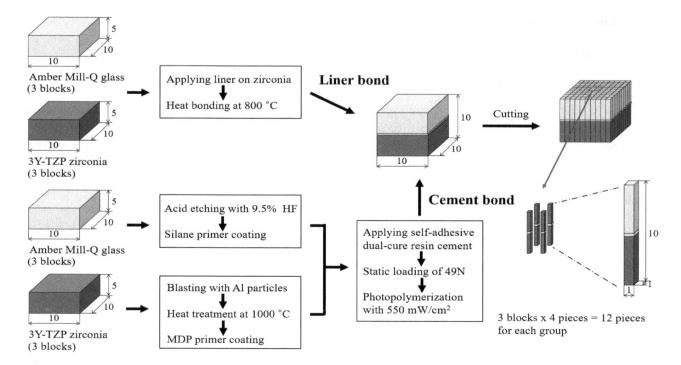

Figure 1. Schematic summary for the preparation process of specimens for the microtensile bond test.

2.2. Fracture Test for Implant-Supported Crowns

2.2.1. Preparation of Implant-Supported Crowns

The mandibular right first molar was scanned using a D900L scanner (3Shape, Copenhagen, Denmark) to create an implant-supported crown. Twenty ceramic crowns were produced by milling a lithium disilicate-reinforced glass ceramic block using CAD/CAM milling machine (CEREC MC, Sirona, Salzburg, Austria) to make 10 samples per group for the liner-bonded and cement-bonded groups. The internal aspect of each crown was acid-etched for bonding to a zirconia abutment presenting with a diameter of 4 mm and length of 8 mm. The bonding was performed using the same method as described in the section of the bond strength test for each liner-bonded and cement-bonded group. The zirconia abutments were connected to the titanium link abutments (SRN-SURO-H, GeoMedi Co, Ltd., Uiwang, Gyeonggi, Korea) with a dual-cure resin cement after applying an MDP containing primer.

The prepared crowns were coated with a thin layer of e.max Ceram glaze paste (Ivoclar/Vivadent, Schaan, Liechtenstein) and glazed in an electric furnace (Programat EP3000/G2). The temperature was raised to 730 °C at a rate of 35 °C/min and held for 1 min. For the liner-bonded group (MLG: Milled, liner-bonded and glazed), the ceramic crowns were glazed following the bonding with the zirconia abutments. However, for the cement-bonded group (MGC: Milled, glazed, and cement-bonded), the ceramic crowns were glazed prior to bonding to the abutments.

2.2.2. Fracture Test of Implant-Supported Crown

The prepared ceramic crown/abutment specimens were connected to titanium implant analogs (Geo 3D Analog, GeoMedi Co, Ltd., Uiwang, Gyeonggi, Korea) with titanium abutment screws and tightened to 30 N·cm twice at 30 seconds interval using a torque gauge (9810P, Aikoh Engineering Co, Higashiosaka, Osaka, Japan) [27]. The screw access holes were filled with a light-activated composite resin (Filteck[TM] Z350 XT, 3M ESPE, MN, USA), and the prepared specimens were immersed in distilled water at 37 °C for 24 h.

The crowns were supported and secured to a base retainer and loaded axially to fracture in a universal testing machine (Universal testing machine 4201, Instron, Canton, MA, USA). The compression load was transferred through a 5 mm diameter steel ball positioned in the central fossa of the crown.

The load was applied at a crosshead speed of 0.5 mm/min and continued to the point of fracture, and the fracture load of each ceramic crown was recorded [28,29]. The initial chipping strength was determined at the point when the load value showed slightly transient drop.

2.3. Surface Analysis

High-resolution field emission scanning electron microscopy (HR FE-SEM in KBSI Jeonju, SU8230, Hitachi, Japan) was used to investigate the topography of the liner-bonded surface, cross-sectional bonded interfaces, and fractured surfaces after etching with a 9.5% hydrofluoric acid gel for 30 s. The liner layer was removed with a 5% hydrofluoric acid solution for 30 min to identify the effects of liner treatment on zirconia ceramic. The distribution of the chemical elements at the bonded interface was analyzed using an energy dispersive X-ray spectrometer (EDS, Bruker, Germany), and the crystal structure on the liner-bonded surface was investigated by X-ray diffraction (XRD, Dmax III-A type, Rigaku, Japan).

2.4. Statistical Analysis

The statistical analysis was conducted by SPSS software (version 12.0, SPSS, Chicago, IL, USA). A Student's t-test was conducted to investigate significant differences between the experimental results for the 2 test groups ($p < 0.05$). A Weibull analysis was performed with the experimentally measured load-at-failure values for each group of bonded ceramic specimens.

3. Results

The null hypothesis on the microtensile bond strength was rejected. Table 1 summarizes the distribution characteristics of the Weibull analysis for the microtensile bond strength test. The Weibull modulus (m) was higher for the liner-bonded group (5.8) than for the cement-bonded group (4.1). The mean values of microtensile bond strength for the liner-bonded group (47.7 MPa) were significantly higher than for the cement-bonded group (19.6 MPa) ($p < 0.05$). In addition, the Weibull distribution showed a matched tendency with a single mode ($r^2 > 0.958$) (Figure 2).

Table 1. Weibull analysis data of a microtensile bond strength test for lithium disilicate-reinforced glass ceramic and zirconia of the liner-bonded group and the cement-bonded group.

Parameter \ Group	Liner-Bonded	Resin Cement-Bonded
m	5.836	4.133
σ_o	50.8	2.36
r^2	0.961	0.958
$\sigma_{f(mean)} \pm$ SD	47.7 ± 8.7	19.6 ± 4.7
$\sigma_{f(min/med/max)}$	32.8/45.5/58.7	10.9/20.6/26.0
N	12	12

where m = Weibull modulus; σ_o = characteristic strength in MPa; r^2 = Weibull distribution regression coefficient squared; $\sigma_{f(mean)}$ = mean fracture strength in MPa; $\sigma_{f(min/med/max)}$ = minimum, median and maximum fracture strength in MPa; and N=number of samples.

The heat-bonding with the liner was found to induce a chemical interaction with the milled zirconia ceramic abutment. A large number of pores was found in the reaction layer of liner bonding, altering the surface topography of the zirconia ceramic (Figure 3a,b). The zone of the chemical reaction was measured approximately 3 μm across the interface of the bonding of the zirconia ceramic (Figure 3d,e).

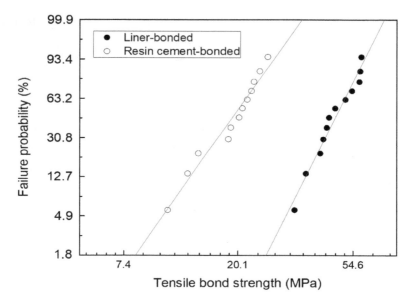

Figure 2. Weibull plots of a microtensile bond strength test for lithium disilicate-reinforced glass ceramic and zirconia of the liner-bonded group and the cement-bonded group.

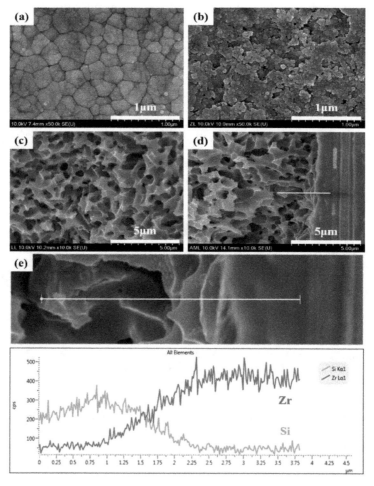

Figure 3. High-resolution field emission scanning electron microscopy (HR FE-SEM) images of the zirconia ceramic specimen demonstrating (**a**) crystal structure after sintering at 1450 °C, (**b**) its alteration of surface morphology with liner treatment (liner removed with acid etching with a 5% hydrofluoric acid solution for 30 min after a fracture test), (**c**) liner-bonded zirconia surface, and (**d**) cross-sectional view of liner-bonded interfacial interaction zone, and (**e**) energy dispersive X-ray spectrometer (EDS) line analysis data of Si and Zr after acid etching with 9.5% hydrofluoric acid gel for 30 s.

The chemical reaction of the liner against the zirconia abutment was confirmed by XRD diffraction analysis, where the peaks were noted as corresponding to lithium metasilicate (Li_2SiO_3) and zirconium silicate ($ZrSiO_4$), as well as zirconia (ZrO_2) and silica (SiO_2) (Figure 4).

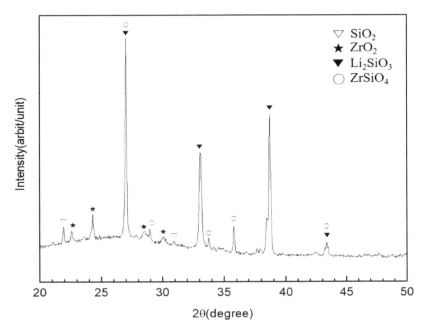

Figure 4. XRD diffraction analysis of the lithium disilicate-reinforced liner-bonded interface of the zirconia ceramic.

The interfacial layer created by the liner-bonding was found to be more consistent than that created by the cement-bonding. The liner-bonded interfacial layer was thicker with a higher mean value and standard deviation (33.6 ± 5.2 μm) than the cement-bonded interfacial layer (13.3 ± 1.6 μm) (Figure 5). Neither a pore nor a gap was noted in the liner-bonded interfacial zone, whereas numerous micro-pores and micor-gaps were found in the cement-bonded interfacial layer.

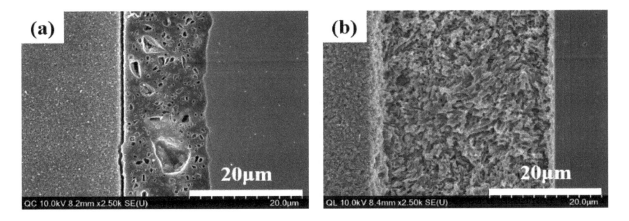

Figure 5. HR FE-SEM images of bonded interface between lithium disilicate-reinforced glass ceramic and zirconia for (**a**) the cement-bonded group and (**b**) the liner-bonded group.

When the debonded surfaces of the liner-bonded and liner-bonded groups were visually evaluated with high magnification images of HR FE-SEM, the mode of failure of the liner-bonded group was mixed with cohesive fracture propagated through the liner (Figure 6). In contrast, the mode of failure of the cement-bonded group was adhesive where the fracture occurred at the interface between the zirconia ceramic and the cement layer (Figure 7).

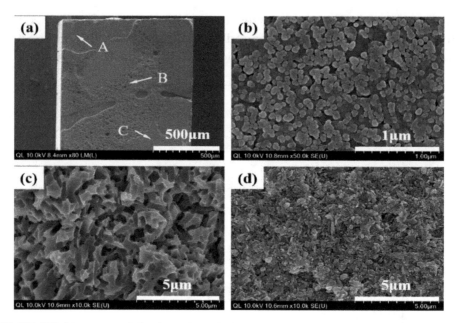

Figure 6. HR FE-SEM images of the liner-bonded group demonstrating mode of failure with the microtensile bond strength test. (**a**) Fracture surface of specimen demonstrating inhomogeneous pattern of fracture, (**b**) magnification of point A demonstrating that the zirconia surface layer reacted with the liner, (**c**) the magnification of point B demonstrating the microstructure of the liner, and (**d**) the magnification of point C demonstrating the presence of needle-shaped lithium disilicate crystals in the lithium disilicate-reinforced glass ceramic.

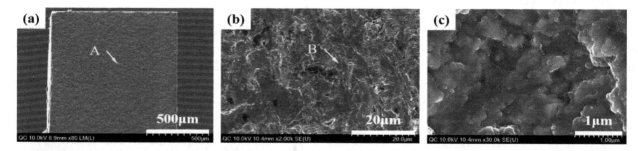

Figure 7. HR FE-SEM images of the cement-bonded group demonstrating mode of failure with the microtensile bond strength test. (**a**) Fractured surface of specimen demonstrating the homogeneous pattern of fracture, (**b**) the magnification of point A demonstrating the irregular structure of the zirconia ceramic, and (**c**) the magnification of point B demonstrating the crystal structure of zirconia.

The null hypothesis was rejected on the initial chipping and fracture strengths but accepted on the fracture strength. The mean values and standard deviations of the initial chipping strength and fracture strength of implant-supported glass ceramic crowns bonded to zirconia ceramic abutments were 843.8 ± 317.5 N and 1929.6 ± 191.1 N for the liner-bonded (MLG) groups and 341.0 ± 90.2 N and 1711.1 ± 275.4 N for the resin cement-bonded (MGC) group (Figure 8). The initial chipping strength of the MLG group was significantly higher than that of the MGC group ($p < 0.05$), although no significant difference was found in the fracture strength.

When the fractured surfaces of the lithium disilicate-reinforced glass ceramic crown and the zirconia ceramic abutment were visually evaluated with a high magnification images of HR FE-SEM, the mode of failure of the MLG group was mixed with adhesive and cohesive fractures propagated through the liner (Figures 9 and 10b–d). However, the mode of failure was adhesive in the MGC group, and the fractures consistently occurred at the interface between the cement layer and the zirconia ceramic abutment (Figures 9 and 10e,f).

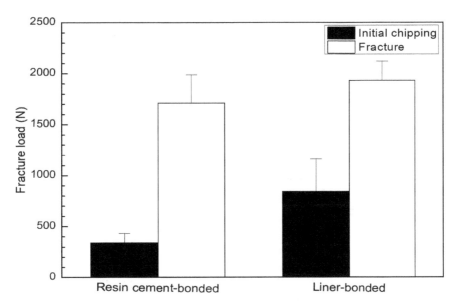

Figure 8. Graphical illustration for initial chipping and fracture strengths of crowns for the resin cement-bonded and liner-bonded groups.

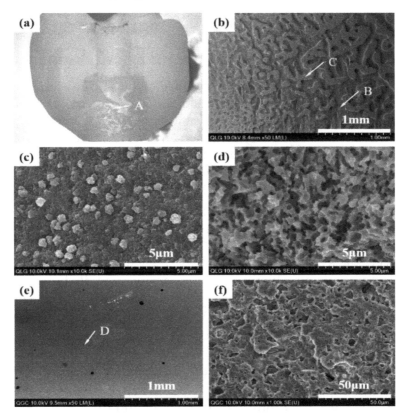

Figure 9. Photographic (**a**) and HR FE-SEM images of the lithium disilicate-reinforced glass ceramic crown that demonstrate the mode of failure; (**b**) the magnification of point A for the (milled, liner-bonded and glazed) MLG group: Inhomogeneous pattern of fracture surface; (**c**) the magnification of point B: Cohesive fracture occurred through the liner; (**d**) the magnification of point C: Adhesive fracture occurred at the interface with liner, and (**e**) magnification of point A for the milled, glazed, and cement-bonded (MGC) group: Homogeneous pattern of fracture surface; (**f**) the magnification of point D: Cement layer indicating adhesive fracture occurred at the interface with the zirconia ceramic abutment.

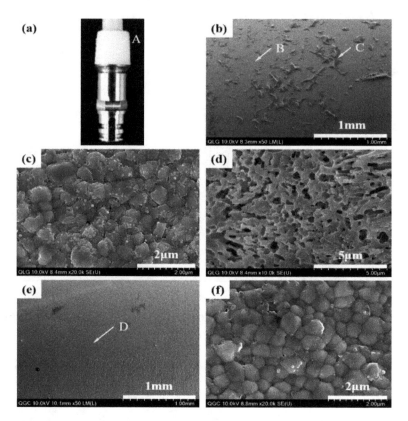

Figure 10. Photographic (**a**) and HR FE-SEM images (**b**–**d**) of the zirconia ceramic abutment; (**b**) the magnification of point A for the MLG group: Inhomogeneous pattern of fracture surface; (**c**) the magnification of point B: Adhesive fracture occurred at the interface with liner; (**d**) the magnification of point C: Cohesive fracture occurred through the liner; (**e**) the magnification of point A for the MGC group: Homogeneous pattern of fracture surface; (**f**) the magnification of point D: Zirconia crystals indicating that an adhesive fracture occurred at the interface with resin cement.

4. Discussion

The liner-bonded ceramic crowns were superior to the cement-bonded ceramic crowns in developing a higher resistance to fracture. The bond strength of the lithium disilicate-reinforced glass ceramic to the zirconia ceramic was higher when the bonding was established with the lithium-disilicate liner than with an adhesive cement. The mean values of microtensile bond strength for liner bond and cement bond were 19.6 and 47.7 MPa, respectively, in this study. As an ideal biomaterial would have bonding forces included in the interval of 5–50 MPa, even if these values are mostly theoretical, both the liner and cement bond tested in this study exhibited bond strength within these limits [30]. The liner-bonded ceramic crowns resisted a higher loading without demonstrating a chipping than the cement-bonded crowns, although no significant difference was found in the fracture strength between the liner-bonded group and the cement-bonded-group. As confirmed in Figures 3 and 5, the strong chemical bonding between the lithium disilicate liner and the zirconia ceramic was induced in the liner-bonded group, but there were lots of pores in the cement and mircro-gaps at the interface of the lithium disilicate-reinforced glass ceramic and cement in the cement-bonded group. Thus, it can be explained that the lower chipping strengths of the cement-bonded crowns than those of the liner-bonded crowns resulted from the stress concentration at defects of the interface when compression load was applied to the crown [31].

The bonding of ceramic restorations commonly involves acid etching and/or sandblasting procedures [32,33]. In the previous studies, it was reported that the shear bond strength of pre-sintered zirconia and the veneering porcelain did not change by conditioner treatment, but the failure mode was improved after thermal cycling [32]. It was also identified that the sandblasted zirconia surfaces had significantly higher shear bond strengths than non-treated and chemically etched surfaces without thermocycling, irrespective of conditioner treatment, and the highest shear bond strength and improved failure mode was confirmed by the application of both conditioner treatment and sandblasting [33]. Zirconia ceramics do not demonstrate the typical undercut features created by acid etching since they have chemical stability and almost no glass matrix. The silane treatment is not as effective as in silicate ceramics. The zirconia ceramics are usually roughened using an air-borne particle abrasion technology [34,35]. This procedure exposes sharp asperities of surface structures and increases surface area for bonding [36,37]. The resin cement should wet the surface and adhere to the irregular surface of ceramic restoration. This type of bonding relies on the surface characteristics of ceramic restorations, as well as the wettability and chemical compositions of resin cements, including the mechanisms of polymerization. According to Dérand et al. and Lüthy et al., the implant-supported zirconia restorations can fail at the interface when bonding is established with resin cements containing only 2,2-bis[p-(2′-hydroxy-3′-methacryloxypropoxy)phenylene]propane (bis-GMA) or 1,6-bis(methacryloxy-2-ethoxycarbonylamino)-2,4,4-trimethylhexane (UDMA) monomer [38,39]. In another study, it was identified that the shear bond strength of resin cements containing MDP of a zirconia ceramic was significantly improved by the application of a zirconia primer on both polished and blasted zirconia surfaces when comparing the results of the non-treatment of zirconia primer [40].

The one-piece system of zirconia abutments was found to present with some degree of misfit at the implant–abutment interface because of the challenge of the manufacturing process of the ceramic abutment [41,42]. Under loading, these abutments can induce an abrasion with micromotion at the implant–abutment interface [43]. The abutment screw can be loosened and lead to a bacterial colonization at the interface [6,44], as well a fracture failure of the implant-supported restoration.

The two-piece system of zirconia abutments involves using a titanium base to establish an interfacial connection with similar materials to the implant to avoid possible complications resulting from the use of dissimilar materials [18,22]. These abutments were found to demonstrate a higher bond strength when the abutment was roughened with 110 μm alumina particles at 2.5 atm, coated with a ceramic primer, and bonded with a dual-cure self-adhesive resin cement [45]. However, the increased bond strength was possible when the titanium base was included when roughening the zirconia core by sandblasting. The bonded interface was intimate without demonstrating a gap between the abutment and cement layer. According to Ebert et al. [46], the retention of cement-bonded zirconia abutments was significantly higher when the bonded interfacial gap was less than 30 μm.

The fracture resistance was higher when the zirconia abutment was designed to receive the support of the titanium base [17]. Gehrke et al. [7] used CAD/CAM technology to design zirconia abutments connected to an internal-hex titanium implant. The test specimens were thermocycled and cyclic loaded to fracture. They found that the two-piece system sustained a significantly higher fracture load than the one-piece system. Though the axial force generated during chewing typically does not exceed 220 N [47], the threshold for failure is estimated to be approximately 400 N according to the research conducted by Andersson et al. [48] and Att et al. [44].

Sandblasting is a common method of surface treatment used to bond zirconia ceramic restorations. The effect of this mechanical method, however, is limited to creating desired undercut features and increasing bond strength because of the dense polycrystalline structure of the zirconia ceramic [49,50]. However, the heat-bonding with the lithium disilicate liner was found to induce a chemical bonding to the zirconia ceramic, as indicated by the alteration of the crystal structure of zirconia at the interface of bonding. The zone of the chemical interaction with bonding revealed components of Si and Zr oxides which agreed with the previous research conducted by Jang et al. [31] and Aboushelib et al. [51].

The mode of failure was mixed with cohesive fracture propagated through the liner in the MLG group, whereas the failure was adhesive at the bonded interface of the ceramic and resin cement in the MGC group. The cement layer was thin at the interface and contained numerous pores and gaps. Meanwhile, no gap or pore was noted at the interface of the heat-bonding with the liner. These characteristics of bonding and mode of failure might have played a critical role in developing a higher fracture resistance of the implant-supported glass ceramic crown combined with a two-piece system of a zirconia abutment produced by a CAD/CAM procedure. However, a clinical study is yet to be conducted to determine the clinical success of the glass ceramic crown bonded to the zirconia abutment by means of heat-bonding with the liner.

5. Conclusions

The bond strength and fracture resistance of a milled lithium disilicate-reinforced glass ceramic bonded to a milled zirconia ceramic are affected by the modification of bonding procedures. The bond strength and fracture resistance were significantly higher when the bonding was established by means of heat-bonding with the lithium-disilicate liner than by a resin cement. The pattern of interfacial failure for the liner-bonded group was mixed with the fracture propagated through the liner. However, after visual inspection, the cement-bonded group demonstrated an adhesive failure at the interface of bonding. The results of this study suggest that heat-bonding with the liner can be an alternative to bond CAD/CAM-produced glass ceramic crowns to zirconia ceramic abutments in order to reduce the risk of crown dislodgement and fracture.

Author Contributions: Conceptualization, T.-S.B.; data curation, Y.-S.J. and J.-J.L.; formal analysis, Y.-S.J. and S.-H.O.; investigation, Y.-S.J., S.-H.O. and T.-S.B.; supervision, M.-H.L. and T.-S.B.; validation, Y.-S.J., M.-H.L. and T.-S.B.; writing–original draft, Y.-S.J. and S.-H.O.; writing–review and editing, Y.-S.J. and W.-S.O.

Acknowledgments: This study has reconstructed the data for dissertation of doctor of Sang-Hun Oh. Yong-Seok Jang and Sang-Hoon Oh contributed equally to this work and are considered as joint first author.

References

1. Sailer, I.; Sailer, T.; Stawarczyk, B.; Jung, R.E.; Hämmerle, C.H.F. In vitro study of the influence of the type of connection on the fracture load of zirconia abutments with internal and external implant-abutment connections. *Int. J. Oral Maxillofac. Implant.* **2009**, *24*, 850–858.
2. Wadhwani, C.; Piñeyro, A.; Avots, J. An Esthetic Solution to the Screw-Retained Implant Restoration: Introduction to the Implant Crown Adhesive Plug: Clinical Report. *J. Esthet. Restor. Dent.* **2011**, *23*, 138–143. [CrossRef] [PubMed]
3. Wilson, T.G., Jr. The positive relationship between excess cement and peri-implant disease: A prospective clinical endoscopic study. *J. Periodontol.* **2009**, *80*, 1388–1392. [CrossRef] [PubMed]
4. Sailer, I.; Zembic, A.; Jung, R.E.; Hämmerle, C.H.F.; Mattiola, A. Single-tooth implant reconstructions: Esthetic factors influencing the decision between titanium and zirconia abutments in anterior regions. *Eur. J. Esthet. Dent.* **2007**, *2*, 3.
5. Zembic, A.; Sailer, I.; Jung, R.E.; Hämmerle, C.H.F. Randomized-controlled clinical trial of customized zirconia and titanium implant abutments for single-tooth implants in canine and posterior regions: 3-year results. *Clin. Oral Implant. Res.* **2009**, *20*, 802–808. [CrossRef] [PubMed]
6. Nakamura, K.; Kanno, T.; Milleding, P.; Ortengren, U. Zirconia as a dental implant abutment material: A systematic review. *Int. J. Prosthodont.* **2010**, *23*, 4.
7. Gehrke, P.; Johannson, D.; Fischer, C.; Stawarczyk, B.; Beuer, F. In vitro fatigue and fracture resistance of one- and two-piece CAD/CAM zirconia implant abutments. *Int. J. Oral Maxillofac. Implant.* **2015**, *30*, 546–554. [CrossRef]
8. Kosmač, T.; Oblak, Č.; Marion, L. The effects of dental grinding and sandblasting on ageing and fatigue behavior of dental zirconia (Y-TZP) ceramics. *J. Eur. Ceram. Soc.* **2008**, *28*, 1085–1090. [CrossRef]
9. Denry, I.; Kelly, J.R. State of the art of zirconia for dental applications. *Dent. Mater.* **2008**, *24*, 299–307. [CrossRef]
10. Park, J.I.; Lee, Y.; Lee, J.H.; Kim, Y.L.; Bae, J.M.; Cho, H.W. Comparison of fracture resistance and fit accuracy of customized zirconia abutments with prefabricated zirconia abutments in internal hexagonal implants. *Clin. Implant. Dent. Relat. Res.* **2013**, *15*, 769–778. [CrossRef]
11. Hamilton, A.; Judge, R.B.; E Palamara, J.; Evans, C. Evaluation of the fit of CAD/CAM abutments. *Int. J. Prosthodont.* **2013**, *26*, 370–380. [CrossRef] [PubMed]

12.	Martínez-Rus, F.; Ferreiroa, A.; Özcan, M.; Bartolomé, J.F.; Pradíes, G. Fracture resistance of crowns cemented on titanium and zirconia implant abutments: A comparison of monolithic versus manually veneered all-ceramic systems. *Int. J. Oral Maxillofac. Implant.* **2012**, *27*, 6.

13.	Klotz, M.W.; Taylor, T.D.; Goldberg, A.J. Wear at the titanium-zirconia implant-abutment interface: A pilot study. *Int. J. Oral Maxillofac. Implant.* **2011**, *26*, 970–975.

14.	Stimmelmayr, M.; Edelhoff, D.; Güth, J.-F.; Erdelt, K.; Happe, A.; Beuer, F. Wear at the titanium–titanium and the titanium–zirconia implant–abutment interface: A comparative in vitro study. *Dent. Mater.* **2012**, *28*, 1215–1220. [CrossRef] [PubMed]

15.	Foong, J.K.; Judge, R.B.; Palamara, J.E.; Swain, M.V. Fracture resistance of titanium and zirconia abutments: An in vitro study. *J. Prosthet. Dent.* **2013**, *109*, 304–312. [CrossRef]

16.	Elsayed, A.; Wille, S.; Al-Akhali, M.; Kern, M. Comparison of fracture strength and failure mode of different ceramic implant abutments. *J. Prosthet. Dent.* **2017**, *117*, 499–506. [CrossRef]

17.	Elsayed, A.; Wille, S.; Al-Akhali, M.; Kern, M. Effect of fatigue loading on the fracture strength and failure mode of lithium disilicate and zirconia implant abutments. *Clin. Oral Implant. Res.* **2018**, *29*, 20–27. [CrossRef]

18.	Gehrke, P.; Alius, J.; Fischer, C.; Erdelt, K.J.; Beuer, F. Retentive strength of two-piece CAD/CAM zirconia implant abutments. *Clin. Implant. Dent. Relat. Res.* **2014**, *16*, 920–925. [CrossRef]

19.	Truninger, T.C.; Stawarczyk, B.; Leutert, C.R.; Sailer, T.R.; Hämmerle, C.H.; Sailer, I. Bending moments of zirconia and titanium abutments with internal and external implant–abutment connections after aging and chewing simulation. *Clin. Oral Implant. Res.* **2012**, *23*, 12–18. [CrossRef]

20.	Hjerppe, J.; Lassila, L.V.J.; Rakkolainen, T.; Narhi, T.; Vallittu, P.K. Load-bearing capacity of custom-made versus prefabricated commercially available zirconia abutments. *Int. J. Oral Maxillofac. Implant.* **2011**, *26*, 1.

21.	Canullo, L. Clinical outcome study of customized zirconia abutments for single-implant restorations. *Int. J. Prosthodont.* **2007**, *20*, 5.

22.	Canullo, L.; Coelho, P.G.; Bonfante, E.A. Mechanical testing of thin-walled zirconia abutments. *J. Appl. Oral Sci.* **2013**, *21*, 20–24. [CrossRef]

23.	Cheng, C.-W.; Yang, C.-C.; Yan, M. Bond strength of heat-pressed veneer ceramics to zirconia with various blasting conditions. *J. Dent. Sci.* **2018**, *13*, 301–310. [CrossRef]

24.	Yue, X.; Hou, X.; Gao, J.; Bao, P.; Shen, J. Effects of MDP-based primers on shear bond strength between resin cement and zirconia. *Exp. Ther. Med.* **2019**, *17*, 3564–3572. [CrossRef] [PubMed]

25.	Sato, T.; Anami, L.; Melo, R.; Valandro, L.; Bottino, M. Effects of Surface Treatments on the Bond Strength Between Resin Cement and a New Zirconia-reinforced Lithium Silicate Ceramic. *Oper. Dent.* **2016**, *41*, 284–292. [CrossRef]

26.	Mahmoodi, N.; Hooshmand, T.; Heidari, S.; Khoshro, K. Effect of sandblasting, silica coating, and laser treatment on the microtensile bond strength of a dental zirconia ceramic to resin cements. *Lasers Med. Sci.* **2016**, *31*, 205–211. [CrossRef]

27.	Yilmaz, B.; Gilbert, A.; Seidt, J.; McGlumphy, E.; Clelland, N. Displacement of Implant Abutments Following Initial and Repeated Torqueing. *Int. J. Oral Maxillofac. Implant.* **2015**, *30*, 1011–1018. [CrossRef] [PubMed]

28.	Schriwer, C.; Skjold, A.; Gjerdet, N.R.; Øilo, M. Monolithic zirconia dental crowns. Internal fit, margin quality, fracture mode and load at fracture. *Dent. Mater.* **2017**, *33*, 1012–1020. [CrossRef] [PubMed]

29.	Mores, R.T.; Borba, M.; Corazza, P.H.; Della Bona, Á.; Benetti, P. Influence of surface finishing on fracture load and failure mode of glass ceramic crowns. *J. Prosthet. Dent.* **2017**, *118*, 511–516. [CrossRef] [PubMed]

30.	Scribante, A.; Contreras-Bulnes, R.; Montasser, M.A.; Vallittu, P.K. Orthodontics: Bracket Materials, Adhesives Systems, and Their Bond Strength. *BioMed Res. Int.* **2016**, *2016*, 1–3. [CrossRef]

31.	Jang, Y.-S.; Noh, H.-R.; Lee, M.-H.; Lim, M.-J.; Bae, T.-S. Effect of Lithium Disilicate Reinforced Liner Treatment on Bond and Fracture Strengths of Bilayered Zirconia All-Ceramic Crown. *Materials* **2018**, *11*, 77. [CrossRef] [PubMed]

32.	Sawada, T.; Spintzyk, S.; Schille, C.; Zöldföldi, J.; Paterakis, A.; Schweizer, E.; Stephan, I.; Rupp, F.; Geis-Gerstorfer, J. Influence of Pre-Sintered Zirconia Surface Conditioning on Shear Bond Strength to Resin Cement. *Materials* **2016**, *9*, 518. [CrossRef] [PubMed]

33.	Spintzyk, S.; Yamaguchi, K.; Sawada, T.; Schille, C.; Schweizer, E.; Ozeki, M.; Geis-Gerstorfer, J. Influence of the Conditioning Method for Pre-Sintered Zirconia on the Shear Bond Strength of Bilayered Porcelain/Zirconia. *Materials* **2016**, *9*, 765. [CrossRef]

34. Kern, M.; Wegner, S.M. Bonding to zirconia ceramic: Adhesion methods and their durability. *Dent. Mater.* **1998**, *14*, 64–71. [CrossRef]

35. Blatz, M.B.; Chiche, G.; Holst, S.; Sadan, A. Influence of surface treatment and simulated aging on bond strengths of luting agents to zirconia. *Quintessence Int.* **2007**, *38*, 9.

36. Ramos-Tonello, C.M.; Trevizo, B.F.; Rodrigues, R.F.; Magalhães, A.P.R.; Furuse, A.Y.; Lisboa-Filho, P.N.; Borges, A.F.S.; Tabata, A.S. Pre-sintered Y-TZP sandblasting: Effect on surface roughness, phase transformation, and Y-TZP/veneer bond strength. *J. Appl. Oral Sci.* **2017**, *25*, 666–673. [CrossRef] [PubMed]

37. He, M.; Zhang, Z.; Zheng, D.; Ding, N.; Liu, Y. Effect of sandblasting on surface roughness of zirconia-based ceramics and shear bond strength of veneering porcelain. *Dent. Mater. J.* **2014**, *33*, 778–785. [CrossRef] [PubMed]

38. Dérand, P.; Dérand, T. Bond strength of luting cements to zirconium oxide ceramics. *Int. J. Prosthodont.* **2000**, *13*, 131–135.

39. Lüthy, H.; Loeffel, O.; Hammerle, C. Effect of thermocycling on bond strength of luting cements to zirconia ceramic. *Dent. Mater.* **2006**, *22*, 195–200. [CrossRef]

40. Shin, Y.-J.; Shin, Y.; Yi, Y.-A.; Kim, J.; Lee, I.-B.; Cho, B.-H.; Son, H.-H.; Seo, D.-G. Evaluation of the shear bond strength of resin cement to Y-TZP ceramic after different surface treatments. *Scanning* **2014**, *36*, 479–486. [CrossRef]

41. Baldassarri, M.; Hjerppe, J.; Romeo, D.; Fickl, S.; Thompson, V.P.; Stappert, C.F.J. Marginal accuracy of three implant-ceramic abutment configurations. *Int. J. Oral Maxillofac. Implant.* **2012**, *27*, 3.

42. Smith, N.A.; Turkyilmaz, I. Evaluation of the sealing capability of implants to titanium and zirconia abutments against Porphyromonas gingivalis, Prevotella intermedia, and Fusobacterium nucleatum under different screw torque values. *J. Prosthet. Dent.* **2014**, *112*, 561–567. [CrossRef] [PubMed]

43. Han, J.; Zhao, J.; Shen, Z. Zirconia ceramics in metal-free implant dentistry. *Adv. Appl. Ceram.* **2017**, *116*, 138–150. [CrossRef]

44. Att, W.; Kurun, S.; Gerds, T.; Strub, J.R. Fracture resistance of single-tooth implant-supported all-ceramic restorations: An in vitro study. *J. Prosthet. Dent.* **2006**, *95*, 111–116. [CrossRef] [PubMed]

45. Von Maltzahn, N.F.; Holstermann, J.; Kohorst, P. Retention Forces between Titanium and Zirconia Components of Two-Part Implant Abutments with Different Techniques of Surface Modification. *Clin. Implant. Dent. Relat. Res.* **2016**, *18*, 735–744. [CrossRef] [PubMed]

46. Ebert, A.; Hedderich, J.; Kern, M. Retention of zirconia ceramic copings bonded to titanium abutments. *Int. J. Oral Maxillofac. Implant.* **2007**, *22*, 921–927.

47. Proeschel, P.; Morneburg, T. Task-dependence of Activity/Bite-force Relations and its Impact on Estimation of Chewing Force from EMG. *J. Dent. Res.* **2002**, *81*, 464–468. [CrossRef] [PubMed]

48. Andersson, B.; Taylor, Å.; Lang, B.R.; Scheller, H.; Schärer, P.; Sorensen, J.A.; Tarnow, D. Alumina ceramic implant abutments used for single-tooth replacement: A prospective 1-to 3-year multicenter study. *Int. J. Prosthodont.* **2001**, *14*, 432–438. [PubMed]

49. Liu, D.; Matinlinna, J.P.; Pow, E.H. Insights into porcelain to zirconia bonding. *J. Adhes. Sci. Technol.* **2012**, *26*, 1249–1265.

50. Fischer, J.; Grohmann, P.; Stawarczyk, B. Effect of zirconia surface treatments on the shear strength of zirconia/veneering ceramic composites. *Dent. Mater. J.* **2008**, *27*, 448–454. [CrossRef] [PubMed]

51. Aboushelib, M.N.; Kleverlaan, C.J.; Feilzer, A.J. Selective infiltration-etching technique for a strong and durable bond of resin cements to zirconia-based materials. *J. Prosthet. Dent.* **2007**, *98*, 379–388. [CrossRef]

8

Modifications of Dental Implant Surfaces at the Micro and Nano-Level for Enhanced Osseointegration

In-Sung Luke Yeo

Department of Prosthodontics, School of Dentistry and Dental Research Institute, Seoul National University, Seoul 03080, Korea; pros53@snu.ac.kr

Abstract: This review paper describes several recent modification methods for biocompatible titanium dental implant surfaces. The micro-roughened surfaces reviewed in the literature are sandblasted, large-grit, acid-etched, and anodically oxidized. These globally-used surfaces have been clinically investigated, showing survival rates higher than 95%. In the past, dental clinicians believed that eukaryotic cells for osteogenesis did not recognize the changes of the nanostructures of dental implant surfaces. However, research findings have recently shown that osteogenic cells respond to chemical and morphological changes at a nanoscale on the surfaces, including titanium dioxide nanotube arrangements, functional peptide coatings, fluoride treatments, calcium–phosphorus applications, and ultraviolet photofunctionalization. Some of the nano-level modifications have not yet been clinically evaluated. However, these modified dental implant surfaces at the nanoscale have shown excellent in vitro and in vivo results, and thus promising potential future clinical use.

Keywords: surface modification; osseointegration; SLA; TiO$_2$ nanotube; fluoride; photofunctionalization

1. Introduction

The surface quality of titanium (Ti) dental implants, which replace missing teeth, is one of the keys to the long-term clinical success of implants in a patient's mouth [1]. The bone response to the Ti implant surface depends on its surface characteristics: Contact (bone formation on the implant surface towards the bone) and distance osteogenesis occur around micro-roughened Ti surfaces while only distance osteogenesis (bone formation from the old bone toward the implant surface) appear around turned Ti [2]. Although contact osteogenesis seems to require other factors to be triggered, modification of the implant surface is very important to accelerate osseointegration [3].

Ti is known to be stable in biologic responses and not to trigger a foreign body reaction when inserted into the human body [4,5]. Therefore, osseointegration was originally defined as the direct contact between a loaded implant surface and bone at the microscopic level of resolution [1]. Recently, this term has been interpreted from a new point of view: Osseointegration is essentially a demarcation response to a foreign body of Ti when the Ti implant is immobile in bone [6]. This demarcation is immune-driven and is classified as a type IV hypersensitivity [7]. Based on the original definition, the modification of a Ti implant surface implies that the surface would be more biocompatible, thereby increasing the bioaffinity of the hard tissue and accelerating the bone response to the surface. The new standpoint on osseointegration suggests that the modified Ti surface would be recognized more sensitively by the hard tissue, which would isolate this foreign body with a faster and stronger accumulation of bone substances. Thus, the nature of osseointegration is under investigation at present [8]. The detection of the actual bond between the bone and implant surfaces could support the bioaffinitive nature of bone response to the surfaces [9,10]. Only friction and physical contact would exist at the interface if the bony demarcation hypothesis is correct.

To date, implant surfaces have been modified in various ways under the bioaffinity concept for osseointegration. Conventionally, the topography of the surface has been changed at the micro-level

(1–10 μm). At present, some chemical features and nanotechnologies have been added to the surfaces. This review introduces several recent advancements of biocompatible implant surfaces with a few representative micro-roughened modified surfaces. Since most implant surfaces used in the global market have been made of commercially pure Ti (cp-Ti), especially grade 4 cp-Ti, this review is based on the modification of a grade 4 cp-Ti surface.

2. Micro-Roughened Modification

2.1. Sandblasted, Large-Grit, Acid-Etched (SLA) Surface

The computer numerical controlled milling of cp-Ti manufactures screw-shaped endosseous dental implants. The surface machined by this milling procedure, which is now called a turned Ti surface, shows many parallel grooves in scanning electron microscopy (SEM). The turned surface experiences no modification process, which has frequently served as a control to evaluate the biocompatibility of modified surfaces. When an implant is inserted into the bone and the implant surface becomes juxtaposed to the bone, bone healing (or osseointegration) on the surface is known to be fulfilled by two mechanisms: distance and contact osteogenesis [2,11]. In distance osteogenesis, new bone starts to be formed on the surfaces of bone. The direction of bone growth is from the bone towards the implant surface (Figure 1A). In contact osteogenesis, or de novo bone formation, new bone formation begins on the implant surface. The direction of bone growth is from the implant towards the bone, opposite to that for distance osteogenesis (Figure 1B). When an endosseous implant with a turned surface is placed into the jawbone, only distance osteogenesis occurs, which implies that more time is needed for sufficient osseointegration to withstand masticatory forces [2,12]. The necessity of reduction in the patient's edentulous period has led the modification of an implant surface to accelerate bone healing.

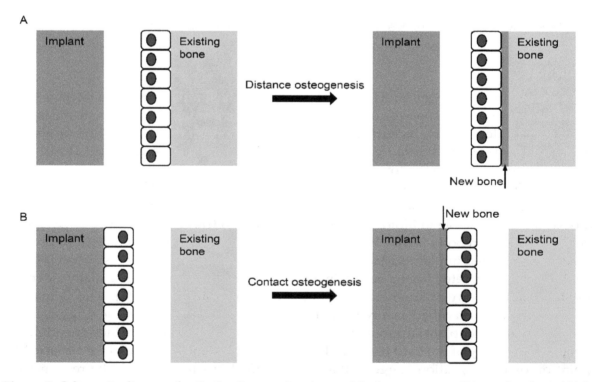

Figure 1. Schematic diagram for the healing mechanisms of the bone surrounding an implant. (**A**) In distance osteogenesis, the direction of bone formation is from the existing bone to the implant; (**B**) in contact osteogenesis, however, the direction is opposite, from the implant to the existing bone, which is known not to occur on the turned Ti (Titanium) surface without any modification.

The traditional approach to the surface modification of a Ti implant has been roughening at the micro-level. One of the most successful surfaces in clinical dentistry is the sandblasted, large-grit, and acid-etched (or SLA) surface. An SLA Ti surface is made by sandblasting the turned Ti surface with large-grit particles, the sizes of which range from 250 μm to 500 μm in general, and by acid-etching the blasted surface. The acids for etching are usually strong acids including hydrochloric, sulfuric, and nitric acids. SEM shows topographically changed irregularities on the SLA surface, with large dips, small micropits, sharp edges, and pointed tips. Sa, one of the surface parameters defined as the arithmetic mean height of the surface, is approximately 1.5 μm to 2 μm. Osteogenic cells migrate to the roughened Ti surface through the fibrin clot that is formed at the peri-implant site after bone drilling for implant insertion, and these cells appear to recognize the irregularities of the SLA surface as lacunae to be filled with bone materials [2,13]. Contact osteogenesis occurs as the osteogenic cells secrete a bone matrix. The occurrence of both contact and distance osteogenesis accelerates the osseointegration on the SLA surface compared to the turned surface.

The Ti surface of a dental implant is originally hydrophobic [14]. Water (H_2O) is considered to have initial contact with the implant surface when the implant is inserted into the bone [15]. Therefore, there have been attempts to add hydrophilicity to an SLA surface, since hydrophilicity is expected to help accelerate the bone healing process [14,16]. A dental implant with a hydrophilic SLA surface, commercially called SLActive (Institute Straumann AG, Basel, Switzerland), is made with a water rinse of the original SLA implant in a nitrogen chamber and a packaging technique of storing the implant in an isotonic sodium chloride solution with no atmospheric contact, and this hydrophilic implant is being clinically used in the global market [17].

Regardless of whether an SLA surface is hydrophobic or hydrophilic, this dental implant surface has shown excellent long-term clinical results [18–22]. A previous 10-year retrospective study investigating more than 500 SLA Ti implants concluded that both the survival and success rates were 97% or higher [18]. The 10-year survival rate of SLA Ti implants was reported to be higher than 95%, even in periodontally compromised patients, although strict periodontal interventions were applied to these patients [20]. Similar results were found in 10-year prospective studies investigating the survival rates of dental implants with SLA surfaces [19,21,22]. This modified surface, roughened at the micro-scale, is one of the dental implant surfaces that has been most frequently tested in clinics for the longest period.

2.2. Anodic Oxidation

The genuine biocompatible surface on the Ti dental implant is Ti oxide (TiO_2), not Ti itself, which is spontaneously formed when the Ti surface is exposed to the atmosphere. However, this Ti oxide layer is very thin (a few nm in thickness) and is imperfect with defects [23]. Also, chemically unstable Ti^{3+} and Ti^{2+} are known to exist in the oxide layer [24]. Therefore, there have been several techniques developed to thicken and stabilize the Ti oxide layer, which is considered to increase the biocompatibility of the surface [25–27]. When Ti becomes the anode under an electric potential in an electrochemical cell, Ti is oxidized to be Ti^{4+}, and the TiO_2 layer is able to be thickened and roughened [15]. Topographically, the oxidized Ti surface for a dental implant has many volcano-like micropores with various sizes, which are observed in SEM. The surface characteristics of the anodized Ti surface depend on the applied potential, surface treatment time, concentrations, and types of electrolytes [15,27]. The arithmetic mean height of this surface, or Sa, is evaluated to be approximately 1 to 1.5 μm for dental use [28–31].

Osteogenic cells appear to recognize the topography of a dental implant surface although we do not yet know which surface topography is more proper in bone healing, or if the irregularities of the SLA surface are more effective for the osteogenic cell response than the microporous structure of the anodized surface [32]. To date, no in vivo model has found any significant differences in bone responses to the microtopographies of Ti dental implant surfaces [33,34]. What is definitely known about implant surface topography is that the cp-Ti surfaces topographically modified at the microscale accelerate osseointegration more than the turned surface, and these modified surfaces show superior results to the turned surface during in vitro, in vivo, and clinical studies.

The anodically oxidized Ti surface has shown superior results to the turned surface in various in vitro tests and in vivo histomorphometry [31,34–36]. A previous meta-analytic study reported lower failure rates of the oxidized Ti implants than those of the turned implants from the included 38 clinical investigations [37]. A prior retrospective and a 10-year prospective study concluded that that success rates were higher than 95% for the TiUnite surface (Brånemark System, Nobel Biocare, Göteborg, Sweden), which is a trade name for the oxidized Ti surface [38,39]. However, a recent 20-year randomized controlled clinical trial notably reported a similar marginal bone loss between micro-roughened and turned Ti implants [40]. This clinical study used an identical implant design with an implant-abutment connection structure and internal friction connection [40]. Identifying which of the two factors (surface characteristics and implant design) is a major contributor to the long-term clinical success of dental implants needs to be thoroughly investigated, although higher success or survival rates have been steadily published for Ti dental implants with modified surfaces at the micro-scale, compared to the turned implant [19,41,42].

3. Molecular Modification

3.1. TiO$_2$ Nanotube

Anodic oxidation is extended to the modification of a Ti dental implant at the nanoscale (1–100 nm). The electric current of the electrochemical cell, temperature, the pH values of electrolyte solutions, the electrolytes, oxidation voltage, and oxidation time affect the nanotopographies of the Ti surface [43,44]. In an electrochemical cell composed of Ti at the anode and platinum (or Ti) at the cathode, the TiO$_2$ layer is normally formed on the Ti implant surface of the anode [43]. In an appropriate fluoride-based electrolyte, the nano-morphology of the TiO$_2$ layer is changed, and the aligned TiO$_2$ nanotube layer is developed (Figure 2) [43].

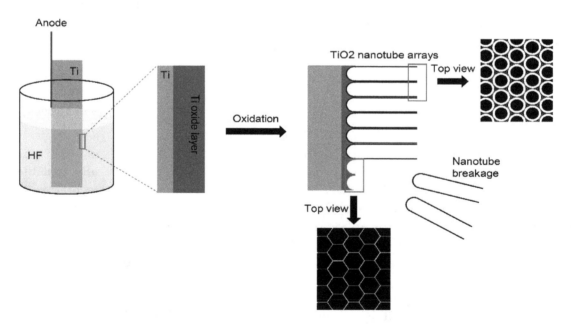

Figure 2. Schematic diagram showing the formation of TiO$_2$ nanotube arrays. In the electrolyte solution containing hydrogen fluoride (HF), regular tube structures are formed on the Ti surface of the anode at a nanoscale. When the structures are viewed on top, the circular forms of the tubules are found via scanning electron microscopy. The binding between the nanotube arrays and Ti surface is generally weak, and breakdown is frequent at the interface. The morphology underneath the tubes is hexagonal.

In the past, implant surface nanostructures were reported to have no effect on cell responses and bone responses to dental implant surfaces and were thought to depend on the microtopographies of the surfaces [45,46]. Optimal micro-roughness is known at present to be 1.5 μm in Sa and approximately

4 μm in diameter of the surface irregularities [30,47]. However, a previous review article noted that the microtopographies of the dental implant surfaces have a limited influence on the initial responses of the in vivo hard tissue environment [48]. Presently, the nanotopographical features of Ti implant surfaces have been known to be contributors to the initial biologic responses of the hard tissue, including osteoblast activities and osteoclast reactions [44,49].

This modified surface with TiO_2 nanotube arrays is highly biocompatible [44,50,51]. Both osteoblasts and osteoclasts showed maximal cellular responses to Ti surfaces with TiO_2 nanotubes that were 15 nm in diameter [52]. Interestingly, smaller TiO_2 nanotubes, which were approximately 30 nm in diameter, were more effective in the adhesion and growth of mesenchymal stem cells than larger TiO_2 nanotubes that ranged from 70 nm to 100 nm, while the latter TiO_2 nanotubes were more inductive in the differentiation into osteoblast-like cells, although there is contrary to previous studies [52,53]. The modified TiO_2 nanotubular surface showed excellent bone-to-implant contact in the osteoporotic bone in an in vivo study using ovariectomized rats [54].

Another characteristic of this nano-modified surface is a drug delivery effect [55–58]. Drug release from TiO_2 nanotubes is associated with the dimensions of TiO_2 nanotube arrays regardless of the direct release or indirect discharge by nanocarriers [59]. The diameter and length of TiO_2 nanotubes generally increase as the voltage and duration of the oxidation process increase, and the drug release has been found to be effective when the diameter is larger than approximately 100 nm [56,59,60]. A combination of this nano-modified TiO_2 surface and carrier molecules, including micelles, is being actively investigated for drug delivery at a constant rate, unrelated to the drug concentration and release period [57,58,60].

The nanotopography of the TiO_2 nanotubular surface has antibacterial properties alongside delivering antibiotic drugs [61]. Streptococcus mutans, which are associated with the initial formation of biofilm in the oral cavity, were reported to adhere to the TiO_2 nanotube arrays less than to a micro-roughened SLA surface [62]. The hydrophilic properties of TiO_2 nanotubes seems to hinder bacterial adhesion to the nanotubular surface [62]. However, it is notable that many studies have described the wettability of the TiO_2 nanotube arrays, showing conflicting results in cellular and bacterial responses to the nanotubular surface [61,63,64]. Although the hydrophilicity of the TiO_2 nanotube arrays is adjustable, some studies reported that the reduction of bacterial adhesion was due to the hydrophilic properties of the surface, whereas other studies described that such a result was due to the hydrophobic properties [61,63,64]. Further investigation is required to determine the mechanism of bacterial and cellular responses to the wettability of Ti surfaces.

Despite that the modified surface with TiO_2 nanotube arrays has very useful advantages (e.g., high biocompatibility, the capability of drug delivery, and antibacterial properties), this surface has been neither applied nor tested clinically. The mechanical strength between the TiO_2 nanotubes and the base Ti surface is too weak for this surface to be applied to a dental implant [43]. Recently, the hexagonal nano-structure of the base Ti surface was evaluated to be adequate for biologic application when the TiO_2 nanotube arrays are removed from the base surface in order to prevent the delamination of the TiO_2 nanotube coating in an in vivo environment (Figure 2) [44]. The aligned TiO_2 nanotube-layered surface has great potential in biologic and clinical applications [55–57,65]. However, it is necessary to overcome this delamination problem before this TiO_2 nanotubular surface is clinically used in the field of dental implantology.

3.2. Functional Peptides

Water and ions have first contact with the implant surface when the bone is drilled for implant insertion and a screw-shaped endosseous dental implant is placed into the bone. Then, the plasma proteins adhere to the surface through ionic bridges (like a calcium ion linkage), and the fibrin clot is formed. During hemostasis, extracellular matrix (ECM) proteins gradually replace the plasma proteins [15]. The adhesion proteins, including fibronectin and vitronectin (which are also ECM proteins), are recognized by the transmembrane proteins of osteogenic cells like integrins. Through binding of the transmembrane proteins to the osteogenic cells, the cells interact with ECM, which controls the cellular activities for bone healing [66]. Therefore, the bone healing process starts from the adhesion of the osteogenic cells to surfaces, and these adhesion proteins can play a role in accelerating osseointegration into dental implants when the proteins are applied to the implant surfaces. Core amino acid sequences, which are extracted from the original adhesion proteins and still have binding activities to the transmembrane receptors, are very useful in rapid bone healing when the core sequences are treated on the implant surfaces. These core functional peptides are considered to be more promising candidates for implant surface treatment than the original proteins because of the lower antigenicity and simpler adjustability of the peptides [67].

A functional peptide derived from the fibronectin, arginyl-glycyl-aspartic acid sequence, revealed improved histomorphometric results when this peptide was coated on a Ti dental implant surface and when this peptide-treated surface was compared to the uncoated surface [68]. Two functional amino acid sequences derived from another adhesion protein, laminin, showed excellent results as accelerating modifiers for Ti implant surfaces for osseointegration [35,67]. These functional peptides based on the adhesion of osteogenic cells seem to surpass the effects of the microtopographical features of the underlying Ti implant surfaces in bone healing, although further studies are definitely needed [35,69]. The mechanism behind the superior bone cell responses has been tried to be explained, based on the hypothesized tunable allosteric control of the receptor proteins [67,70]. A recent investigation evaluating a functional peptide from vitronectin found a Janus effect of this peptide for bone formation, activating osteoblasts and inhibiting osteoclasts, that is, controlling the osteoporotic environment locally to be favorable for osseointegration [71].

Cytokines, particularly growth factors, are another class of bioactive proteins. Bone morphogenetic proteins (BMPs) are available for bone healing in the field of dental implantology. Human recombinant BMP-2 (rhBMP-2) is used in the global market for bone regeneration. BMP-2 is known to have a direct effect on osteogenic cells to promote bone formation with various interactions between this protein and other bioactive molecules, including osteogenic genes [72,73]. However, these growth factors have many problems to be solved before clinical application to Ti dental implant surfaces. BMP-2 has complicated biologic effects depending on its concentrations and surroundings; osteogenesis, adipogenesis, and chodrogenesis, but osteolysis also occurs [72,74,75]. The rhBMP-2-treated Ti surface was reported to make bone healing around a dental implant faster in an in vivo model [76,77]. However, it is recognizable that growth factors are usually active in free forms, not in bound forms. Therefore, these molecules are ineffective or, if any, limitedly active when the factors are bound or attached to implant surfaces [78]. The cell transmembrane proteins that recognize these growth factors are disengaged in the attachment of the cells [78]. Because of the multiple enigmatic effects of these growth factors on living tissues and the growth factor receptors' lack of involvement in cell adhesion, growth factor-treated implant surfaces have not been used clinically until now.

Although these bioactive molecules, including the adhesion molecules and growth factors, have the potential to be applied to dental implants for accelerated osseointegration, the Ti dental implants on which these molecules are coated have not been clinically tested; there have been no published clinical trials to report the results of such implants. The functional peptides from the adhesion molecules are to be clinically tried and applied in dental implantology in the near future due to the simplicity in their biologic effects and their low probability of side effects. For growth factors, it seems to be necessary to find core amino acid sequences from growth factors to increase the clinical applicability of these factors. Before these derived peptides are clinically tried, further studies are required on release strategies for the molecules from the implant surfaces and on the biologic activities of the core peptides.

3.3. Fluoride Treatment (Cathodic Reduction)

When a Ti implant is a cathode in the hydrofluoric acid solution of an electrochemical cell, a fluoride ion gives an electron to the cathode, where the reduction of a Ti ion occurs. As a result, a trace amount of fluoride ions adheres to the Ti implant surface when the concentration of hydrogen fluoride is low in the solution. This trace amount of fluoride ions is known to primarily affect osteoprogenitor cells and undifferentiated osteoblasts to enhance bone formation, rather than highly differentiated osteoblasts [79,80]. Furthermore, fluoride is helpful for bone mineralization because of its properties that are attractive for calcium [78]. However, fluoride ions are thought to become cytotoxic as the number of ions increases on the Ti implant surface.

Clinically, a modified surface is used as a dental implant surface (Osseospeed, Astra Tech, Dentsply, Waltham, MA, USA), which is fluoride-treated after the grade 4 cp-Ti is sandblasted with TiO$_2$ particles. This fluoride-modified surface has a very low amount of fluoride, which is difficult to find by energy dispersive spectroscopy, while x-ray photoelectron spectroscopy is able to detect this trace amount [81,82]. The average mean height of this marketed surface has been investigated to be approximately 1.5 μm [30,82]. The fluoride-treated Ti surface has shown stronger binding between the bone and this surface than the control Ti surface without fluoride-treatment [83,84]. However, finding any significant differences in the histomorphometric results has been very rare when the fluoride-treated dental implants have been compared in vivo to other modified implants, including SLA implants, while some previous studies have been found to show more favorable results in bone responses to the fluoride-treated surface than those to its predecessor with no application of fluoride [78,82,85,86].

Dental implants with a fluoride-treated surface have exhibited high rates of success and survival rates in clinical trials. These fluoride-treated implants have supported prosthodontic restorations in edentulous mandibles with a 100% survival rate for ten years [87]. Regardless of the maxilla or the mandible, high survival rates of over 95% have been reported for the surface-modified dental implants in the prospective clinical studies, the observation periods of which are longer than 5 years [87–89]. It is notable and very interesting that these previous clinical studies have consistently reported the vertical loss of bone surrounding the implants of less than 0.5–1 mm, which is interpreted as almost no change of the bone level [40,87,89]. Importantly, these clinical studies used fluoride-treated dental implants with the same implant macro-design, including an identical thread shape and internal friction implant–abutment connection, so care must be taken when interpreting data in comparison studies of the biologic responses between the dental implant systems [82]. It remains uncertain which factor (surface chemistry in fluoride treatment, surface topography, implant–abutment connection tectonics) is a major contributor to the biologic responses in humans to this marketed fluoride-treated dental implant.

3.4. Hydroxyapatite and Other Calcium–Phosphorus Compounds

This idea of hydroxyapatite (HA) coating on a Ti dental implant surface is based on the fact that the main component of bone is HA. HA (Ca$_{10}$(PO$_4$)$_6$(OH)$_2$) is still the most commonly-utilized coating material for Ti dental implant surfaces [90]. HA and other calcium-phosphorus coating materials are basically osteoconductive to the surrounding bone. The biologic features of these materials, such as their biodegradation properties and foreign body reactions, seem to depend on calcium/phosphorus ratios, crystallinities, and coating thicknesses [31,90–93]. Plasma spraying (a conventional atmospheric plasma-spray method) is one of the most widely used methods to coat HA on a Ti implant surface [90]. HA particles that are contained and heated in a plasma flame whose temperature is approximately 15,000 to 20,000 Kelvin are sprayed on the Ti surface, resulting in a HA coating layer that is 50–100 μm in thickness [94]. The spray parameters, including the flame combination and spraying flow rate, affect the chemical and physical features of the HA coating [92].

The HA coating is biocompatible with the hard tissue, showing direct contact with bone and the attachment of osteoblasts on the coating surface [95,96]. Many studies have reported enhanced bone apposition and the prevention of metal-ion release into the bone from metal implants with an HA coated surface [97–101]. However, the HA coating layer has some critical issues to be addressed. Like the TiO$_2$ nanotube arrays, the delamination of the coating layer from the Ti dental implant surface is one of the problems (adhesive failure) [92]. Delaminated or worn HA particles hinder bone healing and provoke inflammation around the implant inserted into the bone [92,102]. The thick coating layer is able to make a breakage inside the layer, especially at the implant in a load-bearing area (cohesive failure) [92]. Recently, a thin calcium–phosphorus coating layer has been achieved and investigated using various coating techniques [76,93,101,103]. Compared to the plasma sprayed HA coating, however, the other calcium–phosphorus coatings are considered to lack long term clinical results [104,105].

The five-year clinical success rate of the HA coated implant has been evaluated to be approximately 95% [106]. However, this success rate has dropped markedly to below 80% after 10 years of implant placement [106–108]. Such a low success rate may result from the above-mentioned problems of the HA coating layer. It is notable, however, that these clinical evaluations resulted from the data of cylindrical implants [107,108]. A previous study using HA coated screw-shaped implants (MicroVent, Zimmer Dental, Carlsbad, CA, USA) reported that the long-term clinical success rate (> 10 years) was higher than 90% [109]. Nevertheless, clinical trials are certainly necessary to evaluate the calcium–phosphorus coating more precisely.

3.5. Photofunctionalization

In 1997, it was determined that the wettability of the TiO_2 surface is increased by ultraviolet (UV) radiation [110]. Originally, the UV-induced TiO_2 surface is amphiphilic—both hydrophilic and oleophilic [110]. However, the enhanced biologic effect of this surface is considered to be caused by the hydrophilic properties. Such hydrophilicity and elimination of hydrocarbon contamination on the TiO_2 surface are known to be the mechanisms behind further activated bone responses to a dental implant in UV-mediated photofunctionalization. The hard tissue affinity drops for an aged Ti surface that has been stored for longer than two weeks [111]. UV irradiation on the Ti implant surface appears to make the Ti surface reactivate, as the implant is freshly made.

UV radiation is subcategorized into three types according to its wavelengths and dermal biologic reactions to the electromagnetic waves: UVA, UVB, and UVC [112]. The wavelengths of UVA range from 320 to 400 nm, and those of UVC range from 200 to 280 nm [113]. Both UVA and UVC contribute to increasing the hydrophilicity of the Ti surface. However, considering the fact that some reports show the promoted osteogenic activities on hydrophobic surfaces, the removal of carbon from the Ti surface, which is caused by UVC, is likely a fundamental mechanism behind excellent osseointegration [114–117]. Strictly, neither UVA nor UVC appears to make a topographic change at the nano-scale on the Ti surface [115,117]. Friction force microscopy shows a nano-scale modification that UV irradiation may produce by converting Ti^{4+} to Ti^{3+} [110]. UV treatment on the Ti surface enhances the adsorption of proteins, such as albumin and fibronectin, which are plasma proteins in the human body [118]. UV-photofunctionalized implant surfaces show improved osteogenic cell attachment, spreading, and proliferation [117]. The antibacterial effects are described for the UV activation of the Ti surface [112]. Faster bone responses to UV-treated Ti surfaces are reported in various in vivo studies, some of which show almost 100% bone-to-implant contact [117–120].

A previous clinical study showed that the stability of implants inserted into the patients' jaw bones increased more rapidly when the implants were UV-photofunctionalized [121]. The retrospective clinical studies concluded that UV-mediated photofunctionalization reduced early implant failure, and the success rate of the photofunctionalized implants was 97.6% during the functional loading period of approximately 2.5 years [122,123]. No prospective long-term clinical study (published in English) evaluating UV-mediated photofunctionalization has yet been found in the field of implant dentistry. However, a prospective clinical evaluation of UV-treated implants over more than 5 years is expected to be published shortly.

3.6. Laser Ablation

For laser ablation, an implant whose collar, or neck area, was treated by laser micromachining to generate nano-channels is used (Laser-Lok, BioHorizons, Birmingham, AL, USA) [124,125].

Laser ablation is also able to produce micro-scale patterns by controlling laser processing parameters [126]. This approach was intended to promote not only fast osseointegration, but also connective tissue attachment [124,127]. The connective tissue fiber direction in the soft tissue attachment is known to be perpendicular to the laser-microtextured Ti implant surface, which is characteristically different from the general orientation of the fibers parallel to implant surfaces [127,128]

This marketed laser-modified surface (Laser-Lok) showed significantly improved bone-to-implant contact in a previous in vivo study, compared to a turned Ti surface [129]. The survival rate was evaluated to be 95.6% in a two-year retrospective multicenter study and to be 94% in another 5-year retrospective controlled study [127,130]. Recently, the prospective three-year results of a randomized clinical trial were reported for single implant-supported restorations with the laser-modified Ti implant surface, where the survival rate was estimated to be 96.1% [131]. Both the hard and soft tissue responses to the laser-modified Ti surface appear to be favorable [127,130–132]. However, long-term prospective clinical results of laser micromachining are still needed.

4. Concluding Remarks

When the bone is prepared for implant placement, surgical trauma provokes bleeding and hemostasis. Moreover, this surgical trauma activates the growth and differentiation factors released from the bone debris and matrix [15]. Surface modification of the Ti dental implant focuses on improving such initial biologic responses to the implant surface. Researchers and dental clinicians anticipate the best performance of the implant surfaces during these initial events and more readily establish these events by changing the physical and chemical properties of the surfaces, thereby boosting the speed and strengthening the quality of the healing process [133]. However, as the long-term clinical studies show, implant-supported prostheses have been used for a long time in patients' mouths. Therefore, the modified surfaces also need to harmonize with the bone remodeling process, which has not yet been investigated. This paper reviews several modified surfaces of dental implants that are widely used in the global market or are highly possible to be clinically used. All these reviewed surfaces are targeted to accelerate early bone responses. The late responses of the hard tissue to the surfaces, including bone remodeling, need to be investigated. Moreover, long-term clinical trials are still required for these implant surfaces.

References

1. Albrektsson, T.; Branemark, P.I.; Hansson, H.A.; Lindstrom, J. Osseointegrated titanium implants. Requirements for ensuring a long-lasting, direct bone-to-implant anchorage in man. *Acta Orthop. Scand.* **1981**, *52*, 155–170. [CrossRef] [PubMed]
2. Davies, J.E. Mechanisms of endosseous integration. *Int. J. Prosthodont.* **1998**, *11*, 391–401. [PubMed]
3. Choi, J.Y.; Sim, J.H.; Yeo, I.L. Characteristics of contact and distance osteogenesis around modified implant surfaces in rabbit tibiae. *J. Periodontal Implant Sci.* **2017**, *47*, 182–192. [CrossRef] [PubMed]
4. Albrektsson, T.; Wennerberg, A. Oral implant surfaces: Part 1–review focusing on topographic and chemical properties of different surfaces and in vivo responses to them. *Int. J. Prosthodont.* **2004**, *17*, 536–543. [PubMed]
5. Kulkarni, M.; Mazare, A.; Gongadze, E.; Perutkova, S.; Kralj-Iglic, V.; Milosev, I.; Schmuki, P.; Iglic, A.; Mozetic, M. Titanium nanostructures for biomedical applications. *Nanotechnology* **2015**, *26*, 062002. [CrossRef]
6. Albrektsson, T.; Jemt, T.; Molne, J.; Tengvall, P.; Wennerberg, A. On inflammation-immunological balance theory-A critical apprehension of disease concepts around implants: Mucositis and marginal bone loss may represent normal conditions and not necessarily a state of disease. *Clin. Implant Dent. Relat. Res.* **2019**, *21*, 183–189. [CrossRef]
7. Albrektsson, T.; Chrcanovic, B.; Molne, J.; Wennerberg, A. Foreign body reactions, marginal bone loss and allergies in relation to titanium implants. *Eur. J. Oral Implantol.* **2018**, *11*, S37–S46.
8. Davies, J.E. INVITED COMMENTARY: Is Osseointegration a Foreign Body Reaction? *Int. J. Prosthodont.* **2019**, *32*, 133–136. [CrossRef]
9. Brunski, J. On Implant Prosthodontics: One Narrative, Twelve Voices - 2. *Int. J. Prosthodont.* **2018**, *31*, s15–s22.

10.   Kwon, T.K.; Choi, J.Y.; Park, J.I.; Yeo, I.L. A Clue to the Existence of Bonding between Bone and Implant Surface: An In Vivo Study. *Mater.* **2019**, *12*, 1187. [CrossRef]

11.   Osborn, J.; Newesely, H. Dynamic aspects of the implant-bone interface. *Dental implants* **1980**, *111*, 123.

12.   Branemark, P.I.; Adell, R.; Breine, U.; Hansson, B.O.; Lindstrom, J.; Ohlsson, A. Intra-osseous anchorage of dental prostheses. I. Experimental studies. *Scand. J. Plast. Reconstr. Surg.* **1969**, *3*, 81–100. [CrossRef] [PubMed]

13.   Sims, N.A.; Gooi, J.H. Bone remodeling: Multiple cellular interactions required for coupling of bone formation and resorption. *Semin. Cell Dev. Biol.* **2008**, *19*, 444–451. [CrossRef] [PubMed]

14.   Rupp, F.; Scheideler, L.; Olshanska, N.; de Wild, M.; Wieland, M.; Geis-Gerstorfer, J. Enhancing surface free energy and hydrophilicity through chemical modification of microstructured titanium implant surfaces. *J. Biomed. Mater. Res. A.* **2006**, *76*, 323–334. [CrossRef] [PubMed]

15.   Yeo, I.-S. Surface modification of dental biomaterials for controlling bone response. In *Bone Response to Dental Implant Materials*; Woodhead Publishing: Cambridge, UK, 2017; pp. 43–64.

16.   Rupp, F.; Scheideler, L.; Rehbein, D.; Axmann, D.; Geis-Gerstorfer, J. Roughness induced dynamic changes of wettability of acid etched titanium implant modifications. *Biomaterials* **2004**, *25*, 1429–1438. [CrossRef] [PubMed]

17.   Wall, I.; Donos, N.; Carlqvist, K.; Jones, F.; Brett, P. Modified titanium surfaces promote accelerated osteogenic differentiation of mesenchymal stromal cells in vitro. *Bone* **2009**, *45*, 17–26. [CrossRef]

18.   Buser, D.; Janner, S.F.; Wittneben, J.G.; Bragger, U.; Ramseier, C.A.; Salvi, G.E. 10-year survival and success rates of 511 titanium implants with a sandblasted and acid-etched surface: A retrospective study in 303 partially edentulous patients. *Clin. Implant Dent. Relat. Res.* **2012**, *14*, 839–851. [CrossRef]

19.   Nicolau, P.; Guerra, F.; Reis, R.; Krafft, T.; Benz, K.; Jackowski, J. 10-year outcomes with immediate and early loaded implants with a chemically modified SLA surface. *Quintessence Int.* **2018**, *50*, 2–12.

20.   Roccuzzo, M.; Bonino, L.; Dalmasso, P.; Aglietta, M. Long-term results of a three arms prospective cohort study on implants in periodontally compromised patients: 10-year data around sandblasted and acid-etched (SLA) surface. *Clin. Oral Implants Res.* **2014**, *25*, 1105–1112. [CrossRef]

21.   Rossi, F.; Lang, N.P.; Ricci, E.; Ferraioli, L.; Baldi, N.; Botticelli, D. Long-term follow-up of single crowns supported by short, moderately rough implants-A prospective 10-year cohort study. *Clin. Oral Implants Res.* **2018**, *29*, 1212–1219. [CrossRef]

22.   Van Velzen, F.J.; Ofec, R.; Schulten, E.A.; Ten Bruggenkate, C.M. 10-year survival rate and the incidence of peri-implant disease of 374 titanium dental implants with a SLA surface: A prospective cohort study in 177 fully and partially edentulous patients. *Clin. Oral Implants Res.* **2015**, *26*, 1121–1128. [CrossRef] [PubMed]

23.   Li, S.M.; Yao, W.H.; Liu, J.H.; Yu, M.; Wu, L.; Ma, K. Study on anodic oxidation process and property of composite film formed on Ti-10V-2Fe-3Al alloy in SiC nanoparticle suspension. *Surf. Coat Tech.* **2015**, *277*, 234–241. [CrossRef]

24.   Hanawa, T. Metal ion release from metal implants. *Mat. Sci. Eng. C-Bio. S.* **2004**, *24*, 745–752. [CrossRef]

25.   Manhabosco, T.M.; Tamborim, S.M.; dos Santos, C.B.; Muller, I.L. Tribological, electrochemical and tribo-electrochemical characterization of bare and nitrided Ti6Al4V in simulated body fluid solution. *Corros. Sci.* **2011**, *53*, 1786–1793. [CrossRef]

26.   Wang, J.W.; Ma, Y.; Guan, J.; Zhang, D.W. Characterizations of anodic oxide films formed on Ti6A14V in the silicate electrolyte with sodium polyacrylate as an additive. *Surf. Coat Tech.* **2018**, *338*, 14–21. [CrossRef]

27.   Zhang, L.; Duan, Y.; Gao, R.; Yang, J.; Wei, K.; Tang, D.; Fu, T. The Effect of Potential on Surface Characteristic and Corrosion Resistance of Anodic Oxide Film Formed on Commercial Pure Titanium at the Potentiodynamic-Aging Mode. *Materials* **2019**, *12*, 370. [CrossRef]

28.   Kwon, T.K.; Lee, H.J.; Min, S.K.; Yeo, I.S. Evaluation of early bone response to fluoride-modified and anodically oxidized titanium implants through continuous removal torque analysis. *Implant Dent.* **2012**, *21*, 427–432. [CrossRef]

29.   Lee, H.J.; Yang, I.H.; Kim, S.K.; Yeo, I.S.; Kwon, T.K. In vivo comparison between the effects of chemically modified hydrophilic and anodically oxidized titanium surfaces on initial bone healing. *J. Periodontal. Implant Sci.* **2015**, *45*, 94–100. [CrossRef]

30.   Wennerberg, A.; Albrektsson, T. On implant surfaces: A review of current knowledge and opinions. *Int. J. Oral Maxillofac. Implants.* **2010**, *25*, 63–74.

31. Yeo, I.S.; Han, J.S.; Yang, J.H. Biomechanical and histomorphometric study of dental implants with different surface characteristics. *J. Biomed. Mater. Res. B. Appl. Biomater.* **2008**, *87*, 303–311. [CrossRef]

32. Cooper, L.F. A role for surface topography in creating and maintaining bone at titanium endosseous implants. *J. Prosthet. Dent.* **2000**, *84*, 522–534. [CrossRef] [PubMed]

33. Koh, J.W.; Kim, Y.S.; Yang, J.H.; Yeo, I.S. Effects of a calcium phosphate-coated and anodized titanium surface on early bone response. *Int. J. Oral Maxillofac. Implants.* **2013**, *28*, 790–797. [CrossRef] [PubMed]

34. Yeo, I.S. Reality of dental implant surface modification: A short literature review. *Open Biomed. Eng. J.* **2014**, *8*, 114–119. [CrossRef] [PubMed]

35. Kang, H.K.; Kim, O.B.; Min, S.K.; Jung, S.Y.; Jang, D.H.; Kwon, T.K.; Min, B.M.; Yeo, I.S. The effect of the DLTIDDSYWYRI motif of the human laminin alpha2 chain on implant osseointegration. *Biomaterials* **2013**, *34*, 4027–4037. [CrossRef]

36. Min, S.K.; Kang, H.K.; Jang, D.H.; Jung, S.Y.; Kim, O.B.; Min, B.M.; Yeo, I.S. Titanium surface coating with a laminin-derived functional peptide promotes bone cell adhesion. *Biomed Res Int* **2013**, *2013*, 638348. [CrossRef]

37. Chrcanovic, B.R.; Albrektsson, T.; Wennerberg, A. Turned versus anodised dental implants: A meta-analysis. *J. Oral Rehabil.* **2016**, *43*, 716–728. [CrossRef]

38. Degidi, M.; Nardi, D.; Piattelli, A. 10-year follow-up of immediately loaded implants with TiUnite porous anodized surface. *Clin. Implant. Dent. Relat. Res.* **2012**, *14*, 828–838. [CrossRef]

39. Shibuya, Y.; Kobayashi, M.; Takeuchi, J.; Asai, T.; Murata, M.; Umeda, M.; Komori, T. Analysis of 472 Branemark system TiUnite implants:a retrospective study. *Kobe J. Med. Sci.* **2010**, *55*, E73–E81.

40. Donati, M.; Ekestubbe, A.; Lindhe, J.; Wennstrom, J.L. Marginal bone loss at implants with different surface characteristics - A 20-year follow-up of a randomized controlled clinical trial. *Clin. Oral Implants Res.* **2018**, *29*, 480–487. [CrossRef]

41. Adell, R.; Lekholm, U.; Rockler, B.; Branemark, P.I. A 15-year study of osseointegrated implants in the treatment of the edentulous jaw. *Int. J. Oral Surg.* **1981**, *10*, 387–416. [CrossRef]

42. Rocci, A.; Rocci, M.; Rocci, C.; Scoccia, A.; Gargari, M.; Martignoni, M.; Gottlow, J.; Sennerby, L. Immediate loading of Branemark system TiUnite and machined-surface implants in the posterior mandible, part II: A randomized open-ended 9-year follow-up clinical trial. *Int. J. Oral Maxillofac. Implants.* **2013**, *28*, 891–895. [CrossRef] [PubMed]

43. Li, T.; Gulati, K.; Wang, N.; Zhang, Z.; Ivanovski, S. Understanding and augmenting the stability of therapeutic nanotubes on anodized titanium implants. *Mater. Sci. Eng. C. Mater. Biol. Appl.* **2018**, *88*, 182–195. [CrossRef] [PubMed]

44. Shin, Y.C.; Pang, K.M.; Han, D.W.; Lee, K.H.; Ha, Y.C.; Park, J.W.; Kim, B.; Kim, D.; Lee, J.H. Enhanced osteogenic differentiation of human mesenchymal stem cells on Ti surfaces with electrochemical nanopattern formation. *Mater. Sci. Eng. C. Mater. Biol. Appl.* **2019**, *99*, 1174–1181. [CrossRef] [PubMed]

45. Rice, J.M.; Hunt, J.A.; Gallagher, J.A.; Hanarp, P.; Sutherland, D.S.; Gold, J. Quantitative assessment of the response of primary derived human osteoblasts and macrophages to a range of nanotopography surfaces in a single culture model in vitro. *Biomaterials* **2003**, *24*, 4799–4818. [CrossRef]

46. Wennerberg, A.; Albrektsson, T. Suggested guidelines for the topographic evaluation of implant surfaces. *Int. J. Oral Maxillofac. Implants.* **2000**, *15*, 331–344.

47. Hansson, S.; Norton, M. The relation between surface roughness and interfacial shear strength for bone-anchored implants. A mathematical model. *J. Biomech.* **1999**, *32*, 829–836. [CrossRef]

48. Mendonca, G.; Mendonca, D.B.; Aragao, F.J.; Cooper, L.F. Advancing dental implant surface technology–from micron- to nanotopography. *Biomaterials* **2008**, *29*, 3822–3835. [CrossRef]

49. Liu, H.; Webster, T.J. Nanomedicine for implants: A review of studies and necessary experimental tools. *Biomaterials* **2007**, *28*, 354–369. [CrossRef]

50. Ahn, T.K.; Lee, D.H.; Kim, T.S.; Jang, G.C.; Choi, S.; Oh, J.B.; Ye, G.; Lee, S. Modification of Titanium Implant and Titanium Dioxide for Bone Tissue Engineering. *Adv. Exp. Med. Biol.* **2018**, *1077*, 355–368.

51. Awad, N.K.; Edwards, S.L.; Morsi, Y.S. A review of TiO$_2$ NTs on Ti metal: Electrochemical synthesis, functionalization and potential use as bone implants. *Mater. Sci. Eng. C. Mater. Biol. Appl.* **2017**, *76*, 1401–1412. [CrossRef]

52. Park, J.; Bauer, S.; Schlegel, K.A.; Neukam, F.W.; von der Mark, K.; Schmuki, P. TiO$_2$ nanotube surfaces: 15 nm–an optimal length scale of surface topography for cell adhesion and differentiation. *Small* **2009**, *5*, 666–671. [CrossRef] [PubMed]

53. Oh, S.; Brammer, K.S.; Li, Y.S.; Teng, D.; Engler, A.J.; Chien, S.; Jin, S. Stem cell fate dictated solely by altered nanotube dimension. *Proc. Natl. Acad. Sci. USA* **2009**, *106*, 2130–2135. [CrossRef]

54. Jiang, N.; Du, P.; Qu, W.; Li, L.; Liu, Z.; Zhu, S. The synergistic effect of TiO$_2$ nanoporous modification and platelet-rich plasma treatment on titanium-implant stability in ovariectomized rats. *Int. J. Nanomed.* **2016**, *11*, 4719–4733.

55. Gulati, K.; Ivanovski, S. Dental implants modified with drug releasing titania nanotubes: Therapeutic potential and developmental challenges. *Expert Opin. Drug Deliv.* **2017**, *14*, 1009–1024. [CrossRef] [PubMed]

56. Kwon, D.H.; Lee, S.J.; Wikesjo, U.M.E.; Johansson, P.H.; Johansson, C.B.; Sul, Y.T. Bone tissue response following local drug delivery of bisphosphonate through titanium oxide nanotube implants in a rabbit model. *J. Clin. Periodontol.* **2017**, *44*, 941–949. [CrossRef] [PubMed]

57. Wang, Q.; Huang, J.Y.; Li, H.Q.; Zhao, A.Z.; Wang, Y.; Zhang, K.Q.; Sun, H.T.; Lai, Y.K. Recent advances on smart TiO$_2$ nanotube platforms for sustainable drug delivery applications. *Int. J. Nanomed.* **2017**, *12*, 151–165. [CrossRef]

58. Yang, W.; Deng, C.; Liu, P.; Hu, Y.; Luo, Z.; Cai, K. Sustained release of aspirin and vitamin C from titanium nanotubes: An experimental and stimulation study. *Mater. Sci. Eng. C. Mater. Biol. Appl.* **2016**, *64*, 139–147. [CrossRef]

59. Hamlekhan, A.; Sinha-Ray, S.; Takoudis, C.; Mathew, M.T.; Sukotjo, C.; Yarin, A.L.; Shokuhfar, T. Fabrication of drug eluting implants: Study of drug release mechanism from titanium dioxide nanotubes. *J. Phys. D. Appl. Phys.* **2015**, *48*, 275401. [CrossRef]

60. Aw, M.S.; Gulati, K.; Losic, D. Controlling drug release from titania nanotube arrays using polymer nanocarriers and biopolymer coating. *J. Biomater. Nanobiotechnol.* **2011**, *2*, 477. [CrossRef]

61. Kunrath, M.F.; Leal, B.F.; Hubler, R.; de Oliveira, S.D.; Teixeira, E.R. Antibacterial potential associated with drug-delivery built TiO$_2$ nanotubes in biomedical implants. *AMB Express.* **2019**, *9*, 51. [CrossRef]

62. Miao, X.; Wang, D.; Xu, L.; Wang, J.; Zeng, D.; Lin, S.; Huang, C.; Liu, X.; Jiang, X. The response of human osteoblasts, epithelial cells, fibroblasts, macrophages and oral bacteria to nanostructured titanium surfaces: A systematic study. *Int. J. Nanomed.* **2017**, *12*, 1415–1430. [CrossRef] [PubMed]

63. Gittens, R.A.; Scheideler, L.; Rupp, F.; Hyzy, S.L.; Geis-Gerstorfer, J.; Schwartz, Z.; Boyan, B.D. A review on the wettability of dental implant surfaces II: Biological and clinical aspects. *Acta Biomater.* **2014**, *10*, 2907–2918. [CrossRef] [PubMed]

64. Kulkarni, M.; Patil-Sen, Y.; Junkar, I.; Kulkarni, C.V.; Lorenzetti, M.; Iglic, A. Wettability studies of topologically distinct titanium surfaces. *Colloids Surf. B Biointerfaces* **2015**, *129*, 47–53. [CrossRef] [PubMed]

65. Kaur, G.; Willsmore, T.; Gulati, K.; Zinonos, I.; Wang, Y.; Kurian, M.; Hay, S.; Losic, D.; Evdokiou, A. Titanium wire implants with nanotube arrays: A study model for localized cancer treatment. *Biomaterials* **2016**, *101*, 176–188. [CrossRef]

66. Stephansson, S.N.; Byers, B.A.; Garcia, A.J. Enhanced expression of the osteoblastic phenotype on substrates that modulate fibronectin conformation and integrin receptor binding. *Biomaterials* **2002**, *23*, 2527–2534. [CrossRef]

67. Yeo, I.S.; Min, S.K.; Kang, H.K.; Kwon, T.K.; Jung, S.Y.; Min, B.M. Identification of a bioactive core sequence from human laminin and its applicability to tissue engineering. *Biomaterials* **2015**, *73*, 96–109. [CrossRef]

68. Ryu, J.J.; Park, K.; Kim, H.S.; Jeong, C.M.; Huh, J.B. Effects of anodized titanium with Arg-Gly-Asp (RGD) peptide immobilized via chemical grafting or physical adsorption on bone cell adhesion and differentiation. *Int. J. Oral Maxillofac. Implants.* **2013**, *28*, 963–972. [CrossRef]

69. Kim, S.; Choi, J.Y.; Jung, S.Y.; Kang, H.K.; Min, B.M.; Yeo, I.L. A laminin-derived functional peptide, PPFEGCIWN, promotes bone formation on sandblasted, large-grit, acid-etched titanium implant surfaces. *Int. J. Oral Maxillofac. Implants.* **2019**, *34*, 836–844. [CrossRef]

70. Motlagh, H.N.; Wrabl, J.O.; Li, J.; Hilser, V.J. The ensemble nature of allostery. *Nature* **2014**, *508*, 331–339. [CrossRef]

71. Min, S.K.; Kang, H.K.; Jung, S.Y.; Jang, D.H.; Min, B.M. A vitronectin-derived peptide reverses ovariectomy-induced bone loss via regulation of osteoblast and osteoclast differentiation. *Cell Death Differ.* **2018**, *25*, 268–281. [CrossRef]

72. Rogers, M.B.; Shah, T.A.; Shaikh, N.N. Turning Bone Morphogenetic Protein 2 (BMP2) on and off in Mesenchymal Cells. *J. Cell Biochem.* **2015**, *116*, 2127–2138. [CrossRef] [PubMed]

73. Song, R.; Wang, D.; Zeng, R.; Wang, J. Synergistic effects of fibroblast growth factor-2 and bone morphogenetic protein-2 on bone induction. *Mol. Med. Rep.* **2017**, *16*, 4483–4492. [CrossRef] [PubMed]

74. Kang, J.D. Another complication associated with rhBMP-2? *Spine J.* **2011**, *11*, 517–519. [CrossRef] [PubMed]

75. Kawaguchi, H.; Jingushi, S.; Izumi, T.; Fukunaga, M.; Matsushita, T.; Nakamura, T.; Mizuno, K.; Nakamura, T.; Nakamura, K. Local application of recombinant human fibroblast growth factor-2 on bone repair: A dose-escalation prospective trial on patients with osteotomy. *J. Orthop. Res.* **2007**, *25*, 480–487. [CrossRef]

76. Choi, J.Y.; Jung, U.W.; Kim, C.S.; Jung, S.M.; Lee, I.S.; Choi, S.H. Influence of nanocoated calcium phosphate on two different types of implant surfaces in different bone environment: An animal study. *Clin. Oral Implants Res.* **2013**, *24*, 1018–1022. [CrossRef]

77. Kim, J.E.; Kang, S.S.; Choi, K.H.; Shim, J.S.; Jeong, C.M.; Shin, S.W.; Huh, J.B. The effect of anodized implants coated with combined rhBMP-2 and recombinant human vascular endothelial growth factors on vertical bone regeneration in the marginal portion of the peri-implant. *Oral Surg. Oral Med. Oral Pathol. Oral Radiol.* **2013**, *115*, e24–e31. [CrossRef]

78. Ellingsen, J.E.; Thomsen, P.; Lyngstadaas, S.P. Advances in dental implant materials and tissue regeneration. *Periodontol. 2000.* **2006**, *41*, 136–156. [CrossRef]

79. Bellows, C.G.; Heersche, J.N.; Aubin, J.E. The effects of fluoride on osteoblast progenitors in vitro. *J. Bone Miner. Res.* **1990**, *5*, S101–S105. [CrossRef]

80. Kassem, M.; Mosekilde, L.; Eriksen, E.F. Effects of fluoride on human bone cells in vitro: Differences in responsiveness between stromal osteoblast precursors and mature osteoblasts. *Eur. J. Endocrinol.* **1994**, *130*, 381–386. [CrossRef]

81. Choi, J.Y.; Lee, H.J.; Jang, J.U.; Yeo, I.S. Comparison between bioactive fluoride modified and bioinert anodically oxidized implant surfaces in early bone response using rabbit tibia model. *Implant Dent.* **2012**, *21*, 124–128. [CrossRef]

82. Choi, J.Y.; Kang, S.H.; Kim, H.Y.; Yeo, I.L. Control variable implants improve interpretation of surface modification and implant design effects on early bone responses: An in vivo study. *Int. J. Oral Maxillofac. Implants.* **2018**, *33*, 1033–1040. [CrossRef] [PubMed]

83. Ellingsen, J.E. Pre-treatment of titanium implants with fluoride improves their retention in bone. *J. Mater. Sci-Mater. M.* **1995**, *6*, 749–753. [CrossRef]

84. Ellingsen, J.E.; Johansson, C.B.; Wennerberg, A.; Holmen, A. Improved retention and bone-to-implant contact with fluoride-modified titanium implants. *Int. J. Oral Max. Impl.* **2004**, *19*, 659–666.

85. Hong, Y.S.; Kim, M.J.; Han, J.S.; Yeo, I.S. Effects of hydrophilicity and fluoride surface modifications to titanium dental implants on early osseointegration: An in vivo study. *Implant Dent.* **2014**, *2*, 529–533. [CrossRef] [PubMed]

86. Taxt-Lamolle, S.F.; Rubert, M.; Haugen, H.J.; Lyngstadaas, S.P.; Ellingsen, J.E.; Monjo, M. Controlled electro-implementation of fluoride in titanium implant surfaces enhances cortical bone formation and mineralization. *Acta Biomater.* **2010**, *6*, 1025–1032. [CrossRef]

87. Windael, S.; Vervaeke, S.; Wijnen, L.; Jacquet, W.; De Bruyn, H.; Collaert, B. Ten-year follow-up of dental implants used for immediate loading in the edentulous mandible: A prospective clinical study. *Clin. Implant Dent. Relat. Res.* **2018**, *20*, 515–521. [CrossRef]

88. Mertens, C.; Steveling, H.G. Early and immediate loading of titanium implants with fluoride-modified surfaces: Results of 5-year prospective study. *Clin. Oral Implants Res.* **2011**, *22*, 1354–1360. [CrossRef]

89. Oxby, G.; Oxby, F.; Oxby, J.; Saltvik, T.; Nilsson, P. Early loading of fluoridated implants placed in fresh extraction sockets and healed bone: A 3- to 5-year clinical and radiographic follow-up study of 39 consecutive patients. *Clin. Implant Dent. Relat. Res.* **2015**, *17*, 898–907. [CrossRef]

90. Xuereb, M.; Camilleri, J.; Attard, N.J. Systematic review of current dental implant coating materials and novel coating techniques. *Int. J. Prosthodont.* **2015**, *28*, 51–59. [CrossRef]

91. Alizadeh-Osgouei, M.; Li, Y.; Wen, C. A comprehensive review of biodegradable synthetic polymer-ceramic composites and their manufacture for biomedical applications. *Bioact. Mater.* **2019**, *4*, 22–36. [CrossRef]

92. Sun, L.; Berndt, C.C.; Gross, K.A.; Kucuk, A. Material fundamentals and clinical performance of plasma-sprayed hydroxyapatite coatings: A review. *J. Biomed. Mater. Res.* **2001**, *58*, 570–592. [CrossRef]

93. You, C.; Yeo, I.S.; Kim, M.D.; Eom, T.K.; Lee, J.Y.; Kim, S. Characterization and in vivo evaluation of calcium phosphate coated cp-titanium by dip-spin method. *Curr. Appl. Phys.* **2005**, *5*, 501–506. [CrossRef]

94. Gupta, A.; Dhanraj, M.; Sivagami, G. Status of surface treatment in endosseous implant: A literary overview. *Indian J. Dent. Res.* **2010**, *21*, 433–438. [CrossRef] [PubMed]

95. Geesink, R.G.; de Groot, K.; Klein, C.P. Bonding of bone to apatite-coated implants. *J. Bone Joint Surg. Br.* **1988**, *70*, 17–22. [CrossRef] [PubMed]

96. Manero, J.M.; Salsench, J.; Nogueras, J.; Aparicio, C.; Padros, A.; Balcells, M.; Gil, F.J.; Planell, J.A. Growth of bioactive surfaces on dental implants. *Implant Dent.* **2002**, *11*, 170–175. [CrossRef] [PubMed]

97. Dalton, J.E.; Cook, S.D. In vivo mechanical and histological characteristics of HA-coated implants vary with coating vendor. *J. Biomed. Mater. Res.* **1995**, *29*, 239–245. [CrossRef]

98. Ducheyne, P.; Healy, K.E. The effect of plasma-sprayed calcium phosphate ceramic coatings on the metal ion release from porous titanium and cobalt-chromium alloys. *J Biomed Mater Res* **1988**, *22*, 1137–1163. [CrossRef]

99. Ducheyne, P.; Hench, L.L.; Kagan, A., II; Martens, M.; Bursens, A.; Mulier, J.C. Effect of hydroxyapatite impregnation on skeletal bonding of porous coated implants. *J. Biomed. Mater. Res.* **1980**, *14*, 225–237. [CrossRef]

100. Oonishi, H.; Yamamoto, M.; Ishimaru, H.; Tsuji, E.; Kushitani, S.; Aono, M.; Ukon, Y. The effect of hydroxyapatite coating on bone growth into porous titanium alloy implants. *J. Bone Joint Surg. Br.* **1989**, *71*, 213–216. [CrossRef]

101. Yeo, I.S.; Min, S.K.; An, Y. Influence of bioactive material coating of Ti dental implant surfaces on early healing and osseointegration of bone. *J. Korean Phys. Soc.* **2010**, *57*, 1717–1720. [CrossRef]

102. Yeung, W.K.; Reilly, G.C.; Matthews, A.; Yerokhin, A. In vitro biological response of plasma electrolytically oxidized and plasma-sprayed hydroxyapatite coatings on Ti-6Al-4V alloy. *J. Biomed. Mater. Res. B Appl. Biomater.* **2013**, *101*, 939–949. [CrossRef]

103. Wennerberg, A.; Jimbo, R.; Allard, S.; Skarnemark, G.; Andersson, M. In vivo stability of hydroxyapatite nanoparticles coated on titanium implant surfaces. *Int. J. Oral Maxillofac. Implants.* **2011**, *26*, 1161–1166.

104. Ostman, P.O.; Wennerberg, A.; Ekestubbe, A.; Albrektsson, T. Immediate occlusal loading of NanoTite tapered implants: A prospective 1-year clinical and radiographic study. *Clin. Implant Dent. Relat. Res.* **2013**, *15*, 809–818. [CrossRef]

105. Oztel, M.; Bilski, W.M.; Bilski, A. Risk factors associated with dental implant failure: A study of 302 implants placed in a regional center. *J. Contemp. Dent. Pract.* **2017**, *18*, 705–709. [CrossRef]

106. Van Oirschot, B.A.; Bronkhorst, E.M.; van den Beucken, J.J.; Meijer, G.J.; Jansen, J.A.; Junker, R. A systematic review on the long-term success of calcium phosphate plasma-spray-coated dental implants. *Odontology* **2016**, *104*, 347–356. [CrossRef]

107. Artzi, Z.; Carmeli, G.; Kozlovsky, A. A distinguishable observation between survival and success rate outcome of hydroxyapatite-coated implants in 5–10 years in function. *Clin. Oral Implants Res.* **2006**, *17*, 85–93. [CrossRef]

108. Binahmed, A.; Stoykewych, A.; Hussain, A.; Love, B.; Pruthi, V. Long-term follow-up of hydroxyapatite-coated dental implants–a clinical trial. *Int. J. Oral Maxillofac. Implants.* **2007**, *22*, 963–968.

109. Schwartz-Arad, D.; Mardinger, O.; Levin, L.; Kozlovsky, A.; Hirshberg, A. Marginal bone loss pattern around hydroxyapatite-coated versus commercially pure titanium implants after up to 12 years of follow-up. *Int. J. Oral Maxillofac. Implants.* **2005**, *20*, 238–244.

110. Wang, R.; Hashimoto, K.; Fujishima, A.; Chikuni, M.; Kojima, E.; Kitamura, A.; Shimohigoshi, M.; Watanabe, T. Light-induced amphiphilic surfaces. *Nature* **1997**, *388*, 431–432. [CrossRef]

111. Att, W.; Hori, N.; Takeuchi, M.; Ouyang, J.; Yang, Y.; Anpo, M.; Ogawa, T. Time-dependent degradation of titanium osteoconductivity: An implication of biological aging of implant materials. *Biomaterials* **2009**, *30*, 5352–5363. [CrossRef]

112. Flanagan, D. Photofunctionalization of dental implants. *J. Oral Implantol.* **2016**, *42*, 445–450. [CrossRef]

113. Clydesdale, G.J.; Dandie, G.W.; Muller, H.K. Ultraviolet light induced injury: Immunological and inflammatory effects. *Immunol. Cell Biol.* **2001**, *79*, 547–568. [CrossRef]

114. Aita, H.; Att, W.; Ueno, T.; Yamada, M.; Hori, N.; Iwasa, F.; Tsukimura, N.; Ogawa, T. Ultraviolet light-mediated photofunctionalization of titanium to promote human mesenchymal stem cell migration, attachment, proliferation and differentiation. *Acta Biomater.* **2009**, *5*, 3247–3257. [CrossRef]

115. Jain, S.; Williamson, R.S.; Marquart, M.; Janorkar, A.V.; Griggs, J.A.; Roach, M.D. Photofunctionalization of anodized titanium surfaces using UVA or UVC light and its effects against Streptococcus sanguinis. *J. Biomed. Mater. Res. B Appl. Biomater.* **2018**, *106*, 2284–2294. [CrossRef]

116. Jansen, E.J.; Sladek, R.E.; Bahar, H.; Yaffe, A.; Gijbels, M.J.; Kuijer, R.; Bulstra, S.K.; Guldemond, N.A.; Binderman, I.; Koole, L.H. Hydrophobicity as a design criterion for polymer scaffolds in bone tissue engineering. *Biomaterials* **2005**, *26*, 4423–4431. [CrossRef]

117. Ogawa, T. Ultraviolet photofunctionalization of titanium implants. *Int. J. Oral Maxillofac. Implants.* **2014**, *29*, e95–e102. [CrossRef]

118. Aita, H.; Hori, N.; Takeuchi, M.; Suzuki, T.; Yamada, M.; Anpo, M.; Ogawa, T. The effect of ultraviolet functionalization of titanium on integration with bone. *Biomaterials* **2009**, *30*, 1015–1025. [CrossRef]

119. Park, K.H.; Koak, J.Y.; Kim, S.K.; Han, C.H.; Heo, S.J. The effect of ultraviolet-C irradiation via a bactericidal ultraviolet sterilizer on an anodized titanium implant: A study in rabbits. *Int. J. Oral Maxillofac. Implants.* **2013**, *28*, 57–66. [CrossRef]

120. Lee, J.B.; Jo, Y.H.; Choi, J.Y.; Seol, Y.J.; Lee, Y.M.; Ku, Y.; Rhyu, I.C.; Yeo, I.L. The effect of ultraviolet photofunctionalization on a titanium dental implant with machined surface: An in vitro and in vivo study. *Materials* **2019**, *12*, 2078. [CrossRef]

121. Hirota, M.; Ozawa, T.; Iwai, T.; Ogawa, T.; Tohnai, I. Implant stability development of photofunctionalized implants placed in regular and complex cases: A case-control study. *Int. J. Oral Maxillofac. Implants.* **2016**, *31*, 676–686. [CrossRef]

122. Funato, A.; Yamada, M.; Ogawa, T. Success rate, healing time, and implant stability of photofunctionalized dental implants. *Int. J. Oral Maxillofac. Implants.* **2013**, *28*, 1261–1271. [CrossRef]

123. Hirota, M.; Ozawa, T.; Iwai, T.; Ogawa, T.; Tohnai, I. Effect of photofunctionalization on early implant failure. *Int. J. Oral Maxillofac. Implants.* **2018**, *33*, 1098–1102. [CrossRef]

124. Asensio, G.; Vazquez-Lasa, B.; Rojo, L. Achievements in the Topographic Design of Commercial Titanium Dental Implants: Towards Anti-Peri-Implantitis Surfaces. *J. Clin. Med.* **2019**, *8*, 1982. [CrossRef]

125. Smeets, R.; Stadlinger, B.; Schwarz, F.; Beck-Broichsitter, B.; Jung, O.; Precht, C.; Kloss, F.; Grobe, A.; Heiland, M.; Ebker, T. Impact of Dental Implant Surface Modifications on Osseointegration. *Biomed. Res. Int.* **2016**, *2016*, 6285620. [CrossRef]

126. Souza, J.C.M.; Sordi, M.B.; Kanazawa, M.; Ravindran, S.; Henriques, B.; Silva, F.S.; Aparicio, C.; Cooper, L.F. Nano-scale modification of titanium implant surfaces to enhance osseointegration. *Acta Biomater.* **2019**, *94*, 112–131. [CrossRef]

127. Iorio-Siciliano, V.; Matarasso, R.; Guarnieri, R.; Nicolo, M.; Farronato, D.; Matarasso, S. Soft tissue conditions and marginal bone levels of implants with a laser-microtextured collar: A 5-year, retrospective, controlled study. *Clin. Oral Implants Res.* **2015**, *26*, 257–262. [CrossRef]

128. Degidi, M.; Piattelli, A.; Scarano, A.; Shibli, J.A.; Iezzi, G. Peri-implant collagen fibers around human cone Morse connection implants under polarized light: A report of three cases. *Int. J. Periodontics Restorative Dent.* **2012**, *32*, 323–328.

129. Nevins, M.; Kim, D.M.; Jun, S.H.; Guze, K.; Schupbach, P.; Nevins, M.L. Histologic evidence of a connective tissue attachment to laser microgrooved abutments: A canine study. *Int. J. Periodontics Restorative Dent.* **2010**, *30*, 245–255.

130. Guarnieri, R.; Placella, R.; Testarelli, L.; Iorio-Siciliano, V.; Grande, M. Clinical, radiographic, and esthetic evaluation of immediately loaded laser microtextured implants placed into fresh extraction sockets in the anterior maxilla: A 2-year retrospective multicentric study. *Implant Dent.* **2014**, *23*, 144–154. [CrossRef]

131. Guarnieri, R.; Grande, M.; Ippoliti, S.; Iorio-Siciliano, V.; Riccitiello, F.; Farronato, D. Influence of a Laser-Lok Surface on Immediate Functional Loading of Implants in Single-Tooth Replacement: Three-Year Results of a Prospective Randomized Clinical Study on Soft Tissue Response and Esthetics. *Int. J. Periodontics Restorative Dent.* **2015**, *35*, 865–875. [CrossRef]

132. Farronato, D.; Mangano, F.; Briguglio, F.; Iorio-Siciliano, V.; Riccitiello, F.; Guarnieri, R. Influence of Laser-Lok surface on immediate functional loading of implants in single-tooth replacement: A 2-year prospective clinical study. *Int. J. Periodontics Restorative Dent.* **2014**, *34*, 79–89. [CrossRef]

133. Kunrath, M.F.; Hubler, R. A bone preservation protocol that enables evaluation of osseointegration of implants with micro- and nanotextured surfaces. *Biotech. Histochem.* **2019**, *94*, 261–270. [CrossRef]

9

Survival Probability, Weibull Characteristics, Stress Distribution and Fractographic Analysis of Polymer-Infiltrated Ceramic Network Restorations Cemented on a Chairside Titanium Base: An In Vitro and In Silico Study

João P. M. Tribst [1,*], Amanda M. O. Dal Piva [1], Alexandre L. S. Borges [1], Lilian C. Anami [2], Cornelis J. Kleverlaan [3] and Marco A. Bottino [1]

[1] Department of Dental Materials and Prosthodontics, São Paulo State University (Unesp/SJC), Institute of Science and Technology, São José dos Campos 12245-000, Brazil; amodalpiva@gmail.com (A.M.O.D.P.); alexandre.borges@unesp.br (A.L.S.B.); marco.bottino@unesp.br (M.A.B.)

[2] Department of Dentistry, Santo Amaro University (UNISA), São Paulo 04743-030, Brazil; lianami@gmail.com

[3] Department of Dental Materials Science, Academic Centre for Dentistry Amsterdam (ACTA), Universiteit van Amsterdam and Vrije Universiteit, 1081 LA Amsterdam, The Netherlands; c.kleverlaan@acta.nl

* Correspondence: joao.tribst@gmail.com

Abstract: Different techniques are available to manufacture polymer-infiltrated ceramic restorations cemented on a chairside titanium base. To compare the influence of these techniques in the mechanical response, 75 implant-supported crowns were divided in three groups: CME (crown cemented on a mesostructure), a two-piece prosthetic solution consisting of a crown and hybrid abutment; MC (monolithic crown), a one-piece prosthetic solution consisting of a crown; and MP (monolithic crown with perforation), a one-piece prosthetic solution consisting of a crown with a screw access hole. All specimens were stepwise fatigued (50 N in each 20,000 cycles until 1200 N and 350,000 cycles). The failed crowns were inspected under scanning electron microscopy. The finite element method was applied to analyze mechanical behavior under 300 N axial load. Log-Rank ($p = 0.17$) and Wilcoxon ($p = 0.11$) tests revealed similar survival probability at 300 and 900 N. Higher stress concentration was observed in the crowns' emergence profiles. The MP and CME techniques showed similar survival and can be applied to manufacture an implant-supported crown. In all groups, the stress concentration associated with fractographic analysis suggests that the region of the emergence profile should always be evaluated due to the high prevalence of failures in this area.

Keywords: dental implant–abutment design; dental implants; dental materials; finite element analysis; material testing; ceramics

1. Introduction

Restorations performed using the computer-aided design and manufacturing facility (CAD/CAM) became increasingly popular in dental applications [1]. Due to the wide variety, CAD/CAM materials could be generally divided into two main categories: ceramics and composites [2]. Comparing both categories, indirect composite restorations are more resilient, easier to finish and polish, less abrasive to the antagonist, and allow an easy occlusal adjustment [3]. In contrast, the ceramic restorations present better biocompatibility, superior aesthetics, greater wear resistance and greater color stability [4].

Combining the positive properties of CAD/CAM ceramics and composite materials, a hybrid material was developed, which is also known as a polymer-infiltrated ceramic network (PIC) [5]. This material has a relatively low elastic modulus compared to conventional ceramics [6], besides presenting better marginal integrity and machinability [7]. Among the available CAD/CAM blocks from this new class of materials, the Vita Enamic (Vita Zahnfabrick, Bad Säckingen, Germany) stands out for its better long-term color stability [1] and the ability to deform during a load application prior to fracture [8], which ensures proper aesthetics and strength for the rehabilitation. These characteristics are a consequence of the feldspar ceramic involved in a resin matrix [9] based in urethane dimethacrylate (UDMA) and triethylene glycol dimethacrylate (TEGDMA) [5]. The ceramic portion consists of 58–63% of SiO_2, 20–23% of Al_2O_3, 9–11% of Na_2O, 0.5–2% de B_2O_3, and less than 1% of Zr_2O and CaO [10]. This combination provides adequate wear resistance, flexural strength, and elastic modulus close to dentine tissue [2,11,12]. PICs also have a hardness value between dentin and enamel [11], a maximum fracture load near 2000 N [13], and longitudinal clinical reports with high success rates [14,15]. In observing implant-supported prosthesis, the manufacture of metal–ceramic restorations is defined as the gold standard for prosthetic rehabilitation [16]. However, the monolithic crowns in PIC appear to be a reliable option [16].

Despite the reliability of implant-supported PIC restorations for cemented full-crown design, implant dentistry could present different limitations and aesthetics requirements [17]. Sometimes, the use of a conventional titanium abutment to link the crown and the implant could not be the ideal digital workflow [18]. Since the titanium is a metallic substrate, this abutment can generate a gray zone effect on the peri-implant marginal mucosa [19]. To reduce this effect, the hybrid abutment emerged as an alternative to be used to link the ceramic crown and the implant [20]. The hybrid abutment consists of two parts: a titanium base (Tibase) and ceramic mesostructure. The first one is responsible for keeping the connection between the implant and abutment in metal, and the second one is responsible for improving the peri-implant mucosa aesthetics [20–26]. For this technique, the crown is indicated to be cemented on the mesostructure (two-piece design).

To manufacture the mesostructure, the ceramic blocks containing a central hole (implant-solution CAD/CAM blocks) are required to allow the connection with the Tibase and the screw access to the implant. The literature reports the possibility of performing mesostructures in zirconia, lithium disilicate [20,25,27] and PIC [22–24,28]. The implant solution CAD/CAM blocks also can be machined as a crown without the mesostructure. This approach named one-piece design [29] simplifies the chairside process, requires the use of only one CAD/CAM block, and allows the manufacture of screw-retained crowns [20,28,29]. The comparison of the load-to-fracture of these two designs was performed for zirconia and lithium disilicate restorations [20,26,27]. However, it is well known that dental ceramics fail under fatigue, in consequence of the slow crack growth in stressed areas [30,31]. For this reason, this study investigated the survival probability, Weibull characteristics, and stress distribution of PIC crowns cemented on a chairside titanium base manufactured using different techniques. The null hypothesis was that there would be no difference between the designs for the analyzed parameters.

2. Materials and Methods

2.1. Specimens Preparations

Seventy-five (75) morse-taper implants (Conexão Sistemas de Prótese, Arujá, SP, Brazil) were installed in polyurethane resin, which is a validated material to simulate the bone tissue in in vitro studies due to its elastic behavior and stiffness [32]. For that, the polyurethane resin was manipulated using an identical volume of base and catalyst homogenized in a rubber bowl. The mixture was poured into (25 × 20 mm) polyvinyl chloride cylindrical support. After the complete resin cure, the polyurethane surface was polished with silicon carbide papers (P600 and P1200) under water cooling in an orbital gridding machine (Buehler, Ecomet 250, Lake Bluff, IL, USA). A sequence of surgical drills was used, according to the manufacturer's indication (Conexão Sistemas de Prótese,

Arujá, SP, Brazil), to make a synthetic surgical alveolus perpendicular to the surface and centered in the polyurethane cylinder. In each cylinder, with the aid of a manual torque wrench, the implants (4.1 × 10 mm) were installed (40 N·cm) keeping 3 mm of the implant not embedded in the resin, following the ISO 14801:2016 for mechanical implant testing.

All Tibases (Conexão Sistemas de Prótese, Arujá, Brazil) were sandblasted with 50 μm aluminum oxide (Al_2O_3) particles at a pressure of 1.5 bar, using an implant analog to assist the laboratorial handling. After, they were cleaned in an ultrasonic bath (5 min with isopropyl alcohol) and received a layer of Alloy Primer (Kuraray Noritake Dental Inc., Okayama, Japan) for 60 s. All titanium bases surfaces were gently blow dried, and the screw access holes were protected with a Teflon tape. A thin layer of titanium dioxide-based powder (Ivoclar Vivadent, Schaan, Liechtenstein) was sprayed onto each of the titanium bases for scanning (inEos Blue, inLab SW4.2, Sirona, Benshein, Germany) and subsequent restorations manufacture. The sets were randomly divided into three experimental groups ($n = 25$), according to the prosthesis manufacturing technique.

2.1.1. Crown Cemented on a Mesostructure (CME) Prosthesis Design: Two-Piece Prosthetic Solution Composed by a Crown Cemented on the Hybrid Abutment

In this technique, the first structure to be manufactured is the mesostructure. For that, the inLab software (Sirona Dental Systems, Bensheim, Alemanha) was used to design the mesostructure and its insertion axis. The data were sent to the equipment Cerec inLab (5884742 D329, Sirona for Dental Systems, Benshelm, Germany), and 25 structures were milled using Vita Enamic IS-14 blocks (Vita Zahnfabrik, Bad Säckingen, Germany) that contain a central access hole. The mesostructures were separated from the remaining blocks with the aid of a diamond blade and fine-grained diamond bur under abundant irrigation. Next, the mesostructures were polished with pink (10,000 rpm) and gray rubbers (8000 rpm) from a Vita Enamic Polishing Set (Vita Zahnfabrick) and cleaned in an ultrasonic bath (5 min in distilled water) to remove debris from the polishing rubbers or surface contaminant that may interfere on the adhesive procedure. To complete the hybrid abutment (mesostructure + Tibase), the mesostructure intaglio surface received a silane agent (Clearfill Ceramic Primer, Kuraray Noritake Dental Inc., Okayama, Japan) for 60 s. The self-etching resin cement (Panavia F 2.0, Kuraray Noritake Dental Inc., Okayama, Japan) was manipulated and applied on the Tibase and the mesostructure, which were held in position with 750 g. The excess cement was removed with a microbrush and light cured (Valo, Ultradent Products, South Jordan, UT, USA) following the manufacturer instructions. The hybrid abutments were installed on the implants with 30 N·cm torque. Next, the mesostructures were scanned for conventional full crown preparations. Then, twenty-five (25) crowns were designed, milled in PIC blocks, polished, and cemented on the hybrid abutment (Figure 1). Both cementation lines were polished with the Vita ENAMIC polishing kit at 5000 rpm.

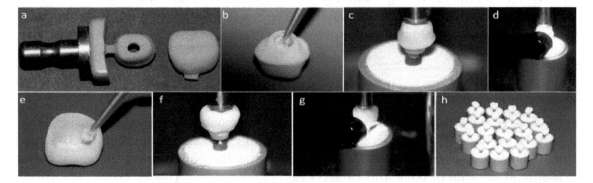

Figure 1. (**a**) Mesostructure machined in implant solution block and monolithic crown machined in conventional block. (**b**) Silanization of the internal surface of the mesostructure. (**c**) Luting of the mesostructure on the titanium base (Tibase) using self-etching resin cement. (**d**) Photoactivation of resin cement. (**e**) Crown silanization. (**f**) Luting of the crown on the mesostructure. (**g**) Light curing. (**h**) Crown cemented on a mesostructure (CME) group crowns completed.

2.1.2. Monolithic Crown (MC) Prosthesis Design: One-Piece Prosthetic Solution Composed by a Crown Direct Cemented on a Titanium Base

In this technique, first, the Tibases were installed on the implants with 30 N·cm torque. Then, the crowns were designed, polished, cleaned, and cemented directly on the Tibases as a conventional abutment. The cementation line was polished with the Vita Enamic polishing kit at 5000 rpm (Figure 2).

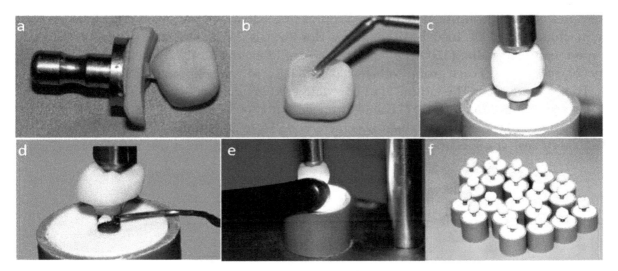

Figure 2. (**a**) Monolithic crown machined in conventional block; (**b**) Silanization of the internal surface of the crown; (**c**) Luting of the crown on the titanium base (Tibase) using self-etching resin cement; (**d**) Removal of excess cement; (**e**) Light curing; (**f**) MC group crowns completed.

2.1.3. MP Prosthesis Design: One-Piece Prosthetic Solution Composed by a Crown Cemented on a Tibase with Screw Access Hole

For the monolithic crown with perforation (MP) group, the crowns were manufactured in one piece using Vita ENAMIC IS-16 blocks (Vita Zahnfabrik, Bad Säckingen, Germany). The crowns with the occlusal perforation were polished, cleaned, and cemented on the Tibases. Through the screw access hole, the sets (crown and Tibase) were positioned on the implants and with a manual torque wrench fixed with 30 N·cm of torque. For each specimen, the screw access hole was conditioned with 5% hydrofluoric acid for 60 s, washed with a water jet for 20 s, and dried with air jets. Then, the bonding agent was applied, and the access was sealed with composite resin. The cementation line and the composite resin interface were polished with a polishing kit (Vita Zahnfabrik, Bad Säckingen, Germany) at 5000 rpm (Figure 3).

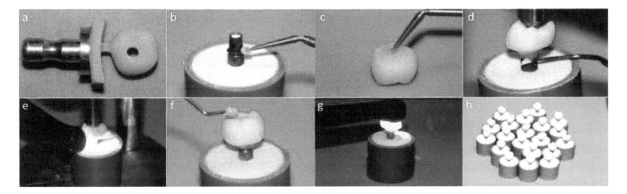

Figure 3. (**a**) Monolithic crown machined in an implant solution block; (**b**) Alloy primer application in the titanium base (Tibase); (**c**) Silanization of the internal surface of the crown; (**d**) Removal of excess cement; (**e**) Light curing; (**f**) Sealing of the screw access hole with composite resin; (**g**) Monolithic crown with perforation; (**h**) (MP) group crowns completed.

For all groups, the crowns (Vita ENAMIC, Vita Zahnfabrik, Bad Säckingen, Germany) were manufactured with identical anatomy, minimum occlusal thickness at 1 mm, 0.8 mm cervical wall around the base, 0.4 mm cervical terminus, and 80 μm space for the cement layer.

2.2. Fatigue Test

The specimens were stored in distilled water for a period of 24 h prior to the fatigue test. Five samples of each group were submitted to the single load to fracture test (SLF) in an universal testing machine (EMIC DL 1000, EMIC, São José dos Pinhais, PR; 1 mm/min speed, 1000 kgf load cell). From the mean load value (1200 N), the fatigue profile used in the stepwise test was determined. Twenty (20) specimens of each group were tested until failure in an adapted fatigue tester (Fatigue Tester, ACTA, The Netherlands). The fatigue load was delivered (6 mm diameter, stainless steel, water, 25 °C, 1.4 Hz) on the occlusal fossa [13,33]. The test started with 300 N during 5000 cycles (40% of the SLF). After each step of 20,000 cycles, the load was increased [34] in 50 N until the maximum load of 1200 N and 350,000 cycles. The specimens were checked for cracks and/or fractures in each step (Figure 4).

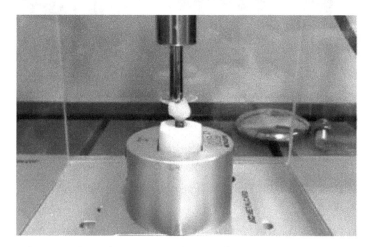

Figure 4. Sample positioned to perform the survival test.

2.3. Fractographic Analysis

The failures were classified according to the patterns obtained after the fatigue test [33,34]. To determine the fracture features methodologically, the ceramic fragments were evaluated to identify the direction of crack propagation and location of the origin [33–35] with the aid of a stereomicroscope (Stereo Discovery.V20, Carl Zeiss, LLC, USA). For that, the regions of interest were divided into quadrants, and the representative specimens were subjected to photomicrographs of greater magnification in each of these quadrants by scanning electron microscopy (SEM). For this, the specimens were cleaned in an ultrasonic bath with isopropyl alcohol for 10 min, dried, gold sputtered, and analyzed under scanning electron microscopy (SEM; Evo LS15, Oberkochen, Carl Zeiss, Germany) to identify the size and origin of the critical defect. The micrographies were merged to enable the crown fractographic analysis overview.

2.4. Nonlinear Finite Element Analysis

The three-dimensional (3D) industrial designs of the implant, Tibase, and prosthetic screw were provided by the manufacturer as stereolitographic files (Conexão Sistemas de Prótese, Arujá, Brazil) and imported to the modeling software (Rhinoceros version 5.0 SR8, McNeel North America, Seattle, WA, USA). Then, through automatic reverse engineering, the polygonal models were converted into 3D models formed by NURBS (Non Uniform Rational Basis Spline). In sequence, a cylinder was created corresponding to the in vitro polyurethane cylinder (20 × 25 mm). Then, the implant was centered perpendicularly to the cylinder, containing 3 mm of exposed threads similar to the in vitro test. A Boolean difference was used to ensure the juxtaposition between these structures. The model finished as a volumetric solid containing an implant, Tibase, screw, and fixation cylinder was tripled to obtain three models with identical geometries.

One specimen from each in vitro group was scanned and exported in STL format. The crowns' 3D models were submitted to the BioCad protocol [36] to perform a volumetric model whose geometry corresponded exactly to the in vitro specimens. Then, this same procedure was repeated to create the mesostructure 3D model. All cement layers were standardized with 80 μm.

For a static structural analysis, the models were checked and imported as a STEP file to the analysis software (ANSYS 17.2, ANSYS Inc., Houston, TX, USA). The contacts were considered nonlinear, containing 0.30 μ friction between the structures in titanium [36]. The number of tangent faces between solids was equivalent to assist the analysis convergence. Through an automatic creation, an initial mesh with tetrahedral elements was created; the absence of mesh defined as obsolete by the software was verified prior to final mesh refinement (Figure 5). The 10% convergence test was used to determine the mesh control to ensure the least possible influence on the results of the mathematical calculation [37–39]. Each piece of material information was inserted for each solid component in isotropic and homogeneous behavior, requiring the modulus of elasticity and Poisson ratio (Table 1) [5,39–41]. During contour definitions, the loading was performed in the occlusal region of the crown. The applied load was 300 N (Figure 5a) on the Z-axis [23]. The fixation location was defined under the surface of the polyurethane cylinder, simulating the sample holder in one plane (Figure 5b). A pre-tension was also applied with 30 N simulating the torque (Figure 5d) during the prosthetic screw tightening [42].

Table 1. Mechanical properties of the materials used in this study.

Material	Elastic Modulus (GPa)	Poisson Ratio	Reference
Titanium	110	0.33	[39]
Polymer infiltrated ceramic	30	0.28	[5]
Polyurethane	3.6	0.3	[40]
Resin cement	18.3	0.3	[41]

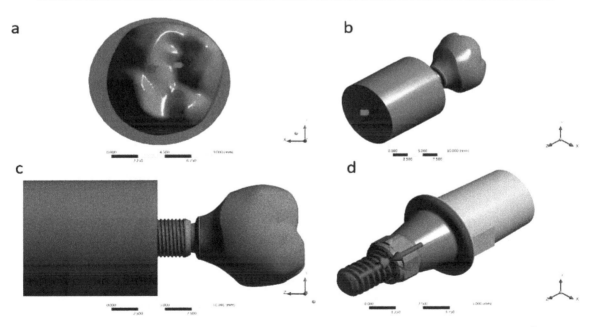

Figure 5. (**a**) Occlusal loading; (**b**) Fixing the system; (**c**) Mesh generated; (**d**) Pre-tension of 30 N·cm.

The composite resin shrinkage for sealing the screw access hole in the MC group was simulated simultaneously in the analysis using the thermal analogy [43]. The solutions were obtained in total deformation, von-Misses stress, maximum principal stress, and microstrain, for each group. The results were presented on an identical scale of values for visual comparison, as well as the absolute values were plotted on graphs for quantitative analysis of the peaks.

2.5. Data Analysis

Survival data were statistically analyzed by Kaplan–Meier and Mantel–Cox tests (Log-Rank and Wilcoxon tests) [44]. Data distribution and reliability analysis were assessed by Weibull analysis associated with two parameters: shape and scale showing the probability distribution of the material to fail in a certain fatigue time using the statistical software (Minitab 16.1.0, State College, PA, USA), with 95% confidence interval. The results obtained in the finite element analysis were exposed and descriptively evaluated through color graphics corresponding to the stress concentration.

3. Results

3.1. Fatigue Test

Weibull analysis showed difference between the mean values of characteristic strength according to the groups (Table 2). Weibull probability plots versus number of cycles reported at the sample failure during the fatigue test are present in Figures 6 and 7. Log-Rank ($p = 0.17$) and Wilcoxon ($p = 0.11$) revealed a similar survival probability between the manufacturing techniques at 300 N and 900 N, according to the confidence interval. However, at 600 N, MP group showed higher survival probability than the MC group, whereas the CME group showed an intermediate behavior (Table 2).

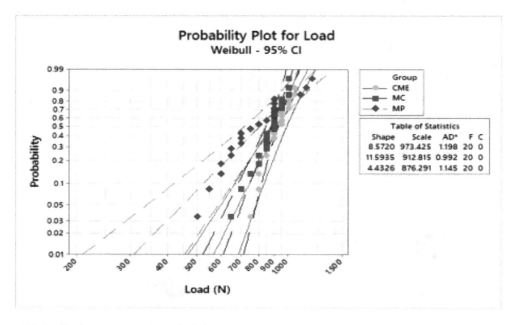

Figure 6. Weibull plot: survival probability versus load (N) reported on sample failure during the fatigue test.

Table 2. Crowns survival in fatigue at different load missions.

Survival Probability (%)		MP	MC	CME
300 N	Upper bound	88	87	85
	Average	84 A	82 A	80 A
	Lower bound	79	77	74
600 N	Upper bound	50	36	40
	Average	44 A	30 B	33 AB
	Lower bound	37	24	27
900 N	Upper bound	7	6	9
	Average	5 A	1 A	6 A
	Lower bound	2	0.5	3

Similar capital letters correspond to no statistical significance between groups in the same row, according to the confidence interval.

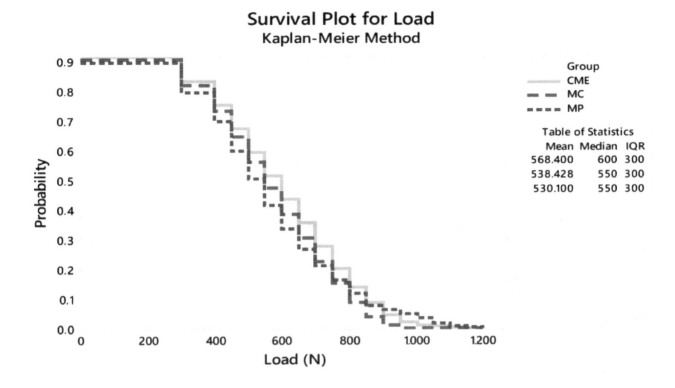

Figure 7. Survival plot using the Kaplan–Meier method.

Regardless of the similar survival and characteristic strength between CME and MP, MP showed lower data variation, being the most reliable technique (Table 3).

Table 3. Weibull modulus (m), characteristic strength (σ), and confidence intervals. The statistical differences were determined based on the confidence interval (CI).

Groups	m (CI)	σ (CI)
MP	8.5 (6.2–1.6)	973.4 (921.9–1027.7)
CME	4.4 (3.2–6.1)	912.8 (877.2–949.8)
MC	11.6 (8.1–16.4)	876.3 (789.1–973.1)

All groups showed cracks, wear facets, and bulk fractures. For the MP group, 15% of the samples presented a bulk fracture in two or more pieces, and 85% of the samples showed chipping failure in the crown emergence profile. For the MC group, 20% of the samples presented a bulk fracture in two or more pieces, and 80% of the samples showed chipping failure in the crown emergence profile. For CME, 20% of the samples showed factures only in the crown exposing the mesostructure, 10% of the samples failed as a bulk fracture with the crack involving the crown and mesostructure, and 70% of the samples failed in the emergence profile without involving the crown (Figure 8). For MC and MP, the fractographic analysis showed that the failure was originated at the cervical area, propagating to the top of the restoration, which was confirmed by the fracture features (Figures 9 and 10). For CME, the specimens in which the fracture was restricted only in the crown, the fractures features suggested the crack propagation direction from the marginal side with several secondary events in the occlusal surface (Figures 11–13).

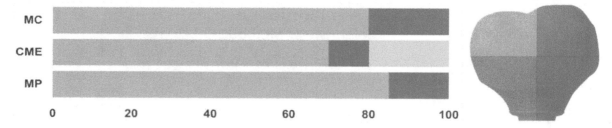

Figure 8. Quantitative analysis of the failures in % regarding the groups and the fracture location. In green, cracks found in the cervical region of the crown. In yellow, cracks found in the occlusal region. In blue, catastrophic failure.

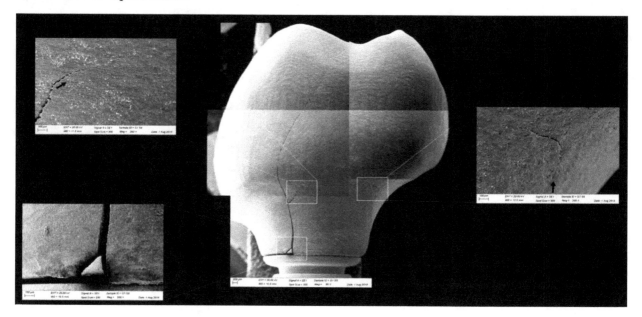

Figure 9. Fractographic analysis of a representative specimen from the MC group. The failure originated in the cervical region and propagated (black arrows) to the top of the restoration without separation of the fractured parts.

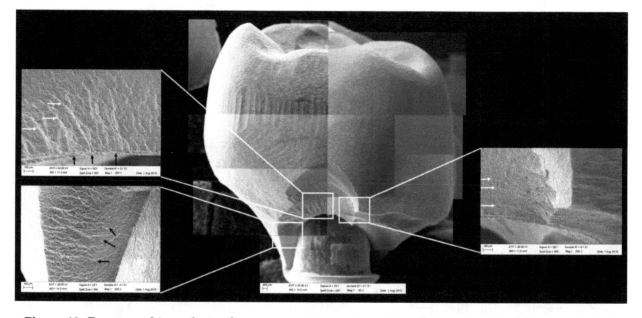

Figure 10. Fractographic analysis of a representative specimen from MP group. The failure originated in the cervical region and propagated to the top of the restoration. The white arrows indicate the hackle lines and the black arrows indicate the twist hackle marks.

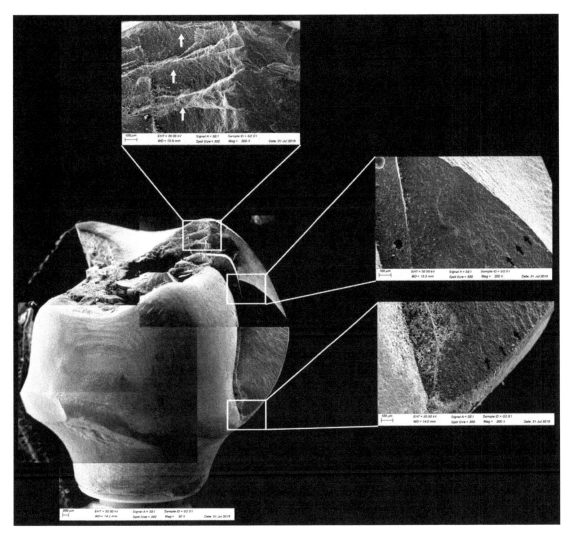

Figure 11. Fractographic analysis of a representative specimen from the CME group. The crown failed without the mesostructure involvement. The white arrows indicate the arrest lines and the black arrows indicate the hackle lines.

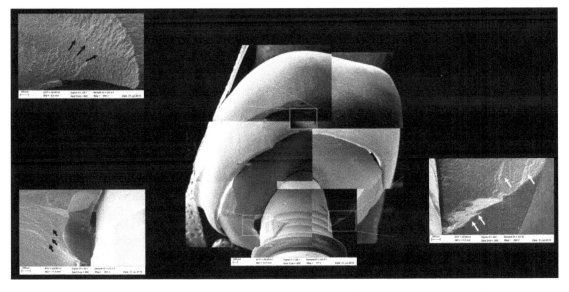

Figure 12. Fractographic analysis of a representative specimen from the CME group. The mesostructure failed without the involvement of the crown. The black arrows indicate the hackle lines, the white arrows indicate the arrest lines, and the red arrows indicate compression curls.

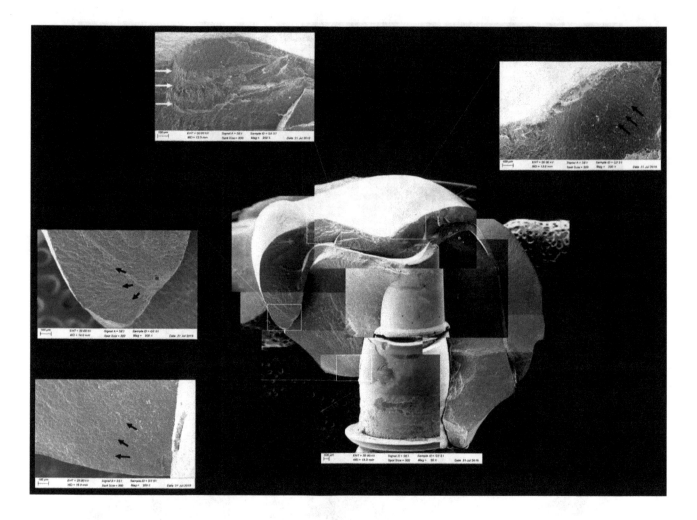

Figure 13. Fractographic analysis of a representative specimen from the CME group. The failure originated in the cervical region and propagated to the top of the restoration. The black arrows indicate the hackle lines, the white arrows indicate the arrest lines, and the red arrows indicate compression curls.

3.2. Nonlinear Finite Element Analysis

Observing the von-Mises failure criterion (Figure 14), which demonstrates the total resulting stress in the structures, it was possible to observe that the cervical region was the most involved regardless of the restoration technique, with the composite resin sealing of the group MP presenting a new stress area as well as the cement layer between the crown and mesostructure for the CME group.

In observing the tensile stress concentration in the crown, the numerical simulation showed a very similar mechanical behavior between the tested groups (Figure 15), with the highest stress concentration in the cervical region of the crown emergence profile. CME also presented stress concentration on the crown intaglio surface, which is compatible with the failure mode of 20% of the samples during the in vitro test (Figure 8). Furthermore, MP specimens showed high stress concentration in the composite resin used to seal the screw access hole. The stress peaks (Figure 16) corroborate with the colorimetric maps of the results (Figures 14 and 15), not allowing to assume a significant difference between the groups (10%).

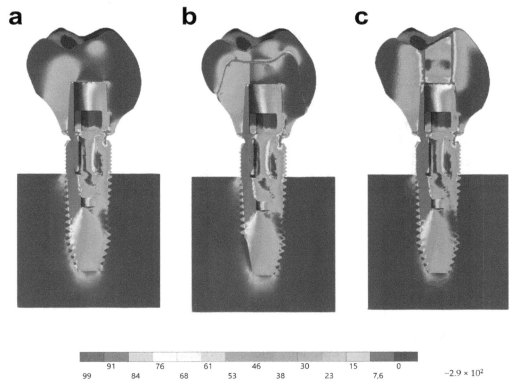

Figure 14. Stress distribution assessed by the von-Mises criterion according to the design of the restoration. **(a)** MC, **(b)** CME, and **(c)** MP.

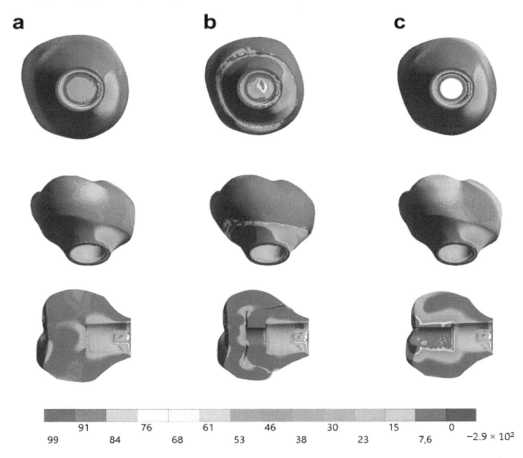

Figure 15. Stress distribution assessed by the maximum principal stress criterion according to the design of the restoration. **(a)** MC, **(b)** CME, and **(c)** MP.

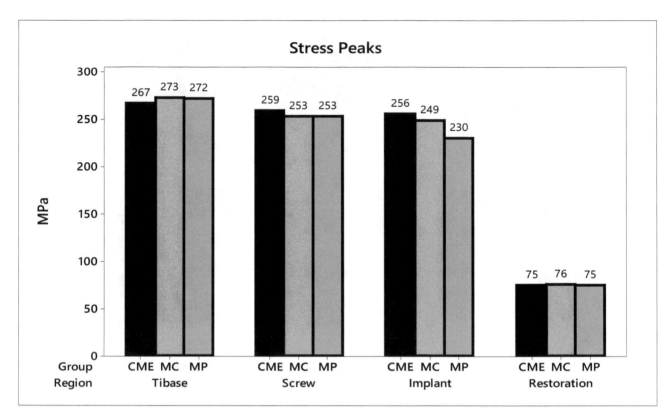

Figure 16. Stress peaks for each structure regarding the different groups. The restoration stress was calculated using the maximum principal stress criterion and the metallic structures using von-Mises criterion.

4. Discussion

This study evaluated the biomechanical behavior and survival probability of implant-supported polymer-infiltrated ceramic (PIC) restorations manufactured using different techniques. The results demonstrated that there is no difference between the groups for the stress distribution and that the reliability was similar between the groups at 300 N and 900 N. Therefore, we partially accept the null hypothesis.

The survival probability of restorations using Tibase as a connection between the implant and the crown is still scarce in the scientific literature [28,45,46]. The indication of this technique depends on the use of CAD/CAM blocks for implant solution that present a connective hole (screw access hole) created by the manufacturer [25,28]. According to the ceramic block size, it is possible to perform a two-piece restoration containing the mesostructure and the crown or a one-piece restoration [15,20,21,26–28,46]. These two restorative techniques were simulated in the present study, respectively, for the CME and MP groups.

The use of mesostructure to build the hybrid abutment to replace the conventional titanium abutments has already been reported [21,26,45]. Up to date, in vitro [26,47,48] and in vivo [49] studies and case reports [50,51] reported the use of lithium disilicate or polycrystalline ceramics to manufacture the mesostructure. Meanwhile, one case report [15] and in silico investigations [22–25] showed the possibility to manufacture the hybrid abutment using PIC material cemented on a Tibase, as performed in this study. Other authors [15] clinically evaluated the CME and MP groups using PIC. The authors suggested that the MP design has a disadvantage in aesthetics compared to the CME due to the presence of the screw access hole filled with composite resin. A literature review [28] suggested the possibility of using PIC to perform a mesostructure; however, the authors affirmed that the lack of longitudinal data does not allow its indication as the material first choice. Based on this, the present study results should assist the clinicians with understanding the biomechanical behavior of this treatment modality.

Comparing the restorative modalities evaluated in the present study, it was possible to observe that there is no difference between CME and MP, which are restorations created using implant solution CAD/CAM blocks and a Tibase. Both designs have already been compared for restorations made with different ceramic material [45]. The authors evaluated 10 anterior lithium disilicate restorations performed for each group and fatigued at 20 Hz until fracture [45], and they found that the MP design was statistically superior. In the present study, 20 restorations were manufactured for each group, the fatigue was adjusted to a maximum of 1.4 Hz, and the survival of MP and CME were not statistically different when PIC is the restorative material. In addition, this study used a posterior total crown with axial loads in order to restrict the failures only in the ceramic material, which was the object of the study.

The literature is not concise regarding the best protocol to use the Tibase. For example, another study [21] compared lithium disilicate anterior crowns using CME and MP techniques. However, the authors only performed the load to fracture using an universal testing machine with $n = 8$ specimens per group. The authors did not find any statistical difference between both designs, corroborating the findings for survival in the present study. Other study evaluated the load to failure of lithium disilicate and zirconia CME versus lithium disilicate MP crowns after aging [27]. Ten specimens per design were submitted to 2000 thermocycles (5–55 °C, water) and mechanical fatigue (150 N, 2 Hz, 100,000 cycles) aging. The authors observed that the lithium disilicate MP presented higher fracture load than a lithium silicate crown cemented on a mesostructure also in lithium silicate or in zirconia.

Still comparing different designs for using a Tibase, previous research [26] compared CME versus MP made in zirconia and lithium disilicate with $n = 8/gr$. The authors simulated premolars fatigued with 1.2 million thermomechanical cycles associated with 120 N load. After aging, the crowns were tested under an SLF test. Besides the cracks in the ceramic crown, the authors found plastic deformation on the Tibase, screw, and implant. This occurred as a consequence of the static load during compression test, which did not allow the slow crack growth in the ceramic material; this is the mechanism of failure for dental ceramics. For example, if the subject of the study is the ceramic design, it should be ideal that the test could provide the predominance of failures in this region, i.e., it will be possible to understand the restoration weakness and to promote new restorative designs. For this reason, the present study performed the stepwise test to determine at which load step the material has the highest probability of failure.

According to the literature [52], the screw access hole for retrieving ceramic implant-supported screw-retained crowns may decrease their fracture resistance. To prove this statement, the authors tested ceramic crowns in six different groups: monolithic zirconia, veneered zirconia, and lithium disilicate with and without screw access holes. The authors did not use a Tibase; instead, they used a custom abutment and the screw access hole was performed during the crown manufacturing, unlike implant-solution CAD/CAM blocks that already present the perforation. The results of the present study do not agree with these authors [52], because analyzing a ceramic restoration on fatigue, the screw access hole sealed with composite resin does not increase the generated stresses in the cervical region or decrease the restoration characteristic strength. Supporting the results found in the present study, previous authors [20,21,45] reported that groups with screw access holes showed similar load to failure to the groups without access holes. In addition, the authors suggested that perforated crowns may be even more resilient than groups without the access hole. The present study did not find any influence of the access hole on the strength characteristic; however, MP showed higher reliability than MC, corroborating with Roberts and Bailey (2018) [27].

According to a literature review [46] describing the possibilities and limitations of metal-free implant-supported single-tooth restorations, the authors described that one of the main advantages in using a Tibase in a digital workflow is the possibility of performing an adequate emergence profile in the crown. The emergence profile of an implant-supported prosthesis plays an important role in achieving esthetics, which are obtained when the clinician uses a properly concave abutment to mold the soft tissues for an adequate esthetic profile [53]. When improperly designed, the abutment emergence profile will compromise the cervical area blood supply, ultimately resulting in a loss of health and volume of the peri-implant tissues. For that reason, the emergence profile in an implant-supported restoration should be narrow to allow a higher volume of soft tissue [54]. Up to date, there has not been any in vitro study that created a restoration design that presents a concave emergence profile in the cervical area during the hybrid abutment testing [20,21,26,45]. During the present experiment, the 3D designs were created with this concern to simulate the most realistic shape of a restoration surrounded by a well-prepared soft tissue.

Observing the stresses analysis with the finite element method, it is possible to observe that the region of the emergence profile is the area of highest stress concentration in the restoration. This occurred probably due to the increase in the peri-implant soft tissue volume that requires the reduction on the restorative material in that region [15,53,54]. Therefore, the cervical area is the critical area of this restorative modality, since it is located near the fulcrum point of the crown and also because it has the smallest ceramic volume. The finite element method to observe the mechanical behavior of implant-supported single crowns associated with hybrid abutments has previously been reported for studies that compared different combinations of ceramic materials [22–24]. Therefore, it has been reported that to reduce the stress in the cervical region of the emergence profile, a flexible material should be used [22]. It is also recommended to use PIC to decrease the stress generated on the crown intaglio surface for CME design [24]. However, the present study demonstrated that MP restorations using only one CAD/CAM block for restoration are very similar to CME groups for the stress concentration in the cervical region. Moreover, the previous studies that simulated this restoration design [22–24] were not accompanied by in vitro experiments such as the present study, demonstrating that in fact, the region of stress concentration coincides with the possible failure origin observed in the fractographic analysis. At the occlusal region, the stress difference was caused by the composite polymerization shrinkage between the groups. Despite this, in the in vitro test, the survival was similar between the groups, and the failures were located at the cervical area.

The fractographic analysis followed the recommendations of the ADM (Academy of Dental Materials) guidance [55]. Thus, in a systematic protocol, all fractured restorations were observed under stereomicroscope to identify fracture features that could indicate the crack direction propagation. In this sense, the main failure mode observed was the crack/fracture of the cervical region in the emergence profile, while a smaller percentage of samples failed radially by splitting the crown into two or more pieces. However, for the CME group, different failure modes were also observed due to the presence of a second cement layer (between the mesostructure and the crown). In this group, in addition to failures in the cervical region, some specimens presented only crown fractures without mesostructure involvement. Some specimens presented mesostructure fracture without crown involvement, and two samples allowed the crack to propagate and separate the crown and mesostructure as a monolithic block. These failure modes in CME design have also been observed by previous studies that analyzed these restoration designs with other materials [26,27]. A fractographic analysis performed on failed zirconia mesostructure with Tibase during clinical use showed the same fracture pattern with the direction of crack propagation from the cervical area to occlusal [29], suggesting that the methods of the present study could provide failure modes similar to those found clinically.

In observing SEM micrographies, it was possible to note that all failures originated from the crown cervical region and spread toward the occlusal region. Secondary effects (damages) in the occlusal third near the compression region were also observed; however, they did not show fracture features that could suggest that the failure could have been originated in this region. It is important that the fractographic analysis is performed dividing each region of interest of the fractured restoration, analyzing each one in higher magnifications. This methodology is widely used to evaluate fractured dental crowns [56], disk-shaped specimens [55], and even for implant-supported crowns with Tibase [29] to assist in understanding how the failure occurred.

The higher variability of the failure modes observed for CME was reflected in the larger data variability in the Weibull test, increasing the slope of the data distribution line and the Weibull modulus.

Therefore, due to the possible different failure modes in this group, it has lower reliability, and therefore its clinical behavior is less predictable. However, its characteristic strength is not inferior to that of the MP and MC groups, which does not contraindicate this design as an option. The Weibull test approach has already been used for studies with dental ceramics [34] and dental implants [16], and it has been used as a statistic method to understand the relationship of data variation and final strength during fatigue [57].

Considering the reliability of the restoration itself, the lowest characteristic strength calculated was 789 N, which is about 34% less than the maximum fracture load initially calculated to determine the load variation in the fatigue test. This only reinforces that the slow crack growth during fatigue decreases the ultimate strength of ceramic restorations and should be taken into consideration during the experimental design of the test [16,31]. The Kaplan–Meier curve showed that the survival probability of the restorations decreases as the load increases, being less than 6% at 900 N, regardless of the design.

For this paper, the MC group simulated the use of a monolithic non-perforated crown as if the Tibase was a conventional abutment for cemented crowns. Although this design survived as well as the CME group and presented an adequate stress concentration, this design does not follow the manufacturer's recommendation [15]. The Tibase is not indicated as a conventional abutment because of the height of the platform, which cannot allow the complete removal of the resin cement from the cervical area in oral medium [15]. This group was created to elucidate whether the difference between the CME and MP groups would be due to the screw access hole of MP group or, due to the second cement layer on the CME design. No difference was calculated between these groups, suggesting that according to the manufacturer's recommendation, both techniques can create crowns of equal geometry, and the same clinical indication is correct. It is noteworthy that there was no loss of the composite resin used to seal the screw access of the MP group, which is not uncommon to be observed clinically for metal–ceramic crowns. Further studies evaluating the interface and bond strength between implant solutions CAD/CAM blocks and composite resin should be performed.

5. Conclusions

Using a digital workflow, the survival of an implant-supported restoration with PIC does not depend on the technique used to make it. The stress concentrations associated with fractographic analysis suggest that the emergence profile of the restoration should always be evaluated due to the high prevalence of failures in this area.

Author Contributions: All authors discussed and agreed upon the idea and made scientific contributions. Conceived and designed the study: J.P.M.T., A.M.O.D.P., L.C.A., C.J.K. and M.A.B. Data acquisition: J.P.M.T. and A.L.S.B. Experiment performing: J.P.M.T., A.M.O.D.P. and C.J.K. Writing the article: J.P.M.T., A.M.O.D.P. and L.C.A. Critical revision and final approval of the article: A.L.S.B., C.J.K. and M.A.B. All authors have agreed to the published version of the manuscript.

Acknowledgments: The authors would like to thank São Paulo Research Foundation (FAPESP) with the grants n° 17/09104-4, n° 18/07404-3 and n° 17/23059-1.

References

1. Sagsoz, O.; Demirci, T.; Demirci, G.; Sagsoz, N.P.; Yildiz, M. The effects of different polishing techniques on the staining resistance of CAD/CAM resin-ceramics. *J. Adv. Prosthodont.* **2016**, *8*, 417–422. [CrossRef] [PubMed]

2. Coldea, A.; Swain, M.V.; Thiel, N. Mechanical properties of polymer-infiltrated-ceramic-network materials. *Dent. Mater.* **2013**, *29*, 419–426. [CrossRef] [PubMed]

3. Conrad, H.J.; Seong, W.-J.; Pesun, I.J. Current ceramic materials and systems with clinical recommendations: A systematic review. *J. Prosthet. Dent.* **2007**, *98*, 389–404. [CrossRef]

4. Denry, I.; Kelly, J. Emerging ceramic-based materials for dentistry. *J. Dent. Res.* **2014**, *93*, 1235–1242. [CrossRef]

5. Ramos, N.D.C.; Campos, T.M.B.; De La Paz, I.S.; Machado, J.P.B.; Bottino, M.A.; Cesar, P.F.; Melo, R. Microstructure characterization and SCG of newly engineered dental ceramics. *Dent. Mater.* **2016**, *32*, 870–878. [CrossRef]

6. Curran, P.; Cattani-Lorente, M.; Wiskott, H.W.A.; Durual, S.; Scherrer, S.S. Grinding damage assessment for CAD-CAM restorative materials. *Dent. Mater.* **2017**, *33*, 294–308. [CrossRef]

7. Goujat, A.; Abouelleil, H.; Colon, P.; Jeannin, C.; Pradelle, N.; Seux, D.; Grosgogeat, B. Mechanical properties and internal fit of 4 CAD-CAM block materials. *J. Prosthet. Dent.* **2017**, *119*, 384–389. [CrossRef]

8. Awada, A.; Nathanson, D. Mechanical properties of resin-ceramic CAD/CAM restorative materials. *J. Prosthet. Dent.* **2015**, *114*, 587–593. [CrossRef]

9. Della Bona, A.; Corazza, P.H.; Zhang, Y. Characterization of a polymer-infiltrated ceramic-network material. *Dent. Mater.* **2014**, *30*, 564–569. [CrossRef]

10. Gracis, S.; Thompson, V.P.; Ferencz, J.L.; Silva, N.R.; Bonfante, E.A. A new classification system for all-ceramic and ceramic-like restorative materials. *Int. J. Prosthodont.* **2015**, *28*, 227–235. [CrossRef]

11. Dirxen, C.; Blunck, U.; Preissner, R. Clinical Performance of a New Biomimetic Double Network Material. *Open Dent. J.* **2013**, *7*, 118–122. [CrossRef] [PubMed]

12. Homaei, E.; Farhangdoost, K.; Tsoi, J.K.-H.; Matinlinna, J.P.; Pow, E.H.N. Static and fatigue mechanical behavior of three dental CAD/CAM ceramics. *J. Mech. Behav. Biomed. Mater.* **2016**, *59*, 304–313. [CrossRef] [PubMed]

13. De Kok, P.; Kleverlaan, C.J.; De Jager, N.; Kuijs, R.; Feilzer, A.J. Mechanical performance of implant-supported posterior crowns. *J. Prosthet. Dent.* **2015**, *114*, 59–66. [CrossRef] [PubMed]

14. Peampring, C. Restorative management using hybrid ceramic of a patient with severe tooth erosion from swimming: A clinical report. *J. Adv. Prosthodont.* **2014**, *6*, 423–426. [CrossRef] [PubMed]

15. Kurbad, A. Final restoration of implants with a hybrid ceramic superstructure. *Int. J. Comput. Dent.* **2016**, *19*, 257–279.

16. Bonfante, E.A.; Suzuki, M.; Lorenzoni, F.C.; Sena, L.A.; Hirata, R.; Bonfante, G.; Coelho, P.G. Probability of survival of implant-supported metal ceramic and CAD/CAM resin nanoceramic crowns. *Dent. Mater.* **2015**, *31*, e168–e177. [CrossRef]

17. Glauser, R.; Sailer, I.; Wohlwend, A.; Studer, S.; Schibli, M.; Schärer, P. Experimental zirconia abutments for implant-supported single-tooth restorations in esthetically demanding regions: 4-year results of a prospective clinical study. *Int. J. Prosthodont.* **2004**, *17*, 285–290.

18. Aboushelib, M.N.; Salameh, Z. Zirconia implant abutment fracture: Clinical case reports and precautions for use. *Int. J. Prosthodont.* **2009**, *22*, 616–619.

19. Prestipino, V.; Ingber, A. All-Ceramic Implant Abutments: Esthetic Indications. *J. Esthet. Restor. Dent.* **1996**, *8*, 255–262. [CrossRef]

20. Elsayed, A.; Wille, S.; Al-Akhali, M.; Kern, M. Comparison of fracture strength and failure mode of different ceramic implant abutments. *J. Prosthet. Dent.* **2017**, *117*, 499–506. [CrossRef]

21. Elsayed, A.; Wille, S.; Al-Akhali, M.; Kern, M. Effect of fatigue loading on the fracture strength and failure mode of lithium disilicate and zirconia implant abutments. *Clin. Oral Implant. Res.* **2017**, *29*, 20–27. [CrossRef] [PubMed]

22. Tribst, J.P.M.; Piva, A.M.D.O.D.; Borges, A.L.S.; Bottino, M.A. Influence of crown and hybrid abutment ceramic materials on the stress distribution of implant-supported prosthesis. *Rev. de Odontol. da UNESP* **2018**, *47*, 149–154. [CrossRef]

23. Tribst, J.P.M.; Piva, A.M.D.O.D.; Borges, A.L.S.; Bottino, M.A. Different combinations of CAD/CAM materials on the biomechanical behavior of a two-piece prosthetic solution. *Int. J. Comput. Dent.* **2019**, *22*, 171–176. [PubMed]

24. Tribst, J.P.M.; Piva, A.M.O.D.; Özcan, M.; Borges, A.L.S.; Bottino, M.A. Influence of Ceramic Materials on Biomechanical Behavior of Implant Supported Fixed Prosthesis with Hybrid Abutment. *Eur. J. Prosthodont. Restor. Dent.* **2019**, *27*, 76–82. [PubMed]

25. Tribst, J.P.M.; Piva, A.M.D.O.D.; Anami, L.C.; Borges, A.L.S.; Bottino, M. A Influence of implant connection on the stress distribution in restorations performed with hybrid abutments. *J. Osseointegration* **2019**, *11*, 507–512.

26. Nouh, I.; Kern, M.; Sabet, A.E.; AboelFadl, A.K.; Hamdy, A.M.; Chaar, M.S. Mechanical behavior of posterior all-ceramic hybrid-abutment-crowns versus hybrid-abutments with separate crowns-A laboratory study. *Clin. Oral Implant. Res.* **2018**, *30*, 90–98. [CrossRef]

27. Roberts, E.E.; Bailey, C.W.; Ashcraft-Olmscheid, D.L.; Vandewalle, K.S. Fracture Resistance of Titanium-Based Lithium Disilicate and Zirconia Implant Restorations. *J. Prosthodont.* **2018**, *27*, 644–650. [CrossRef]

28. Edelhoff, D.; Schweiger, J.; Prandtner, O.; Stimmelmayr, M.; Güth, J.-F. Metal-free implant-supported single-tooth restorations. Part I: Abutments and cemented crowns. *Quintessence Int.* **2019**, *50*, 176–184.

29. Øilo, M.; Arola, D. Fractographic analyses of failed one-piece zirconia implant restorations. *Dent. Mater.* **2018**, *34*, 922–931. [CrossRef]

30. Scherrer, S.S.; Cattani-Lorente, M.; Vittecoq, E.; De Mestral, F.; Griggs, J.A.; Wiskott, H.A. Fatigue behavior in water of Y-TZP zirconia ceramics after abrasion with 30μm silica-coated alumina particles. *Dent. Mater.* **2010**, *27*, e28–e42. [CrossRef]

31. De Melo, R.M.; Pereira, C.; Ramos, N.D.C.; Feitosa, F.; Piva, A.M.D.O.D.; Tribst, J.P.M.; Ozcan, M.; Jorge, A.O.C.; Özcan, M. Effect of pH variation on the subcritical crack growth parameters of glassy matrix ceramics. *Int. J. Appl. Ceram. Technol.* **2019**, *16*, 2449–2456. [CrossRef]

32. Miyashiro, M.; Suedam, V.; Neto, R.T.M.; Ferreira, P.M.; Rubo, J.H. Validation of an experimental polyurethane model for biomechanical studies on implant supported prosthesis - tension tests. *J. Appl. Oral Sci.* **2011**, *19*, 244–248. [CrossRef] [PubMed]

33. Ramos, G.F.; Monteiro, E.; Bottino, M.; Zhang, Y.; De Melo, R.M.; Bottino, M.A. Failure probability of three designs of zirconia crowns. *Int. J. Periodontics Restor. Dent.* **2015**, *35*, 843–849. [CrossRef] [PubMed]

34. Anami, L.C.; Lima, J.; Valandro, L.F.; Kleverlaan, C.; Feilzer, A.; Bottino, M.A. Fatigue Resistance of Y-TZP/Porcelain Crowns is Not Influenced by the Conditioning of the Intaglio Surface. *Oper. Dent.* **2016**, *41*, E1–E12. [CrossRef]

35. Bottino, M.A.; Rocha, R.F.V.; Anami, L.C.; Özcan, M.; Melo, R.M. Fracture of Zirconia Abutment with Metallic Insertion on Anterior Single Titanium Implant with Internal Hexagon: Retrieval Analysis of a Failure. *Eur. J. Prosthodont. Restor. Dent.* **2016**, *24*, 164–168.

36. Idogava, H.T.; Noritomi, P.Y.; Daniel, G.B. Numerical model proposed for a temporomandibular joint prosthesis based on the recovery of the healthy movement. *Comput. Methods Biomech. Biomed. Eng.* **2018**, *21*, 1–9. [CrossRef]

37. Alkan, I.; Sertgöz, A.; Ekici, B. Influence of occlusal forces on stress distribution in preloaded dental implant screws. *J. Prosthet. Dent.* **2004**, *91*, 319–325. [CrossRef]

38. Tribst, J.P.M.; Piva, A.M.D.O.D.; De Melo, R.M.; Borges, A.L.S.; Bottino, M.A.; Ozcan, M. Short communication: Influence of restorative material and cement on the stress distribution of posterior resin-bonded fixed dental prostheses: 3D finite element analysis. *J. Mech. Behav. Biomed. Mater.* **2019**, *96*, 279–284. [CrossRef]

39. Benzing, U.R.; Gall, H.; Weber, H. Biomechanical aspects of two different implant-prosthetic concepts for edentulous maxillae. *Int. J. Oral Maxillofac. Implant.* **1995**, *10*, 188–198.

40. Souza, A.; Xavier, T.; Platt, J.; Borges, A.L.S. Effect of Base and Inlay Restorative Material on the Stress Distribution and Fracture Resistance of Weakened Premolars. *Oper. Dent.* **2015**, *40*, 158–166. [CrossRef]

41. Singh, S.V.; Gupta, S.; Sharma, D.; Pandit, N.; Nangom, A.; Satija, H. Stress distribution of posts on the endodontically treated teeth with and without bone height augmentation: A three-dimensional finite element analysis. *J. Conserv. Dent.* **2015**, *18*, 196–199. [CrossRef] [PubMed]

42. Tribst, J.P.M.; De Melo, R.M.; Borges, A.L.S.; Souza, R.O.D.A.E.; Bottino, M.A. Mechanical Behavior of Different Micro Conical Abutments in Fixed Prosthesis. *Int. J. Oral Maxillofac. Implant.* **2016**, *33*, 1199–1205. [CrossRef] [PubMed]

43. Correia, A.; Tribst, J.P.M.; Matos, F.D.S.; Platt, J.A.; Caneppele, T.M.F.; Borges, A.L.S. Polymerization shrinkage stresses in different restorative techniques for non-carious cervical lesions. *J. Dent.* **2018**, *76*, 68–74. [CrossRef] [PubMed]

44. Bewick, V.; Cheek, L.; Ball, J. Statistics review 12: Survival analysis. *Crit. Care* **2004**, *8*, 389–394. [CrossRef] [PubMed]

45. Kaweewongprasert, P.; Phasuk, K.; Levon, J.A.; Eckert, G.J.; Feitosa, S.; Valandro, L.F.; Bottino, M.C.; Morton, D. Fatigue Failure Load of Lithium Disilicate Restorations Cemented on a Chairside Titanium-Base. *J. Prosthodont.* **2018**, *28*, 973. [CrossRef] [PubMed]

46. Edelhoff, D.; Schweiger, J.; Prandtner, O.; Stimmelmayr, M.; Güth, J.-F. Metal-free implant-supported single-tooth restorations. Part II: Hybrid abutment crowns and material selection. *Quintessence Int.* **2019**, *50*, 260–269.

47. Bidra, A.S.; Rungruanganunt, P. Clinical Outcomes of Implant Abutments in the Anterior Region: A Systematic Review. *J. Esthet. Restor. Dent.* **2013**, *25*, 159–176. [CrossRef]

48. Sailer, I.; Asgeirsson, A.G.; Thoma, D.S.; Fehmer, V.; Aspelund, T.; Ozcan, M.; Pjetursson, B.E. Fracture strength of zirconia implant abutments on narrow diameter implants with internal and external implant abutment connections: A study on the titanium resin base concept. *Clin. Oral Implant. Res.* **2018**, *29*, 411–423. [CrossRef]

49. Mehl, C.; Gaßling, V.; Schultz-Langerhans, S.; Açil, Y.; Bähr, T.; Wiltfang, J.; Kern, M. Influence of Four Different Abutment Materials and the Adhesive Joint of Two-Piece Abutments on Cervical Implant Bone and Soft Tissue. *Int. J. Oral Maxillofac. Implant.* **2016**, *31*, 1264–1272. [CrossRef]

50. Pitta, J.; Fehmer, V.; Sailer, I.; Hicklin, S.P. Monolithic zirconia multiple-unit implant reconstructions on titanium bonding bases. *Int. J. Comput. Dent.* **2018**, *21*, 163–171.

51. Adolfi, D.; Tribst, J.P.M.; Adolfi, M.; Piva, A.M.D.O.D.; Saavedra, G.D.S.F.A.; Bottino, M.A. Lithium Disilicate Crown, Zirconia Hybrid Abutment and Platform Switching to Improve the Esthetics in Anterior Region: A Case Report. *Clin. Cosmet. Investig. Dent.* **2020**, *12*, 31–40. [CrossRef] [PubMed]

52. Hussien, A.N.M.; Rayyan, M.M.; Sayed, N.M.; Segaan, L.G.; Goodacre, C.J.; Kattadiyil, M.T. Effect of screw-access channels on the fracture resistance of 3 types of ceramic implant-supported crowns. *J. Prosthet. Dent.* **2016**, *116*, 214–220. [CrossRef] [PubMed]

53. Steigmann, M.; Monje, A.; Chan, H.; Wang, H.-L. Emergence profile design based on implant position in the esthetic zone. *Int. J. Periodontics Restor. Dent.* **2014**, *34*, 559–563. [CrossRef] [PubMed]

54. Schoenbaum, T.R.; Swift, E.J. Abutment Emergence Contours for Single-Unit Implants. *J. Esthet. Restor. Dent.* **2015**, *27*, 1–3. [CrossRef] [PubMed]

55. Scherrer, S.S.; Lohbauer, U.; Della Bona, A.; Vichi, A.; Tholey, M.; Kelly, J.R.; Van Noort, R.; Cesar, P.F. ADM guidance—Ceramics: Guidance to the use of fractography in failure analysis of brittle materials. *Dent. Mater.* **2017**, *33*, 599–620. [CrossRef] [PubMed]

56. Lohbauer, U.; Belli, R.; Cune, M.S.; Schepke, U. Fractography of clinically fractured, implant-supported dental computer-aided design and computer-aided manufacturing crowns. *SAGE Open Med. Case Rep.* **2017**, *5*, 1–9. [CrossRef]

57. Quinn, J.B.; Quinn, G.D. A practical and systematic review of Weibull statistics for reporting strengths of dental materials. *Dent. Mater.* **2009**, *26*, 135–147. [CrossRef]

10

Axial Displacements and Removal Torque Changes of Five Different Implant-Abutment Connections under Static Vertical Loading

Ki-Seong Kim and Young-Jun Lim *

Department of Prosthodontics and Dental Research Institute, School of Dentistry, Seoul National University, Seoul 03080, Korea; namsang0249@nate.com
* Correspondence: limdds@snu.ac.kr

Abstract: The aim of this study was to examine the settling of abutments into implants and the removal torque value under static loading. Five different implant-abutment connections were selected (Ext: external butt joint + two-piece abutment; Int-H2: internal hexagon + two-piece abutment; Int-H1: internal hexagon + one-piece abutment; Int-O2: internal octagon + two-piece abutment; Int-O1: internal octagon + one-piece abutment). Ten implant-abutment assemblies were loaded vertically downward with a 700 N load cell at a displacement rate of 1 mm/min in a universal testing machine. The settling of the abutment was obtained from the change in the total length of the entire implant-abutment unit before and after loading using an electronic digital micrometer. The post-loading removal torque value was compared to the initial torque value with a digital torque gauge. The settling values and removal torque values after 700 N static loading were in the following order, respectively: Ext < Int-H1, Int-H2 < Int-O2 < Int-O1 and Int-O2 < Int-H2 < Ext < Int-H1, Int-O1 ($\alpha = 0.05$). After 700 N vertical static loading, the removal torque values were statistically different from the initial values, and the post-loading values increased in the Int-O1 group and Int-H1 group ($\alpha = 0.05$) and decreased in the Ext group, Int-H2 group, and Int-O2 group ($\alpha = 0.05$). On the basis of the results of this study, it should be taken into consideration that a loss of the preload due to the settling effect can lead to screw loosening during a clinical procedure in the molar region where masticatory force is relatively greater.

Keywords: dental implants; implant-abutment connection; settling effect; static loading; removal torque

1. Introduction

Attempts have been made to understand the factors that could compromise the settling effect of different implant abutment connections [1,2]. Various implant elements including the implant-abutment interface, the types of abutments, the screw characteristics, and the cyclic loading condition have all been shown to influence settling into implants and a loss of preload [3,4].

Loosening of the abutment screws and fixture failure in implant-supported restorations reportedly occur more frequently in the premolar and molar areas than in the incisor region [5,6]. This may result from differences in masticatory force and prosthetic design. Occlusion can be critical for implant longevity due to the nature of the potential load created by tooth contacts. The mechanism and vector of force transferred by posterior teeth differ from those of anterior teeth because posterior teeth have a stronger biting force in the vertical direction. Furthermore, these forces are produced by the action of the masticatory muscles [7].

The various forces that are exerted upon dental implants during function differ in magnitude and direction. In natural dentition, the periodontal ligament has the capacity to absorb stress and allow for tooth movement, but the bone-implant interface has little capacity to allow for the movement of an implant [8,9]. The force is distributed primarily along the crest of the ridge due to the lack of micromovement of implants [10].

Cyclic loading, which simulates functional loading, can significantly influence the overall intimacy of the settling of abutments into implants and their mechanical interlocking at the bone–implant interface [2]. However, cyclic loading is not the only factor that could influence the settling phenomenon in posterior teeth. Cyclic loading and the static loading are two independent conditions, and both can affect the settling of abutments into implants after occlusal loading.

In particular, vertical forces generated on implants in the posterior region are greatest at the implant-abutment interface. This means that vertical masticatory forces can affect settling into implants and a loss of preload after occlusal static loading.

Bruxism or clenching can create destructive lateral stresses and overloading when it transfers force to the supporting bone [11]. Parafunctional movements exert a greater maximum occlusal force than natural mastication. Van Eijden measured the mean magnitudes of a maximal vertical bite force in normal dentition without implants as follows: 469 ± 85 N at the canine region, 583 ± 99 N at the second premolar region, and 723 ± 138 N at the second molar region [12]. These results were comparable to the mean maximum bite force of 738 ± 209 N measured by Braun et al. [13]. In addition, Morneburg and Pröschel investigated vertical masticatory forces in vivo on implant-supported fixed partial dentures and found a mean total masticatory force of 220 N with a maximum of 450 N [14]. On the basis of these findings, the present study evaluated the degree of settling and compared preload loss using the removal torque values before and after 700 N static vertical loading.

The aim of this study was to evaluate the settling of abutments into implants and removal torque values of five different implant-abutment connections that differ significantly in macroscopic geometry after static vertical loading at 700 N.

2. Materials and Methods

2.1. Implant-Abutment Systems Selection and Study Protocol

One external and two internal connection implant systems from the Osstem Implant (Osstem Co., Seoul, Korea) were selected for the study. The abutment–implant assemblies were divided into five groups according to the implant connection designs and abutment types (Table 1, Figure 1).

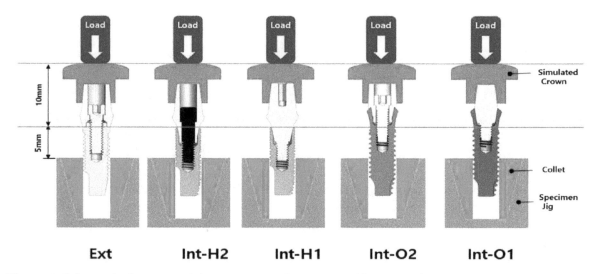

Figure 1. Schematic drawing of the test setup. Ext: external hexagon fixture + Cemented abutment; Int-H2: internal hexagon fixture + two-piece abutment; Int-H1: internal hexagon fixture + one-piece abutment; Int-O2: internal octagon fixture + two-piece abutment; Int-O1: internal octagon fixture + one-piece abutment.

Table 1. Characteristics of experimental implant-abutment systems.

Group	Ext	Int-H2	Int-H1	Int-O2	Int-O1
Implant system	US II	GS II		SS II	
Implant/abutment interface	External butt joint	11° taper internal hexagon		8° morse taper internal octagon	
Abutment type	Cemented (two-piece)	Transfer (two-piece)	Rigid (one-piece)	Comocta (two-piece)	Solid (one-piece)
Abutment material	Ti CP-Gr 3	Ti CP-Gr 3	Ti-6Al-4V	Ti CP-Gr 3	Ti-6Al-4V
Abutment diameter	Ø5.0	Ø5.0	Ø5.0	Ø4.3	Ø3.5
Abutment gingival height	2 mm	2 mm	2 mm	-	-
Abutment height (H_A)	5.5 mm	5.5 mm	5.5 mm	4 mm	4 mm
Abutment screw	Ta	WC/C Ta	-	Ta	-
Fixture material	Ti CP-Gr 4	Ti CP-Gr 4		Ti CP-Gr 4	
Fixture diameter	Ø4.0	Ø4.0	Ø4.0	Ø4.1	Ø4.1
Fixture height(H_F)	11.4 mm	11.5 mm	11.5 mm	11.5 mm	11.5 mm
Feature					

Ext: external hexagon fixture + Cemented abutment; Int-H2: internal hexagon fixture + two-piece abutment; Int-H1: internal hexagon fixture + one-piece abutment; Int-O2: internal octagon fixture + two-piece abutment; Int-O1: internal octagon fixture + one-piece abutment; Ta: titanium alloy; WC/C Ta: tungsten carbide/carbon-coated titanium alloy; H_A: Abutment height; H_F: fixture height.

Ext: External butt joint + Cemented abutment (two-piece)
Int-H2: Internal hexagon + Transfer abutment (two-piece)
Int-H1: Internal hexagon + Rigid abutment (one-piece)
Int-O2: Internal octagon + Comocta abutment (two-piece)
Int-O1: Internal octagon + Solid abutment (one-piece)

Ten implant-abutment assemblies were constructed for each group (total $n = 50$). Each assembly was held in a vise during the torque tightening procedure. The desired torque was applied to the abutment screw with a digital torque gauge (MGT12, MARK-10 Co., Hicksville, NY, USA).

The schematic diagram of experimental design based on protocol sequence is presented in Figure 2. Each abutment was tightened into the corresponding implant at 30 Ncm torque twice at 10 minute intervals. Ten minutes after the second tightening, the initial removal torque was measured with a digital torque gauge (MGT12E, Mark-10 corp, Hicksville, NY, USA). Each assembly was secured again at 30 Ncm torque, and the total length of the implant-abutment assembly was measured with an electronic digital micrometer (no. 293-561-30, Mitutoyo, Japan). After the initial measurement of the total length, a metal cap fabricated to reproduce the crown was mounted on the abutment of the assembly and the entire unit was fixed in a loading jig (Figure 3). The loading jig was designed to withstand a 700 N vertical static force applied to the implant-abutment assembly. All the specimens were tested in a universal testing machine (Instron 8841, Instron Corp., Mass, Norwood MA, USA) under 700 N vertical static loading, corresponding to the maximum biting force in posterior teeth [12,13].

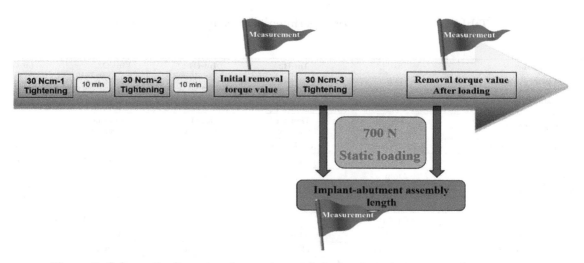

Figure 2. Schematic diagram of experimental design based on protocol sequence.

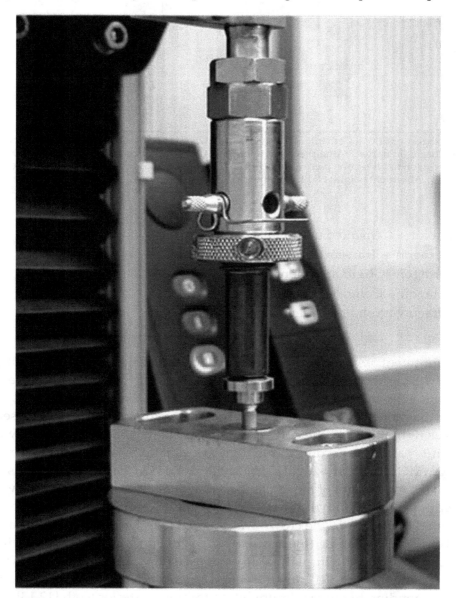

Figure 3. Loading machine and customized jig (Instron 8841, Instron Corp., Mass, Norwood MA, USA).

At the completion of static loading, the total length and removal torque of each implant-abutment specimen were measured in the same manner. The settling value of the abutment was calculated from the changes in the total lengths of the implant-abutment assembly before and after loading. The measurements were accurate up to 0.001 mm (1 μm) and the same operator performed all of the specimen preparations and testing in random order. The details of the experimental protocol and the overall outcomes between the magnitude of applied torque and the axil displacement of abutments into implants in external and internal implant-abutment connections were reported in previous studies [1,2].

2.2. Statistical Analysis

One-way ANOVA and Tukey's honestly significant difference (HSD) tests were used to analyze settling lengths and removal torque of the five implant-abutment systems before and after 700 N vertical static loading. A paired t-test was performed to compare the initial and post-loading removal torques for each implant connection system. $p < 0.05$ was considered to represent a statistically significant difference.

3. Results

The mean lengths and settling values of the specimen groups after vertical static loading are presented in Tables 2 and 3 and Figure 4. After 700 N static loading, there were statistically significant differences in the settling values in the Ext group (0.8 ± 0.45 μm), Int-H1 group (10.2 ± 0.84 μm), Int-H2 group (11.2 ± 0.84 μm), Int-O2 group (19.2 ± 4.21 μm), and Int-O1 group (25.6 ± 2.97 μm) ($\alpha = 0.05$). In the internal octagon groups with an 8° Morse taper interface, there were greater increases compared with those seen in the other groups. A multiple comparison test by Tukey's HSD exhibited differences in the settling values in each group after 700 N static loading in the following order: Ext < Int-H1, Int-H2 < Int-O2 < Int-O1 (see Tables 2 and 3).

Table 2. Mean total lengths and standard deviations of the implant-abutment specimens before and after 700 N static loading.

Group	Ext (mm)	Int-H2 (mm)	Int-H1 (mm)	Int-O2 (mm)	Int-O1 (mm)
Tightening torque 30 Ncm-③ *	18.6096 ±0.0054	18.9624 ±0.0153	19.0456 ±0.0261	18.9564 ±0.0222	18.9992 ±0.0041
Load 700 N Static **	18.6088 ±0.0054	18.9512 ±0.0151	19.0354 ±0.0266	18.9372 ±0.0222	18.9736 ±0.0035

* Additional tightening at 30 Ncm after measuring the initial removal torque after the second 30 Ncm tightening.
** After 700 N vertical static loading.

Table 3. Mean settling values after 700 N static loading in each group and multiple comparisons using Tukey's honestly significant difference (HSD).

Group	Settling Values Mean ± SD (μm)	Group Comparisons †
Ext	0.8 ± 0.45	
Int-H2	11.2 ± 0.84	Ext < Int-H1, Int-H2 < Int-O2 < Int-O1
Int-H1	10.2 ± 0.84	
Int-O2	19.2 ± 4.21	
Int-O1	25.6 ± 2.97	Settling value = (total lengths of the implant-abutment assemblies at 30 Ncm-③) minus (total lengths of the implant-abutment assemblies after 700 N static loading)

† Tukey's HSD method was performed for between group comparisons ($p < 0.05$).

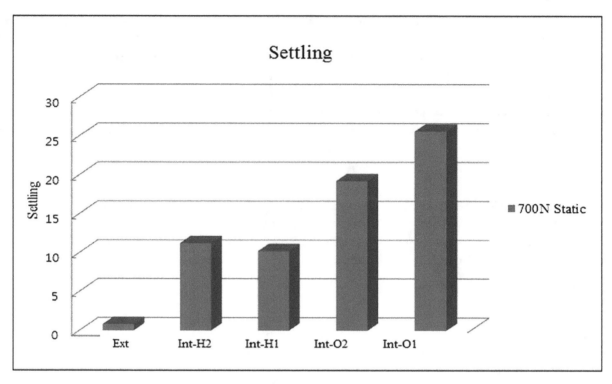

Figure 4. Settling of abutments into the implants after static loading (μm).

The mean values of removal torque after loading are presented in Tables 4–6 and Figure 5. After 700 N static loading, the Int-O1 group exhibited the highest removal torque of 39.64 ± 4.28 Ncm. The other groups are shown in the following decreasing order: Int-H1 (36.38 ± 6.25 Ncm), Ext (22.78 ± 0.40 Ncm), Int-H2 (11.62 ± 0.56 Ncm), and Int-O2 (1.14 ± 0.40 Ncm). Using Tukey's HSD, the specific group-wise comparisons in the post-loading removal torque values were as follows: Int-O2 < Int-H2 < Ext < Int-H1, Int-O1.

Table 4. Multiple comparisons of mean values of initial removal torque and removal torque after 700 N static loading.

Test	Group ($n = 5$)	Tightening Torque (Ncm)	Removal Torque (Ncm)	Significance †
Initial removal torque	Ext	30	24.22 ± 0.81	Int-H2 < Ext, Int-O2 < Int-H1 < Int-O1
	Int-H2	30	21.22 ± 1.04	
	Int-H1	30	27.44 ± 0.92	
	Int-O2	30	25.38 ± 1.86	
	Int-O1	30	30.54 ± 0.56	
Removal torque after 700N static loading	Ext	30	22.78 ± 0.40	Int-O2 < Int-H2 < Ext < Int-H1, Int-O1
	Int-H2	30	11.62 ± 0.56	
	Int-H1	30	36.38 ± 6.25	
	Int-O2	30	1.14 ± 0.40	
	Int-O1	30	39.64 ± 4.28	

† Tukey's HSD method was performed for between group comparisons ($p < 0.05$).

Table 5. Comparison of the mean values of initial and post-loading removal torque in each group.

Group	Initial R/T [a]	R/T after Static Load [b]	Significance †
Ext	24.22 ± 0.81	22.78 ± 0.40	*
Int-H2	21.22 ± 1.04	11.62 ± 0.56	**
Int-H1	27.44 ± 0.92	36.38 ± 6.25	NS
Int-O2	25.38 ± 1.86	1.14 ± 0.40	*
Int-O1	30.54 ± 0.56	39.64 ± 4.28	*

[a] Removal torque values before loading; [b] Removal torque values 700 N static loading; † Paired t-test was performed to compare the removal torque values before and after loading: NS, not significant; * $p < 0.01$; ** $p < 0.001$.

Table 6. Comparisons of the mean values of initial removal torque and removal torque after static loading in each group.

Group	Removal Torque	t/P Value
Ext	Initial / after 700 N static loading	6.279 /0.003 *
Int-H2	Initial / after 700 N static loading	16.204 /0.000 *
Int-H1	Initial / after 700 N static loading	−3.313 /0.030 *
Int-O2	Initial / after 700 N static loading	6.413 /0.003 *
Int-O1olid	Initial / after 700 N static loading	−4.768 /0.009 *

* indicates values that were statistically different ($p < 0.05$).

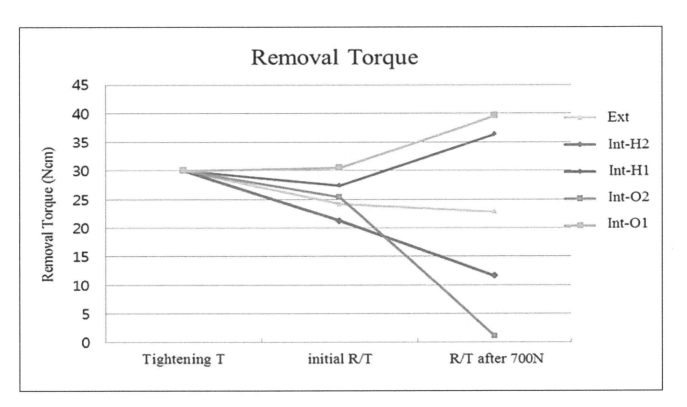

Figure 5. Removal torque (Ncm) after 700 N static loading.

In cases in which one-piece abutments were used for the internal connection system (Int-H1 group and Int-O1 group), the removal torque was increased compared to the initial removal torque. In cases where two-piece abutments were used for the internal connection system (Int-H2 group and Int-O2 group), after 700 N vertical static loading, the removal torque was decreased compared to the initial removal torque to a greater extent. In the Int-O2 group in particular, the abutment screw nearly came loose from the abutment. After 700 N loading, the removal torque value also exhibited a small but significant decrease in the Ext group (Table 6).

4. Discussion

Along with the expanded indications for implants and the changing clinical protocols, the relationship between implant design and load distribution at the implant–bone interface has become an important issue. The inadequate interaction between these two factors may result in both mechanical and biologic complications such as screw loosening and peri-implant bone loss. Whether an implant prosthesis is placed in function after an undisturbed healing period or immediately after placement, the biomechanical environment is, thereafter, a critical factor that influences implant duration and bone preservation. Loads applied to teeth and implants during physiologic oral functions including chewing, clenching, swallowing, or grinding may vary because the anchorage of natural and artificial abutments in the jaw is not of the same type and quality [15].

Most of the studies related to axial displacement [1–3] are on the magnitude of tightening torque and the duration of cyclic loading, and few studies have applied with static loading. Ko et al. [4] reported that axial displacement and reverse torque loss occurred at significantly low levels after the cyclic and static loading in the case of wide-type implants of 5.0 mm diameter. In addition, the CAD/CAM (Computer Aided Design/Computer Aided Manufacturing) customized abutments, which are currently in the spotlight, may show differences in the fabricating process from the stock abutments produced by manufacturers. Therefore, using implant fixtures and abutments made by the same manufacturer, we wanted to prove that axial displacement could occur even at static loading of 700 N, and the difference comes from different connection types.

For osseointegrated dental implants, previous studies have revealed that occlusal interferences and parafunctional activities may lead to mechanical and biologic complications [16]. Many investigators have attempted to evaluate maximum bite forces. Typical maximum bite force magnitudes exhibited by adults are affected by age, sex, degree of edentulism, bite location, and especially parafunction. In centric occlusion involving swallowing and clenching, forces are transmitted bilaterally, predominantly by molars and premolars. For a single tooth or implant in the molar region, the greatest forces occur along the axial direction [17]. Therefore, the results of this study showed the settling effect in relation to a loss of removal torque after 700 N vertical static loading, corresponding to the maximum masticatory force.

The settling effect after 700 N loading showed a clinical association between screw loosening with a loss of preload and an increase in friction. The results followed a similar pattern with cyclic loading in our previous study [2]. The Ext group showed the lowest settling due to its flat platform interface. Likewise, the internal hexagon and octagon groups had statistically greater settling due to their tapered interface. In particular, the internal octagon group with an 8° Morse taper showed the highest settling value compared to the internal hexagon group with an 11° taper.

The removal torque values after 700 N vertical static loading may be influenced by the amount of settling and the type and configuration characteristics of the abutment used. When a two-piece abutment, as seen in the Int-H2 and Int-O2 groups, is used, the screw joint connection is based on the tension mechanism, where a screw may become loose due to a loss of preload by settling. Therefore, the settling effect of the Int-H2 and Int-O2 groups produced a significant decrease in the removal torque even to the extent of the loss of the abutment screw in the Int-O2 group. On the other hand, when a one-piece abutment is used, the main retention mechanism is friction. As a result, the settling effect of the one-piece abutment in the Int-H1 and Int-O1 groups created a greater compressive force at the implant-abutment interface, which resulted in the increased post-loading values of removal torque.

The metal cap used in this experimental protocol was inserted into the abutment by friction only, and without dental cement. The simulated crown had a gap between the abutment and the metal cap in order to prevent any forces from being transferred to the abutment during the removal of the crown. However, because the margin of the crown was seated on the fixture in the original internal octagon design, there was no such space. Consequently, this discrepancy may have led to greater settling values than the actual value due to the lack of a vertical stop. In addition, this study could not use the direct method as described by Haack et al., where the change in the preload was evaluated by measuring the length of an elongated screw [18]. Therefore, further studies are warranted to evaluate the actual measurement of an elongated screw as a value of tightening torque.

5. Conclusions

The current study strived to gain a better understanding of the nature of the implant-abutment screw joint on the basis of the settling effect and removal torque. On the basis of the findings of this study, in the molar region where masticatory force is relatively greater, a loss of preload due to the axial displacement and the possibility of screw loosening should be taken into account in clinical procedures.

The clinical implication of this study is that when the implant fixture of a regular platform with a diameter of 4.0 mm is placed in the posterior molar region, the settling of abutments into implants caused by the vertical force may cause a problem of lowering the occlusion after the prosthesis is mounted.

Author Contributions: Conceptualization, writing—Original draft preparation, data curation, K.-S.K.; supervision, visualization, validation, writing—Review and editing, Y.-J.L. All authors have read and agreed to the published version of the manuscript.

References

1. Kim, K.S.; Lim, Y.J.; Kim, M.J.; Kwon, H.B.; Yang, J.H.; Lee, J.B.; Yim, S.H. Variation in the total lengths of abutment/implant assemblies generated with a function of applied tightening torque in external and internal implant-abutment connection. *Clin. Oral Implants Res.* **2011**, *22*, 834–839. [CrossRef] [PubMed]
2. Kim, K.S.; Han, J.S.; Lim, Y.J. Settling of abutments into implants and changes in removal torque in five different implant-abutment connections. Part 1: Cyclic loading. *Int. J. Oral Maxillofac. Implants* **2014**, *29*, 1079–1084. [CrossRef] [PubMed]
3. Lee, J.H.; Lee, W.; Huh, Y.H.; Park, C.J.; Cho, L.R. Impact of Intentional Overload on Joint Stability of Internal Implant-Abutment Connection System with Different Diameter. *J. Prosthodont.* **2019**, *28*, e649–e656. [CrossRef] [PubMed]
4. Ko, K.H.; Huh, Y.H.; Park, C.J.; Cho, L.R. Axial displacement in cement-retained prostheses with different implant-abutment connections. *Int. J. Oral Maxillofac. Implants* **2019**, *34*, 1098–1104. [CrossRef] [PubMed]
5. Bianco, G.; Di Raimondo, R.; Luongo, G.; Paoleschi, C.; Piccoli, P.; Piccoli, C.; Rangert, B. Osseointegrated implant for single-tooth replacement: A retrospective multicenter study on routine use in private practice. *Clin. Implant Dent. Relat. Res.* **2000**, *2*, 152–158. [CrossRef] [PubMed]
6. Palmer, R.M.; Palmer, P.J.; Smith, B.J. A 5-year prospective study of Astra single tooth implants. *Clin. Oral Implants Res.* **2000**, *11*, 179–182. [CrossRef] [PubMed]
7. Dean, J.S.; Throckmorton, G.S.; Ellis, E., III; Sinn, D.P. A preliminary study of maximum voluntary bite force and jaw muscle efficiency in pre-orthognathic surgery patients. *J. Oral Maxillofac. Surg.* **1992**, *50*, 1284–1288. [CrossRef]
8. Koyano, K.; Esaki, D. Occlusion on oral implants: Current clinical guidelines. *J. Oral Rehabil.* **2015**, *42*, 153–161. [CrossRef] [PubMed]
9. Kim, Y.; Oh, T.; Misch, C.E.; Wang, H.L. Occlusal considerations in implant therapy: Clinical guidelines with biomechanical rationale. *Clin. Oral Implants Res.* **2005**, *1*, 26–35. [CrossRef] [PubMed]
10. Rieger, M.R.; Mayberry, M.; Brose, M.O. Finite element analysis of six endosseous implants. *J. Prosthet. Dent.* **1990**, *63*, 671–676. [CrossRef]
11. Misch, C.E. The effect of bruxism on treatment planning for dental implants. *Dent. Today* **2002**, *2*, 76–81.
12. van Eijden, T.M. Three-dimensional analyses of human bite-force magnitude and moment. *Arch. Oral Biol.* **1991**, *36*, 535–539. [CrossRef]

13.   Braun, S.; Hnat, W.P.; Freudenthaler, J.W.; Marcotte, M.R.; Hönigle, K.; Johnson, B.E. A study of maximum bite force during growth and development. *Angle Orthod.* **1996**, *66*, 261–264. [PubMed]
14.   Morneburg, T.R.; Pröschel, P.A. Measurement of masticatory forces and implant loads: A methodologic clinical study. *Int. J. Prosthodont.* **2002**, *15*, 20–27. [PubMed]
15.   Richter, E.J. In vivo vertical forces on implants. *Int. J. Oral Maxillofac. Implants* **1995**, *10*, 99–108. [PubMed]
16.   Chambrone, L.; Chambrone, L.A.; Lima, L.A. Effects of occlusal overload on peri-implant tissue health: A systematic review of animal-model studies. *J. Periodontol.* **2010**, *81*, 1367–1378. [CrossRef] [PubMed]
17.   Rigsby, D.F.; Bidez, M.W.; Misch, C.E. Bone Response to Mechanical Loads. In *Contemporary Implant Dentistry*, 2nd ed.; Misch, C.E., Ed.; Mosby: St. Louis, Missouri, USA, 1998; pp. 317–328.
18.   Haack, J.E.; Sakaguchi, R.L.; Sun, T.; Coffey, J.P. Elongation and preload stress in dental implant abutment screws. *Int. J. Oral Maxillofac. Implants* **1995**, *10*, 529–536. [PubMed]

11

Bone Immune Response to Materials, Part I: Titanium, PEEK and Copper in Comparison to Sham at 10 Days in Rabbit Tibia

Ricardo Trindade [1,*], Tomas Albrektsson [2,3], Silvia Galli [3], Zdenka Prgomet [4], Pentti Tengvall [2] and Ann Wennerberg [1]

[1] Department of Prosthodontics, Faculty of Odontology, The Sahlgrenska Academy, University of Gothenburg, 405 30 Gothenburg, Sweden; ann.wennerberg@odontologi.gu.se
[2] Department of Biomaterials, Institute of Clinical Sciences, University of Gothenburg, 405 30 Gothenburg, Sweden; tomas.albrektsson@biomaterials.gu.se (T.A.); pentti.tengvall@gu.se (P.T.)
[3] Department of Prosthodontics, Faculty of Odontology, Malmö University, 205 06 Malmö, Sweden; silvia.galli@mau.se
[4] Department of Oral Pathology, Faculty of Odontology, Malmö University, 205 06 Malmö, Sweden; zdenka.prgomet@mau.se
* Correspondence: ricardo.bretes.trindade@gu.se

Abstract: Bone anchored biomaterials have become an indispensable solution for the restoration of lost dental elements and for skeletal joint replacements. However, a thorough understanding is still lacking in terms of the biological mechanisms leading to osseointegration and its contrast, unwanted peri-implant bone loss. We have previously hypothesized on the participation of immune mechanisms in such processes, and later demonstrated enhanced bone immune activation up to 4 weeks around titanium implants. The current experimental study explored and compared in a rabbit tibia model after 10 days of healing time, the bone inflammation/immunological reaction at mRNA level towards titanium, polyether ether ketone (PEEK) and copper compared to a Sham control. Samples from the test and control sites were, after a healing period, processed for gene expression analysis (polymerase chain reaction, (qPCR)) and decalcified histology tissue analysis. All materials displayed immune activation and suppression of bone resorption, when compared to sham. The M1 (inflammatory)/M2 (reparative) -macrophage phenotype balance was correlated to the proximity and volume of bone growth at the implant vicinity, with titanium demonstrating a M2-phenotype at 10 days, whereas copper and PEEK were still dealing with a mixed M1- and M2-phenotype environment. Titanium was the only material showing adequate bone growth and proximity inside the implant threads. There was a consistent upregulation of (T-cell surface glycoprotein CD4) CD4 and downregulation of (T-cell transmembrane glycoprotein CD8) CD8, indicating a CD4-lymphocyte phenotype driven reaction around all materials at 10 days.

Keywords: osseointegration; immune system; biomaterials; foreign body reaction; in vivo study

1. Introduction

Recent evidence suggests that biomaterials induce an immunomodulatory interaction with the host, and materials such as titanium or bone substitutes seem not at all inert upon contact with host bone [1]. The ultimate outcome of biomaterial implantation depends on the extent of the ensuing foreign body reaction (FBR) and related immune and inflammatory mechanisms; current scientific efforts are focusing on understanding this complex host reaction, in order to improve the behavior of implanted biomaterials [2]. However, the precise mechanisms of osseointegration are today not fully understood, especially the long-term immune recognition of implants.

The present authors have explored some immunological mechanisms in a previously published review [3], following the hypothesis that osseointegration is nothing but a special type of immune driven foreign body reaction to the implanted material, ending up in bone demarcation at or near the surface [4]. The main hypothesis was that implants are not biologically inert, meaning that the immune/inflammatory system, in this case with emphasis on the immune system, is activated when titanium interacts with host bone—A hypothesis that later was tested and verified in a recent 4 week experimental pilot animal study, where immunological markers representing macrophages, complement, neutrophils, lymphocytes and bone resorption markers were compared in osteotomy sites, with and without the presence of titanium implants [5]: Titanium sites, showed significant up-/or down-regulation of immune (and inflammatory) markers after 28 days, i.e., at a time point well into the bone remodeling phase The immune system was apparently activated through the complement system, displayed M1 (inflammatory) - and M2 (reparative) -macrophages phenotypes, neutrophil cytosolic factor 1 (NCF-1), and down regulation of markers related to osteoclastic activity. Comparatively, at an earlier stage (10 days) only the M2-macrophage (reparative) phenotype was identified around titanium, when compared to the sham site. From earlier studies immune complement is known to become activated at a very early time point around titanium, and materials are then recognized as foreign objects by inflammatory cells [6]. During bone healing, and after the acute inflammatory phase, macrophages and their classically described polarization into M1 (inflammatory) and M2 (reparative) phenotypes dominate, and are considered to be central in the host reaction to implanted biomaterials [7,8], but the precise in vivo mechanisms are still in need of a thorough clarification. Macrophages are also intimately related to bone biology, interacting closely with osteoblasts during bone formation (these macrophages are named Osteomacs), and also fusing into either osteoclasts or material related multinucleated giant cells (named Foreign Body Giant Cells), determining a further important role for macrophages when considering bone borne biomaterials [9].

In the earlier review [3], and pertaining the current manuscript, it was further hypothesized that the reason why different materials may or not achieve osseointegration is probably related, to some extent, to a persistent immune patrolling resulting in a modified inflammatory reaction around the different materials. These two concepts—That materials are not biologically inert and that a specific persistent immune-inflammatory balance or patrolling around different materials largely dictates whether osseointegration occurs or not—Are fundamental to our understanding of longer-term host reactions to materials in bone.

The aim of the present exploratory in vivo study is to test the hypothesis that different materials trigger different early immune/inflammatory responses upon implantation in rabbit bone, and that these different responses may be important for the establishment of osseointegration, or the ultimate lack of it.

2. Materials and Methods

The current study consists of an experiment in the rabbit proximal tibia (metaphysis), comparing bone healing on sites where osteotomies were performed and then either left to heal without the placement of a material (sham site- Sh), or had one of the three test materials placed for comparison: titanium (Ti), copper (Cu) or polyether ether ketone (PEEK). Each rabbit received one site of each group (two sites per tibia): Sh, Ti, Cu and PEEK. Ti and PEEK were placed on the right tibia and a Sham site was produced and Cu was introduced in the other osteotomy on the left tibia. All implants were machined with a turning process, with a threaded 0.6 mm pitch height, 3.75 mm width Branemark MkIII design. The Ti implants were made of commercially pure titanium grade IV. Implant manufacturers: Ti and PEEK implants were produced by Carlsson and Möller, Helsingborg, Sweden; Copper implants were produced by TL Medical Company, Molndal, Sweden.

The sham site also provokes an inflammatory reaction, which is still present at 10 days and is used as a baseline to compare with the immune reaction elicited by each of the different materials.

2.1. Surgical Procedure

This study was performed on 6 mature, female New Zealand White Rabbits ($n = 6$, weight 3 to 4 Kg), with the ethical approval from the Ethics Committee for Animal Research (number 13-011) of the École Nationale Vétérinaire D'Alfors, Maisons-Alfors, Val-de-Marne, France. All care was taken to minimize animal pain or discomfort during and after the surgical procedures. For the surgical procedures, the rabbits were placed under general anesthesia using a mixture of medetomidine (Domitor, Zoetis, Florham Park, NJ, USA), ketamine (Imalgène 1000, Merial, Lyon, France) and diazepam (Valium, Roche, Basel, Switzerland) for induction, then applying subcutaneous buprenorphine (Buprecare, Animalcare, York, UK) and intramuscular Meloxicam (Metacam; Boehringer Ingelheim Vetmedica, Inc., Ridgefield, CT, USA). A single incision was performed in the internal knee area on each side and the bone exposed for osteotomies and insertion of implants in the sites mentioned above. The surgical site was sutured with a resorbable suture (Vicryl 3-0, Ethicon, Cincinnati, OH, USA) and hemostasis achieved. Following surgery, Fentanyl patches (Duragesic, Janssen Pharmaceutica, Beerse, Belgium) were applied.

The osteotomies were produced with a sequence of increasing diameter twist drills, from 2 mm to 3.15 mm width, and a final countersink bur prepared the cortical part of the bone. The implants used were 3.75 mm in diameter.

The rabbits were housed in separate cages and were allowed to move and eat freely. At 10 days, the rabbits were sacrificed with a lethal injection of sodium pentobarbital (Euthasol, Virbac, Fort Worth, TX, USA). The 6 animals had the implants removed through unscrewing. On 4 of those animals, bone was collected with a 2 mm twist drill from the periphery of the Sh, Ti, Cu and PEEK sites on the most distal portion, and then processed for Gene Expression Analysis through quantitative polymerase chain reaction (qPCR). The 6 animals had the test sites then removed en bloc for histological processing.

2.2. Gene Expression Analysis—qPCR

The bone samples for gene expression analysis were collected from the distal side of the osteotomies of all four groups (following the removal of the implant from the implant sites), with a 2 mm twist drill that removed both cortical and marrow bone in the full length of the osteotomy, to enable the study of the 2 mm peri-implant bone area of each of the Sh, Ti, Cu and PEEK sites. The samples were immediately transferred to separate sterile plastic recipients containing RNA*later* medium (Ambion, Inc., Austin, TX, USA), for preservation. The samples were then refrigerated first at 4 °C and then stored at −20 °C until processing.

2.3. mRNA Isolation

Samples were homogenized using an ultrasound homogenizer (Sonoplus HD3100, Brandelin, Berlin, Germany) in 1 mL PureZOL and total RNA was isolated via column fractionalization using the Aurum™ Total RNA Fatty and Fibrous Tissue Kit (Bio-Rad Laboratories Inc., Hercules, CA, USA) following the manufacturer's instructions. All the samples were DNAse treated using an on-column DNAse I contained in the kit to remove genomic DNA. The RNA quantity for each sample was analyzed in the NanoDrop 2000 Spectrophotometer (Thermo Scientific, Wilmington, NC, USA). BioRad iScript cDNA synthesis kit (Bio-Rad Laboratories Inc., Hercules, CA, USA) was then used to convert mRNA into cDNA, following the manufacturer's instructions.

qPCR primers (Tataa Biocenter, Gothenburg, Sweden) were designed following the National Center of Biotechnology Information (NCBI) Sequence database, including the local factors chosen in order to characterize the immune, inflammatory and bone metabolic pathways (Tables 1 and 2). All primers had an efficiency between 90 and 110%.

Table 1. Gene sequences.

Primer	Forward Sequence	Reverse Sequence	Accession nr/Transcript ID
NCF-1	TTCATCCGCCACATTGCCC	GTCCTGCCACTTCACCAAGA	NM_001082102.1
CD68	TTTCCCCAGCTCTCCACCTC	CGATGATGAGGGGCACCAAG	ENSOCUT00000010382
CD11b	TTCAACCTGGAGACTGAGAACAC	TCAAACTGGACCACGCTCTG	ENSOCUT00000001589
CD14	TCTGAAAATCCTGGGCTGGG	TTCATTCCCGCGTTCCGTAG	ENSOCUT00000004218
ARG1	GGATCATTGGAGCCCCTTTCTC	TCAAGCAGACCAGCCTTTCTC	NM_001082108.1
IL-4	CTACCTCCACCACAAGGTGTC	CCAGTGTAGTCTGTCTGGCTT	ENSOCUT00000024099
IL-13	GCAGCCTCGTATCCCCAG	GGTTGACGCTCCACACCA	ENSOCUT00000000154
M-CSF	GGAACTCTCGCTCAGGCTC	ACATTCTTGATCTTCTCCAGCAAC	ENSOCUT00000030714
OPG	TGTGTGAATGCGAGGAAGGG	AACTGTATTCCGCTCTGGGG	ENSOCUT00000011149
RANKL	GAAGGTTCATGGTTCGATCGG	CCAAGAGGACAGGCTCACTTT	ENSOCUT00000024354
TRAP	TTACTTCAGTGGCGTGCAGA	CGATCTGGGCTGAGACGTTG	NM_001081988.1
CathK	GGAACCGGGGCATTGACTCT	TGTACCCTCTGCATTTGGCTG	NM_001082641.1
PPAR-γ	CAAGGCGAGGGCGATCTT	ATGCGGATGGCGACTTCTTT	NM_001082148.1
C3	ACTCTGTCGAGAAGGAACGGG	CCTTGATTTGTTGATGCTGGCTG	NM_001082286.1
C3aR1	CATGTCAGTCAACCCCTGCT	GCGAATGGTTTTGCTCCCTG	ENSOCUT00000007435
CD46	TCCTGCTGTTCACTTTCTCGG	CATGTTCCCATCCTTGTTTACACTT	ENSOCUT00000033915
CD55	TGGTGTTGGGTGGAGTGACC	AGAGTGAAGCCTCTGTTGCATT	ENSOCUT00000031985
CD59	ACCACTGTCTCTCCTCCCAAGT	GCAATCTTCATACCGCCAACA	NM_001082712.1
C5	TCCAAAACTCTGCAACCTTAACA	AAATGCTTTGACACAACTTCCA	ENSOCUT00000005683
C5aR1	ACGTCAACTGCTGCATCAACC	AGGCTGGGGAGAGACTTGC	ENSOCUT00000029180
CD3	CCTGGGGACAGGAAGATGATGAC	CAGCACCACACGGGTTCCA	NM_001082001.1
CD4	CAACTGGAAACATGCGAACCA	TTGATGACCAGGGGGAAAGA	NM_001082313.2
CD8	GGCGTCTACTTCTGCATGACC	GAACCGGCACACTCTCTTCT	ENSOCUT00000009383
CD19	GGATGTATGTCTGTCGCCGT	AAGCAAAGCCACAACTGGAA	ENSOCUT00000028895
GAPDH	GGTGAAGGTCGGAGTGAACGG	CATGTAGACCATGTAGTGGAGGTCA	NM_001082253.1
ACT-β	TCATTCCAAATATCGTGAGATGCC	TACACAAATGCGATGCTGCC	NM_001101683.1
LDHA	TGCAGACAAGGAACAGTGGA	CCCAGGTAGTGTAGCCCTT	NM_001082277.1

NCF-1, neutrophil cytosolic factor 1; CD68, macrosialin; CD11b, macrophage marker; CD14, monocyte differentiation antigen CD14; ARG1, Arginase 1; IL-4, Interleukin 4; IL-13, Interleukin 13; M-CSF, colony stimulating factor-macrophage; OPG, osteoprotegerin; RANKL, Receptor activator of nuclear factor kappa-B ligand; TRAP, tartrate resistant acid phosphatase; CathK, cathepsin K; PPAR-γ, peroxisome proliferator activated receptor gamma; C3, complement component 3; C3aR1, complement component 3a receptor 1; CD46, complement regulatory protein; CD55, decay accelerating factor for complement; CD59, complement regulatory protein; C5, complement component 5; C5aR1, complement component 5a receptor 1; CD3, T-cell surface glycoprotein CD3; CD4, T-cell surface glycoprotein CD4; CD8, T-cell transmembrane glycoprotein CD8; CD19, B-lymphocyte surface protein CD19; GAPDH, glyceraldehyde-3-phosphate dehydrogenase; ACT-β, actin beta; LDHA, lactate dehydrogenase A.

Table 2. Correspondence between studied gene expression and biological entities.

Biological Entity	Gene
Neutrophil	NCF-1
Macrophage	CD68, CD11b, CD14, ARG1
Macrophage fusion	IL-4, IL-13, M-CSF
Bone resorption	OPG, RANKL, TRAP, CathK, PPAR-γ
Complement	Activation: C3, C3aR1, C5, C5aR1 Inhibition: CD46, CD55, CD59
T-lymphocytes	CD3, CD4, CD8
B-lymphocytes	CD19
Reference genes	GAPDH, ACT-β, LDHA

2.4. Amplification Process

Five μL of SsoAdvanced SYBR™ Green Supermix (Bio-Rad Laboratories Inc., Hercules, CA, USA) and 1 μL of cDNA template together with 0.4 μM of forward and reverse primer were used in the qPCR reaction. Each cDNA sample was performed on duplicates. The thermal cycles were performed on the CFX Connect Real-Time System (Bio-Rad Laboratories Inc., Hercules, CA, USA). The CFX Manager Software 3.0 (Bio-Rad, Hercules, CA, USA) was used for the data analysis.

Three genes (GAPDH, ACT-β, LDHA) were selected as reference genes using the geNorm algorithm integrated in the CFX Manager Software. A quantification cycle (Cq) value of the chosen reference genes (Tables 1 and 2) was used as control; hence the mean Cq value of each target gene (Table 1) was normalized against the reference gene's Cq, giving the genes' relative expression.

For calculation of fold change, the $\Delta\Delta Cq$ was used, comparing mRNA expressions from the different groups. Significance was set at $p < 0.05$ and the regulation threshold at $\times 2$-fold change.

2.5. Decalcified Bone Histology

After removal of the implants from the studied Sh, Ti, Cu and PEEK sites on the 6 subjects, bone was removed en bloc and preserved in 10% formalin (4% buffered formaldehyde, VWR international, Leuven, Belgium) during 48 h for fixation. Samples were decalcified in ethylene diamine tetra-acetic acid (10% unbuffered EDTA; Milestone Srl, Sorisole, Italy) for 4 weeks, with weekly substitution of the EDTA solution, dehydrated and embedded in paraffin (Tissue-Tek TEC, Sakura Finetek Europe BV, Leiden, The Netherlands). Samples were sectioned (4 μm thick) with a microtome (Microm HM355S, Thermo Fischer Scientific, Walldorf, Germany) and stained with hematoxylin-eosin (HE) for histological analysis.

2.6. Statistical Analysis

The gene expression statistical analysis was performed using the t test built in the algorithm of the CFX Manager Software 3.0 package (BioRad, Hercules, CA, USA). The gene expression analysis was made pair wise, each material being evaluated against the Sham in each animal.

2.7. Surface Roughness

The surface roughness of each material was measured (following Wennerberg and Albrektsson guidelines (2000)) [10], with a white light 3D optical Profilometer, gbs, smart WLI extended (Gesellschaft für Bild und Signal verarbeitung mbH, Immenau, Germany) using a $50\times$ objective. MountainsMap®Imaging Topography 7.4 (Digital Surf, Besancon, France) software was used to evaluate the data. Surface roughness parameters were calculated after removing errors of form and waviness. A gaussian filter with a size of 50×50 μm was used. The measuring area was 350×220 μm for all measurements, 3 copper, 3 titanium and 3 PEEK implants were measured, each implant on 9 sites (3 tops, 3 valleys and 3 flanks).

In order to characterize the surface in height, spatial and surface enlargement aspects 4 parameters were selected; S_a that describes the average height distribution measured in μm, S_{ds} which is a measure of the density of summits over the measured area, measured in $1/μm^2$, Ssk (skewness) a parameter that describes the asymmetry of the surface deviation from the mean plane and S_{dr} which describes the surface enlargement compared to a totally flat reference area, measured in %.

3. Results

3.1. Gene Expression Analysis

Each material (Ti, Cu and PEEK) was compared against the Sh site for gene expression regarding the immunological reaction after 10 days of healing- and considering that the Sh site itself, also produces an immune-inflammatory reaction. The results show that when comparing Ti sites with Sh sites (Table 3 and Figure 1), ARG1 (M2-macrophage) is statistically significantly and almost 2-fold upregulated, while CD4 (T helper lymphocytes) is 2-fold upregulated and close to statistical significance. This indicates an activation of the immune system already at 10 days around Ti, when compared to Sh. On the other hand, the downregulation of both C3aR1 (complement component 3a receptor 1) and CD8 (T cytotoxic lymphocytes) was more than 2-fold and at a statistically significant level around Ti compared to Sh, which further supports the notion of an immunological involvement in the host response towards titanium, as it probably represents a biological feedback effect following activation of complement factor C3 and T cells at an earlier stage. Furthermore, peroxisome proliferator-activated receptor gamma (PPAR-γ) is significantly downregulated, while RANKL (Receptor activator of nuclear factor kappa-B ligand) and OPG (osteoprotegerin) showed a non-significant downregulation, indicating an environment around Ti where bone resorption is apparently suppressed. Macrophage colony-stimulating factor (M-CSF) is significantly downregulated, indicating suppression of cell (macrophage) fusion around Ti at 10 days, into either osteoclasts or foreign body giant cells (FBGCs).

Table 3. Gene expression Ti vs. Sham.

Marker	Down-Regulation	p-Value
ARG1	1.82	0.0254
CD4	2.03	0.0598
Marker	**Down-Regulation**	**p-Value**
M-CSF	−2.23	0.0004
PPAR-G	−3.07	0.0008
RANKL	−2.24	0.0678
OPG	−1.85	0.5711
C3aR1	−3.55	0.0137
CD8b	−2.80	0.0195

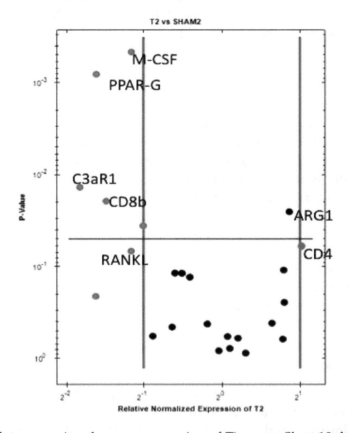

Figure 1. Volcano plot comparing the gene expression of Ti versus Sh at 10 days. Downregulation (vertical green line) and Upregulation (vertical red line) set a ×2 regulation. Statistical significance (horizontal blue line) set at $p < 0.05$—Marker is significant when above blue line.

When comparing PEEK sites with Sh sites (Table 4 and Figure 2), even if not significantly, ARG1 (M2-macrophages), NCF-1 (neutrophils), CD68 (M1-macrophages) and CD4 (T helper cells) are upregulated 2-fold or more around PEEK when compared to Sh sites, indicating early immune activation around PEEK. Downregulation of CD8 (T cytotoxic cell—Significant), complement factors (C3aR1, CD55, CD59 and C5- the last two statistically significant), strongly adds to the notion of immune system involvement in the host reaction towards PEEK implants. The downregulation of PPAR-gamma, RANKL, OPG, TRAP (all statistically significant) and CATHK demonstrates the suppression of bone resorption around PEEK implants after 10 days of insertion in the bone.

Table 4. Gene expression PEEK vs. Sham.

Marker	Down-Regulation	*p*-Value
ARG1	3.11	0.1091
CD68	2.00	0.4304
NCF1	2.61	0.1556
CD4	1.95	0.0771
Marker	**Down-Regulation**	***p*-Value**
PPAR-G	−4.81	0.0009
RANKL	−3.16	0.0286
OPG	−3.13	0.0210
TRAP	−1.91	0.0109
CATHK	−1.75	0.0985
C5	−2.73	0.0044
CD59	−1.87	0.0181
CD55	−1.81	0.0578
C3aR1	−2.84	0.0601
CD8b	−2.86	0.0044

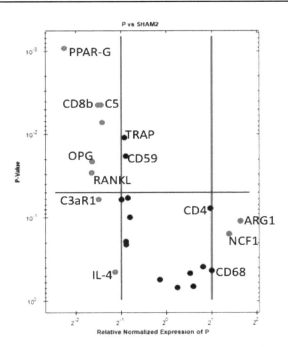

Figure 2. Volcano plot comparing the gene expression of PEEK versus Sh at 10 days. Downregulation (vertical green line) and Upregulation (vertical red line) set a ×2 regulation. Statistical significance (horizontal blue line) set at $p < 0.05$—Marker is significant when above blue line.

Around Copper (Cu) implants, when compared to Sh (Table 5 and Figure 3) at 10 days, ARG1 (M2 macrophage), NCF1 (neutrophils) and CD4 (T helper cells) are statistically significantly upregulated. Furthermore, even if not reaching the statistical significance level of $p < 0.05$, CD19 (B cells), C5aR1 (complement C5 receptor 1), CD68, CD14 and CD11b (the latter three are M1-macrophage markers) are upregulated. These results demonstrate a strong immune activation around Cu upon contact with host bone tissue.

C5, CD59, CD55, CD46 and C3aR1 (complement factors) are downregulated, suggesting a feedback effect following complement activation (which is confirmed by C5aR1 upregulation).

CD8 (T cytotoxic cell) shows a tendency for downregulation around Cu.

The statistically significant downregulation of M-CSF, with the tendency for downregulation of IL-4, even if both not reaching a 2-fold change, suggests that at 10 days of implantation, macrophage fusion into either osteoclasts or FBGCs is suppressed around Cu—Similar to what was observed above around Ti. Additionally, as for Ti and PEEK, bone resorption is suppressed around Cu at 10 days, when compared to Sh, since PPAR-gamma is statistically significantly downregulated and the other bone resorption markers (RANKL, OPG, TRAP and CATHK) show a tendency for downregulation.

Table 5. Gene expression Cu vs. Sham.

Marker	Up-Regulation	p-Value
ARG1	25.74	0.0072
NCF1	3.41	0.0234
CD4	3.11	0.0178
CD19	1.88	0.3768
C5aR1	2.03	0.1021
CD68	1.80	0.4153
CD11b	1.79	0.5131
CD14	1.61	0.6120
Marker	**Down-Regulation**	**p-Value**
PPAR-G	−5.28	0.0001
RANKL	−1.71	0.1301
OPG	−3.74	0.2815
TRAP	−2.25	0.0676
C5	−1.66	0.0007
CD59	−2.01	0.3376
C3aR1	−2.14	0.2071
CD8b	−2.09	0.0906

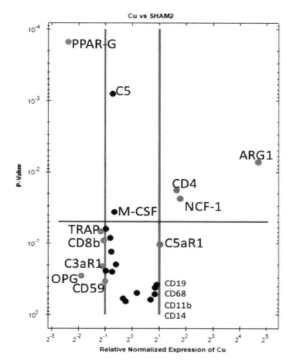

Figure 3. Volcano plot comparing the gene expression of Cu versus Sh at 10 days. Downregulation (vertical green line) and Upregulation (vertical red line) set a ×2 regulation. Statistical significance (horizontal blue line) set at $p < 0.05$—Marker is significant when above blue line.

3.2. Decalcified Bone Histology

Decalcified histological sections of the four groups (Sham and the three different materials) were analyzed at a tissue level. The Sh sites display some bone formation around the osteotomy site, which is decreasing in size after 10 days, as the new bone fills in the osteotomy defect (Figure 4). Ti sites show new bone formation and bone remodeling in the thread areas (Figure 5). Cu sites display no bone formation at the interface of the implant site, showing a division (from the implant area) of a first layer of inflammatory cells with signs of cell lysis and some foreign body giant cells, followed by a proliferative area with parallel aligned fibers to the implant site, which in turn is followed outwards by an area of bone remodeling, more noticeable in areas closer to cortical bone, where osteoblasts and osteoclasts can be observed remodeling the old bone (Figure 6). PEEK sites present very little new bone formation/remodeling areas close to the implant interface, confined to areas in cortical bone proximity, whereas most of the interface presents only a thin proliferative area parallel to the implant site, mostly consisting of fibrous tissue and with very few calcified islands (Figure 7). The cellular components have all been clearly identified, neutrophils, macrophages, osteoclasts, osteoblasts, and also foreign body giant cells. However, quantification has not been performed, as it is not within the scope of the present study.

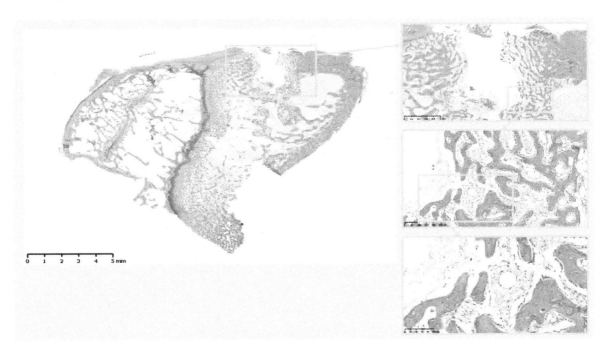

Figure 4. The 10 days Sh site. Bone remodeling with new bone formation around the osteotomy site. Defect is isolated from the marrow space. Scale bars, clockwise: 5 mm, 1 mm, 250 μm and 100 μm.

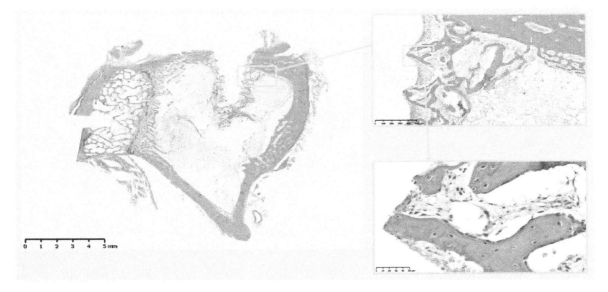

Figure 5. The 10 days Ti site. Bone remodeling and new bone formation around the implant site, isolating it from the marrow space. Scale bars, clockwise: 5 mm, 500 μm and 50 μm.

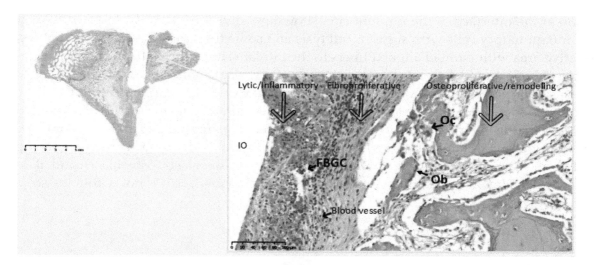

Figure 6. The 10 days Cu site. No bone on the immediate implant vicinity. FBGC, foreign body giant cells; Oc, osteoclast actively remodeling old bone; Ob, Seam of osteoblasts producing new bone (part of the remodeling); IO, Implant/Osteotomy. Reaction to Cu divided in 3 zones, representing the 3 phenomena around implant materials in the bone: From the implant surface Lytic/Inflammatory area, Fibroproliferative area and Osteoproliferative area. The latter two represent an attempt to isolate the material from the marrow cavity. No osseointegration is viable at this time point. Theoretically, around Ti the same phenomena exist, but at a different balance, allowing for osseointegration, through direct bon-to-implant contact. Inflammatory area is highly vascularized. Scale bars 5 mm (left) and 100 μm (right).

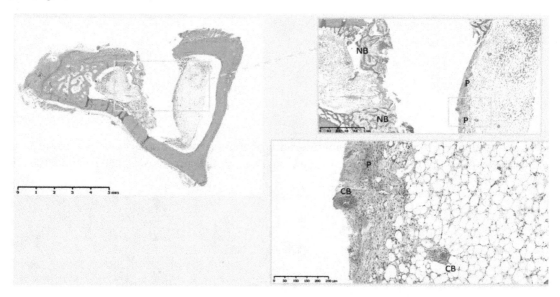

Figure 7. The 10 days PEEK. NB, new bone; forming only in the areas adjacent to cortical bone, while most other interfacial tissue shows no bone formation. P, proliferative area; no visible calcified tissue formation, but for some isolated calcified bone areas (CB, calcified bone). Scale bars, clockwise: 5 mm, 1 mm and 250 μm.

3.3. Surface Roughness

Table 6 shows the results on each material surface roughness analysis. The surface enlargement, which is depending on both height and the density of the surface irregularities, was smallest for the copper implants mostly depending on the lower height deviation compared to titanium and PEEK. Titanium and PEEK had a frequency distribution close to zero, while copper implants had slightly more peaks than pits. In terms of height deviation, titanium demonstrated the roughest surface.

Table 6. Surface roughness analysis.

Surface Roughness	S_a μm Mean	S_{sk} Mean	S_{ds} 1/μm² Mean	S_{dr} % Mean
Copper	0.40	1.2	0.28	47
Titanium	0.75	−0.02	0.25	66
PEEK	0.56	−0.23	0.31	69

S_a, describes the average height distribution measured in μm; S_{ds}, a measure of the density of summits over the measured area, measured in 1/μm²; S_{sk} (skewness), a parameter that describes the asymmetry of the surface deviation from the mean plane; S_{dr}, describes the surface enlargement compared to a totally flat reference area, measured in %.

4. Discussion

The present results demonstrate the immune system activation around Ti, PEEK and Cu once in contact with host bone, after 10 days of implantation- this demonstrates that, eventually, all materials render an immune activation, when in contact with bone.

Macrophage polarization, between M1-macrophage and M2-macrophage phenotypes, has been highlighted as a determining factor in the foreign body reaction, i.e., how host tissues interact with biomaterials [7,8]. M1-macrophages present a pro-inflammatory phenotype, while M2-macrophages have been identified as anti-inflammatory cells, participating in wound healing—Namely in the healing phase of acute inflammation—And also in chronic inflammation associated with immunological diseases, such as Rheumatoid Arthritis and Psoriasis [11]. M1-macrophages are described as induced by interferon-gamma (IFN-γ), while M2 macrophages are described as induced by e.g., IL-4 and IL-13 [8].

One of the main findings in this study is the importance of the M1/M2-macrophage (M1/M2) immunological balance in osseointegration already at this early stage: Titanium displays a reparative/anti-inflammatory M2-macrophage (M2) phenotype (ARG1), whereas Cu and PEEK are still dealing with a mixed pro-inflammatory M1-macrophage (M1) and M2 anti-inflammatory type of reaction (CD68, CD14 and CD11b; ARG1, respectively). The early preferential polarization towards a M2 phenotype around Ti, in the M1/M2 balance, probably explains the event of osseointegration being successful around Ti and not around the other materials—A fact already hypothesized in our previous work [3] and further discussed below.

Another important, and unpredicted, finding is the tilting towards the CD4 T-cell phenotype and suppression of the CD8 T-cell phenotype around all materials, opening a window to further understanding the immune reaction to biomaterials in the bone, by demonstrating the participation of T-cells and indicating an early specific T-cell phenotype (discussed below).

The current results confirm the present authors' previously published results comparing Ti and Sh immune responses, where immune activation around Ti implants was demonstrated in a femur study at 10 days and even more so at 28 days after implantation, i.e., outside the major inflammatory period [12].

For the present experiment, Ti was chosen as an already studied material, and the results of the previous study were confirmed, while PEEK was chosen for its perceived bio-inertness [13] and Cu for its known induction of a stronger inflammatory reaction when in contact with tissues—As demonstrated by Suska et al. 2008 in a rat soft tissue model [14]. As already mentioned, Ti displays mostly a reparative type-2 phenotype (ARG1 and CD4), whereas around Cu (ARG1, NCF1, CD11b, CD68, CD14, C5aR1, CD19) and PEEK (ARG1, CD68, NCF1, CD4) there is still a mixed environment, with pro-inflammatory and anti-inflammatory/reparative elements, which may explain the different bone tissue reaction towards the different materials at a tissue level (supported by the histological findings in this study). Even if some of these markers are not expressed with a statistically significant difference in value, most pass the ×2 threshold in regulation fold-change or are very close to that value; hence, their interpretation is crucial to understand the biological events and the osteoimmunology in relation to the studied materials.

The three materials have shown up-regulation of ARG1, indicating a reparative type-2 anti-inflammatory reaction (M2- macrophages and ILC-2). PEEK and Cu also show a M1-macrophage pro-inflammatory type of reaction, meaning that at 10 days the host tissue is not yet tilting the balance towards a full reparative mode around Cu and PEEK, which may explain, at least in part, the results at tissue level. Hence, the present results confirm the notion of macrophages being central in host reaction to biomaterials, with a decisive role already at 10 days- it would be interesting to study how the biological immune process develops at a later time point, whether it resolves, maintains or increases around Cu and PEEK.

Furthermore, the results show activation of CD4+ T-cells around all materials at 10 days, whereas the CD8+ T-cell phenotype is suppressed. These findings demonstrate the participation of T-cells in the bone healing process around solid biomaterials, although it is not known whether solely an innate or also an adaptive type of immune reaction is present—Classically, the host reaction to biomaterials is perceived as an innate immunological process [5], hence indicating T-cell activity through cytokines, rather than an antigen-antibody interaction. Furthermore, ARG1, which shows a tendency for upregulation in the three materials compared to Sh, is also expressed by type-2 innate lymphoid-cells (ILC-2) [15], supporting an innate immune mechanism. T-helper cells (CD4+) are involved in the regulation of immune responses at many levels, such as interaction with macrophages and the recruitment of neutrophils [16]. Regulatory T-cells (Treg) are also CD4+, and are responsible for suppressing immune inflammatory responses to allow reparative processes, being important, for instance, in halting some forms of autoimmune diseases [17]; hence, upregulation of CD4 most probably indicates an immunologically driven reaction towards tissue repair and proliferation around the studied materials, which has also been suggested by other authors [18].

The statistically significant upregulation of NCF1 around Cu and a similar upregulation around PEEK (even if not statistically significant) already at 10 days, highlights the role of neutrophils in the host-biomaterial interaction; however, in our previous study [5], Ti showed a statistically significant upregulation of NCF1 only after 28 days of healing, which implies a stronger inflammatory reaction around Cu and PEEK at an early stage that may further help dictate a soft tissue formation around these materials, not enabling bone deposition at the implant surface. At an earlier stage in the healing response, neutrophils participate in the inflammatory reaction, although changing phenotype at a later stage in this response, which may be the result of either macrophages inhibiting neutrophil apoptosis for continued neutrophil local performance, or the possible participation in the reparative process, mainly through an enhancing effect on vascularization [19,20]. Vascularization is of particular importance for the early development of tissue around the implants in an attempt to isolate these from the marrow compartment during the foreign body reaction; this is especially important considering that bone is a hypoxic tissue [21].

Complement factors seem mostly suppressed around all of the materials studied, at 10 days. The complement system, however, is complex and self-regulated [22]. The results show that the complement components are mostly downregulated, probably reflecting an inhibitory reaction to an earlier complement activation during the initial healing phase- thus indicating the possible involvement of the complement system from an early time point in the host reaction to implanted materials in the bone.

Furthermore, bone resorption markers were downregulated around all three materials at 10 days, when compared to Sh sites. This demonstrates a bone resorption suppression in the immediate implant environment from an early stage, when compared to our previous study, where this was mostly perceived at a later time point (28 days) around Ti [5]. Hence, a bone forming environment is already being developed around materials from an early healing stage and within the inflammatory period.

Further studies including protein identification techniques are recommended to confirm the gene expression outcomes presented here and rule out possible post-transcriptional or post-translational changes in the biological response.

Copper presents with extensive apoptosis around the surface; one would attribute this to the toxicity of Copper ions, but the surface topography may play an important role in determining the phenotype of Macrophages here: Copper compared to Sham shows an upregulation of ARG1, indicating M2-macrophages already at 10 days (25 times up regulated in Cu, while Ti and PEEK show a less pronounced increase in ARG1, even if also relevant). A possible conclusion is that the chemical aspect of Copper surface is likely a major factor, given the apoptosis seen, but that the surface topography also has to be considered, given that current evidence on M1/M2-macrophage polarization has a clear link to surface topography [8], which relates to our results both on surface analysis and gene expression analysis. Further studies are hence necessary to understand the role of both surface topography and chemistry, which likely differs between different materials. The surface may play a role in the macrophage phenotype, however, in the present study, Cu did not demonstrate an exceptional roughness, rather similar to commercial Ti implants produced with grade 4 Ti. Therefore, the topography may have had an influence but not likely a major one. Recent in vitro studies have shown the effect of surface chemistry and topography in macrophage polarization. Zhang H et al. have demonstrated the surface chemistry immunomodulatory effect of amine silanized titanium, which reduced inflammation and promoted M2 polarization of macrophages [23], while Gao L et al. have demonstrated a M1- to M2-macrophage switch, through surface release of IL-4 [24]. Regarding surface topography, Shayan M et al. have demonstrated both in vitro and in a soft tissue in vivo study, that implant surface nanopatterning is able to selectively polarize macrophages towards M2, hence modulating the immune response to the selected biomaterial [25]. These studies concur with the current bone tissue in vivo experimental results, which demonstrated that different materials modulate the host immune response through the polarization of macrophages, where Ti promotes an early shift to a M2-macrophage phenotype- with the inherent consequences observed at the tissue level, and which may explain the clinical osseointegration seen around Ti implants in bone.

Decalcified histology of specimens from the four groups shows that only Ti develops a structured thread infill of new bone, at 10 days. All the groups form an area of several cell layers clearly isolating the implant material (or osteotomy site in Sh), although Cu and PEEK fail to produce an adequate volume of osseous tissue, showing mostly soft tissue in the interfacial zone. In fact, the present histological results support the published work by Osborne and Newesley (1980), indicating contact osteogenesis around "well tolerated" biomaterials and distance osteogenesis around "less well tolerated" biomaterials [26]. This difference can be explained by the above gene expression analysis, where Ti shows a more reparative environment at such an early stage, when compared to PEEK and Cu.

5. Conclusions/Summary

1. All three materials display immune/inflammatory system activation at 10 days;
2. A more favourable macrophage M1/M2 balance likely leads to a better osseointegration of Ti, as compared to Cu and PEEK:
3. A clearer M2 anti-inflammatory/reparative regulation around Ti at 10 days;
4. A mixture of M1 and M2 (pro- and anti-inflammatory, respectively) regulation around Cu and PEEK (more pronounced around Cu);
5. T-lymphocytes participate in the foreign body reaction to biomaterials at an early stage;
6. T-cells may act through a CD4+ phenotype (T_{helper}/T_{reg}), suppressing the CD8+ $T_{cytotoxic}$ type of reaction at 10 days;
7. The up-regulation of the neutrophil specific factor NCF-1 around Cu and PEEK, indicates a higher inflammatory activity and may in part contribute to an inferior osseointegration on materials other than Ti;
8. Complement system seems predominantly downregulated around materials at 10 days, when compared to the Sh;

9. Bone forming environment (suppression of bone resorption) develops around all three implanted materials at an early stage, and within the inflammatory period;

10. At tissue level, only Ti seems to lead to osseointegration; PEEK and Cu show little or no implant related bone formation (respectively)—Which probably reflects the slightly more pronounced immune activation around the latter materials at this early stage;

11. Surface topography may play a role in macrophage phenotype and on the ultimate tissue level reaction to biomaterials, but further studies are needed.

The present results indicate that Ti osseointegration likely arises from a material-specific inflammatory/immune process leading to a shorter pro-inflammatory period and earlier reparative process, starting still within the inflammatory period and promoting bone apposition on Ti implant surfaces. It is further confirmed that all materials trigger an immune activation, even by materials like PEEK, previously considered as bio-inert. Different materials thus display different inflammatory balances in their vicinity, partly controlled by the immune system. Longer-term studies are necessary to better comprehend the immunobiology and tissue performance beyond the inflammatory period around established and new biomaterials.

Author Contributions: Conceptualization, R.T., T.A., P.T. and A.W.; Methodology, R.T., T.A., P.T. and A.W.; Software, R.T., Z.P., A.W. and S.G.; Validation, R.T. and P.T.; Formal Analysis, R.T. and A.W.; Investigation, R.T. and A.W.; Resources, R.T., P.T., T.A. and A.W.; Data Curation, R.T.; Writing—Original Draft Preparation, R.T. and A.W.; Writing—Review & Editing, P.T., T.A. and A.W.; Visualization, R.T., S.G. and Z.P.; Supervision, A.W., T.A. and P.T.; Project Administration, R.T.; Funding Acquisition, A.W.

References

1. Chen, Z.; Wu, C.; Gu, W.; Klein, T.; Crawford, R.; Xiao, Y. Osteogenic differentiation of bone marrow MSCs by β-tricalcium phosphate stimulating macrophages via BMP2 signalling pathway. *Biomaterials* **2014**, *35*, 1507–1518. [CrossRef] [PubMed]

2. Vishwakarma, A.; Bhise, N.S.; Evangelista, M.B.; Rouwkema, J.; Dokmeci, M.R.; Ghaemmaghami, A.M.; Khademhosseini, A. Engineering immunomodulatory biomaterials to tune the inflammatory response. *Trends Biotechnol.* **2016**, *34*, 470–482. [CrossRef] [PubMed]

3. Trindade, R.; Albrektsson, T.; Tengvall, P.; Wennerberg, A. Foreign body reaction to biomaterials: On mechanisms for buildup and breakdown of osseointegration. *Clin. Implant. Dent. Relat. Res.* **2016**, *18*, 192–203. [CrossRef] [PubMed]

4. Albrektsson, T.; Dahlin, C.; Jemt, T.; Sennerby, L.; Turri, A.; Wennerberg, A. Is marginal bone loss around oral implants the result of a provoked foreign body reaction? *Clin. Implant. Dent. Relat. Res.* **2014**, *16*, 155–165. [CrossRef] [PubMed]

5. Trindade, R.; Albrektsson, T.; Galli, S.; Prgomet, Z.; Tengvall, P.; Wennerberg, A. Osseointegration and foreign body reaction: Titanium implants activate the immune system and suppress bone resorption during the first 4 weeks after implantation. *Clin. Implant. Dent. Relat. Res.* **2018**, *20*, 82–91. [CrossRef] [PubMed]

6. Arvidsson, S.; Askendal, A.; Tengvall, P. Blood plasma contact activation on silicon, titanium and aluminium. *Biomaterials* **2007**, *28*, 1346–1354. [CrossRef]

7. Anderson, J.M.; Jones, J.A. Phenotypic dichotomies in the foreign body reaction. *Biomaterials* **2007**, *28*, 5114–5120. [CrossRef]

8. Sridharan, R.; Cameron, A.R.; Kelly, D.J.; Kearney, C.J.; O'Brien, F.J. Biomaterial based modulation of macrophage polarization: A review and suggested design principles. *Mater. Today (Kidlington)* **2015**, *18*, 313–325. [CrossRef]

9. Miron, R.J.; Bosshardt, D.D. OsteoMacs: Key players around bone biomaterials. *Biomaterials* **2016**, *82*, 1–19. [CrossRef]

10. Wennerberg, A.; Albrektsson, T. Suggested guidelines for the topographic evaluation of implant surfaces. *Int. J. Oral Maxillofac. Implants* **2000**, *15*, 331–344.

11. Porcheray, F.; Viaud, S.; Rimaniol, A.C.; Léone, C.; Samah, B.; Dereuddre-Bosquet, N.; Domont, D.; Gras, G. Macrophage activation switching: An asset for the resolution of inflammation. *Clin. Exp. Immunol.* **2005**, *142*, 481–489. [CrossRef] [PubMed]

12. Anderson, J.M.; Rodriguez, A.; Chang, D.T. Foreign body reaction to biomaterials. *Semin. Immunol.* **2008**, *20*, 86–100. [CrossRef]

13. Johansson, P.; Jimbo, R.; Kjellin, P.; Currie, F.; Chrcanovic, B.R.; Wennerberg, A. Biomechanical evaluation and surface characterization of a nano-modified surface on PEEK implants: A study in the rabbit tibia. *Int. J. Nanomed.* **2014**, *9*, 3903–3911. [CrossRef]

14. Suska, F.; Emanuelsson, L.; Johansson, A.; Tengvall, P.; Thomsen, P. Fibrous capsule formation around titanium and copper. *J. Biomed. Mater. Res. A* **2008**, *85*, 888–896. [CrossRef]

15. Monticelli, L.A.; Buck, M.D.; Flamar, A.L.; Saenz, S.A.; Tait Wojno, E.D.; Yudanin, N.A.; Osborne, L.C.; Hepworth, M.R.; Tran, S.V.; Rodewald, H.R.; et al. Arginase 1 is an innate lymphoid-cell-intrinsic metabolic checkpoint controlling type 2 inflammation. *Nat. Immunol.* **2016**, *17*, 656–665. [CrossRef] [PubMed]

16. Zhu, J.; Paul, W.E. CD4 T cells: Fates, functions, and faults. *Blood* **2008**, *112*, 1557–1569. [CrossRef] [PubMed]

17. Hori, S.; Nomura, T.; Sakaguchi, S. Control of regulatory T cell development by the transcription factor Foxp3. *Science* **2003**, *299*, 1057–1061. [CrossRef]

18. Julier, Z.; Park, A.J.; Briquez, P.S.; Martino, M.M. Promoting tissue regeneration by modulating the immune system. *Acta Biomater.* **2017**, *53*, 13–28. [CrossRef]

19. Soehnlein, O.; Steffens, S.; Hidalgo, A.; Weber, C. Neutrophils as protagonists and targets in chronic inflammation. *Nat. Rev. Immunol.* **2017**, *17*, 248–261. [CrossRef]

20. Christoffersson, G.; Vagesjo, E.; Vandooren, J.; Liden, M.; Massena, S.; Reinert, R.B.; Brissova, M.; Powers, A.C.; Opdenakker, G.; Phillipson, M. VEGF-A recruits a proangiogenic MMP-9-delivering neutrophil subset that induces angiogenesis in transplanted hypoxic tissue. *Blood* **2012**, *120*, 4653–4662. [CrossRef]

21. Taylor, C.T.; Colgan, S.P. Regulation of immunity and inflammation by hypoxia in immunological niches. *Nat. Rev. Immunol.* **2017**, *17*, 774–785. [CrossRef]

22. Ignatius, A.; Schoengraf, P.; Kreja, L.; Liedert, A.; Recknagel, S.; Kandert, S.; Brenner, R.E.; Schneider, M.; Lambris, J.D.; Huber-Lang, M. Complement C3a and C5a modulate osteoclast formation and inflammatory response of osteoblasts in synergism with IL-1β. *J. Cell. Biochem.* **2011**, *112*, 2594–2605. [CrossRef]

23. Zhang, H.; Wu, X.; Wang, G.; Liu, P.; Qin, S.; Xu, K.; Tong, D.; Ding, H.; Tang, H.; Ji, F. Macrophage polarization, inflammatory signaling, and NF-κB activation in response to chemically modified titanium surfaces. *Colloids Surf. B Biointerfaces.* **2018**, *166*, 269–276. [CrossRef]

24. Gao, L.; Li, M.; Yin, L.; Zhao, C.; Chen, J.; Zhou, J.; Duan, K.; Feng, B. Dual-inflammatory cytokines on TiO_2 nanotube-coated surfaces used for regulating macrophage polarization in bone implants. *J. Biomed. Mater. Res. A* **2018**, *106*, 1878–1886. [CrossRef]

25. Shayan, M.; Padmanabhan, J.; Morris, A.H.; Cheung, B.; Smith, R.; Schroers, J.; Kyriakides, T.R. Nanopatterned bulk metallic glass-based biomaterials modulate macrophage polarization. *Acta Biomater.* **2018**, *75*, 427–438. [CrossRef]

26. Osborn, J.F.; Newesly, H. Dynamic aspects of the implant-bone interface. In *Dental Implants, Materials and Systems*; Heimke, G., Ed.; Hanser Verlag: München, Germany, 1980; pp. 111–123, ISBN 978-3446132122.

12

Mechanical and Biological Advantages of a Tri-Oval Implant Design

Xing Yin [1,2], Jingtao Li [1,2], Waldemar Hoffmann [3], Angelines Gasser [3], John B. Brunski [2] and Jill A. Helms [2,*]

[1] State Key Laboratory of Oral Diseases & National Clinical Research Center for Oral Diseases, West China Hospital of Stomatology, Sichuan University, Chengdu 610041, China; yinxing@scu.edu.cn (X.Y.); lijingtao86@163.com (J.L.)

[2] Division of Plastic and Reconstructive Surgery, Department of Surgery, Stanford School of Medicine, Stanford, CA 94305, USA; brunsj6@stanford.edu

[3] Nobel Biocare Services AG, P.O. Box, Zurich-Airport, 8058 Zurich, Switzerland; waldemar.hoffmann@nobelbiocare.com (W.H.); angelines.gasser@nobelbiocare.com (A.G.)

* Correspondence: jhelms@stanford.edu

Abstract: Of all geometric shapes, a tri-oval one may be the strongest because of its capacity to bear large loads with neither rotation nor deformation. Here, we modified the external shape of a dental implant from circular to tri-oval, aiming to create a combination of high strain and low strain peri-implant environment that would ensure both primary implant stability and rapid osseointegration, respectively. Using in vivo mouse models, we tested the effects of this geometric alteration on implant survival and osseointegration over time. The maxima regions of tri-oval implants provided superior primary stability without increasing insertion torque. The minima regions of tri-oval implants presented low compressive strain and significantly less osteocyte apoptosis, which led to minimal bone resorption compared to the round implants. The rate of new bone accrual was also faster around the tri-oval implants. We further subjected both round and tri-oval implants to occlusal loading immediately after placement. In contrast to the round implants that exhibited a significant dip in stability that eventually led to their failure, the tri-oval implants maintained their stability throughout the osseointegration period. Collectively, these multiscale biomechanical analyses demonstrated the superior in vivo performance of the tri-oval implant design.

Keywords: dental implant; osseointegration; alveolar bone remodeling/regeneration; bone biology; finite element analysis (FEA); biomechanics

1. Introduction

Implants have undergone a nearly continual transformation since their inception. Variations in fabrication materials, surface texture, coating, and taper have yielded implants that osseointegrated and are clinically successful [1–5]. Most dental implants, however, still have a circular cross-section, which reflects their origins as titanium screws [6,7].

A non-circular cross-section may have advantages. When placed into a cylindrical osteotomy, conventional implants typically have a uniform bone-implant contact (BIC), and the resulting peri-implant strains are uniformly distributed around its circumference [8]. Although the relationship is not straightforward [9], it is generally presumed that the greater the amount of bone-implant contact (BIC) the better is implant stability [10].

A non-circular, e.g., a tri-oval shaped implant, on the other hand, would be predicted to engage bone on its vertices, or tri-oval maxima, which would provide mechanical stability and result in peri-implant strains concentrated at these regions.

Depending on the extent of tri-ovality, there would also be sites of minimal BIC. An extensive literature has shown that new woven bone first forms in areas where BIC is absent [8,11–14].

In previous studies, we demonstrated that when an implant is placed with high insertion torque (IT), then peri-implant bone is compressed and osteocytes within this bone begin to die [8,15,16].

Some proposed embodiments of dental implants have had non-circular cross-sectional shapes to reduce "friction between the bone and implant during insertion" [17,18]. Once the implant is in place, however, it is not friction but rather peri-implant stresses and strains that appear to be most important: Inserting an implant creates strains in peri-implant tissues [11,19,20], and the magnitude of these strains has a direct, quantifiable impact on the behavior of cells and tissues in the peri-implant environment [20,21].

In areas where an implant contacts bone, the stiff interface stabilizes the implant [15]. There is a biological downside to this relationship, though: if the implant is placed with high IT, then the stiff interfacial bone is compressed to a greater extent, and the result is higher strain. Cells within the bone matrix, i.e., osteocytes, respond to this high strain by dying [8,15,16].

The converse is also true: in areas of low strain, fewer peri-implant osteocytes die and bone resorption is minimal [22]. If the peri-implant bone is "soft", e.g., has a trabecular microstructure, then cells in the low strain environment tend to proliferate. Ultimately, these cells can differentiate into osteoblasts and osseointegration ensues [22].

Once osteocytes have died, necrotic bone is resorbed via an osteoclast-mediated process [8,15]. Thereafter, new bone formation ensues [8,23]. The resorption of dead peri-implant bone, however, jeopardizes implant stability. We speculated that there could be a way to avoid this by purposefully creating a combination of high strain and low strain peri-implant environments that would ensure both mechanical engagement in the surrounding bone, i.e., primary stability, and rapid osseointegration, respectively. In a tri-oval implant design, the maxima regions would theoretically correspond to areas of higher strain and provide initial mechanical stability. The minima regions of the tri-oval design would theoretically correspond to areas of low strain and constitute pro-osteogenic zones where new bone formation would contribute to secondary implant stability. Here, we tested the veracity of this theory by comparing outcomes of tri-oval and round implants placed into healed maxillary sites according to a well-established in vivo mouse model of oral implant osseointegration.

2. Materials and methods

2.1. Implant Design

Implants were manufactured from CP Titanium Grade 4 with a TiUnite surface (Nobel Biocare AB, Goteborg, Sweden). Geometries for round (control) and tri-oval implants are described in Supplemental Table S1.

2.2. Animals and Tooth Extraction Surgeries

Procedures were approved by Stanford Committee on Animal Research (protocol #13146) and conformed to the ARRIVE guidelines. Wild-type C57BL/6 mice (Jackson Laboratory, Bar Harbor, ME, USA, #003291) were housed in a temperature-controlled environment with 12h light/dark cycles. In total, 96 eight-week-old male mice were used.

2.3. Implant Placement, Osteotomy Site Preparation, and Experimental Groups

Extraction of bilateral maxillary 1st molars (mxM1) was performed using forceps. Bleeding was controlled by local pressure. Extraction sockets were allowed to fully heal for four weeks [22]. Pain control was ensured by daily delivery of analgesics. Immediately following surgery mice received sub-cutaneous injections of buprenorphine (0.05–0.1 mg/kg) for analgesia once a day for a total of three days. Animals were fed with regular hard chow diet. Daily monitoring revealed no evidence of prolonged inflammation during healing at the surgical sites. No antibiotics were given to the operated animals.

Following anesthesia, osteotomy sites were produced using a dental engine (NSK, Tokyo, Japan) and a 0.45mm diameter drill bit at 800 rpm (Drill Bit City, Prospect Heights, IL, USA). Aseptic saline was used for irrigation during the drilling process.

A split-mouth design was employed for this study, wherein each mouse received one round implant and one tri-oval implant. See Supplemental Table S2 for the distribution of groups and analyses performed in each group. Implants were placed either below the occlusal plane or at the level of occlusion.

2.4. Implant Insertion Torque Measurement

To compare the insertion torque (IT) of the round and tri-oval implants, two independent experimental setting were performed. In one experimental design, holes (0.45mm diameter) were produced in a uniform block of poplar wood and then round and tri-oval implants were inserted all the way into the wood block. The IT was then recorded by attaching the implants to a miniature torque cell (MRT Miniature Flange Style Reaction Torque Transducer, Interface Inc., Scottsdale, AZ, USA). Poplar wood had an elastic modulus of 10.9 GPa [24], which is on the same order of magnitude as dense bone (e.g., 10–20 GPa) [25].

In another experimental design, the IT was measured directly on mice [26]. Osteotomies (0.45 mm in diameter) were prepared in the healed maxillary tooth extraction sites and the implants were inserted. The animals were sacrificed immediately after implant placement. The mandible was removed to fully expose the inserted implant, and the IT was then measured by connecting the implant to a pre-calibrated hand-held gauge (Tonichi, Tokyo, Japan).

The rationale for comparing insertion torques (IT) of round and trioval implants in wood was not to imply that wood is an excellent substitute test material for bone; rather it was because (a) wood offered a uniform material allowing side-by-side IT tests of round and trioval implants under identical conditions, and (b) the IT tests in wood could be conducted using a sensitive miniature torque transducer that could not be used in vivo.

2.5. Lateral Stability Testing, Finite Element Modeling, and Calculation of Elastic Modulus

A lateral stiffness test (LST) of implants in alveolar bone was carried out using maxillae samples retrieved on PID 0, 3, 7, 14, and 20. The LST was based on an assumed linear relationship between a lateral force exerted on the top of an implant and the resulting lateral displacement of the implant in bone. Our experience with this method, including modeling with finite element analysis indicates that this assumption is valid for displacements in the range of about 0 to 50 μm [15,27].

To carry out LST, the animals were sacrificed and the skulls, with the maxillae removed and sectioned in half sagittally, were submerged in 100% ethanol. The half-maxilla containing the implants was then rigidly clamped to a solid support so that the implant was positioned between a linear actuator (Ultra Motion Digit D-A.083-AB-HT17075-2-K-B/3, Mattituck, NY, USA) equipped with an in-line 10 N force transducer (Honeywell Model 31), and a displacement transducer (MG-DVRT-3, Lord MicroStrain, Williston, VT, USA). A tare load of 0.05 N was applied to one side of the implant while the stylus of the displacement transducer was positioned against the diametrically-opposite side of the implant. Under software command, the actuator was triggered to deliver three cycles of a displacement vs. time waveform with a peak displacement of about 30 μm (Figure 1M). The force was applied, and the resulting lateral displacement of the implant was measured at a consistent height of ~0.5 mm above the crest of the maxillary bone. Previous tests and calculations show that under the force conditions in this test, there is negligible deformation of the titanium implant, meaning that virtually all lateral displacement arises from displacements in the peri-implant tissue. Lateral force and lateral displacement of the implant were recorded and stored to disc for later data analysis and calculation of the ratio between force and displacement, i.e., lateral stiffness (in Newtons/micron).

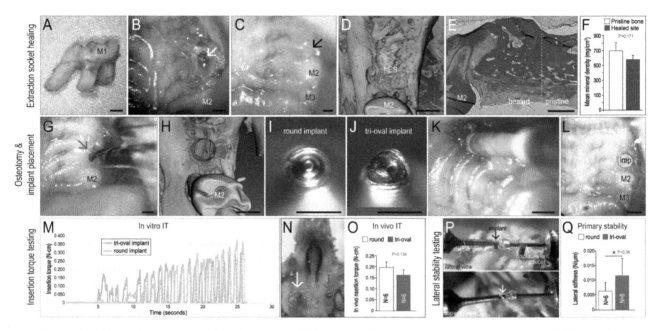

Figure 1. Tri-oval implants placed in type III bone with the same insertion torque exhibit higher primary stability as compared to conventional round implants. (**A**) Maxillary first molars (M1) were extracted from skeletally mature (8-week-old) male mice. (**B**) Intraoral photos of extraction socket (white arrow) and (**C**) Healed extraction site (black arrow). (**D**) Representative micro-CT imaging and (**E**) Representative aniline blue staining of the healed extraction socket on PED28. (**F**) Quantification of mean bone mineral density (BMD) on PED28, where the BMD of the healed extraction site was equivalent to surrounding pristine alveolar bone. (**G**) Osteotomies (0.45 mm dia.; pink arrow) were produced in the healed extraction sites using dental drill. (**H**) Representative micro-CT image of the prepared osteotomy site. (**I**) Geometries of the round and (**J**) tri-oval implants in cross-section. (**K**) Implant placement surgery. (**L**) Implants were positioned at the height of the gingiva. (**M**) In vitro IT testing and (**N**) In vivo IT testing where the white arrow indicates a round implant; blue arrow indicates a tri-oval implant. (**O**) Quantification of in vivo IT for round (white) and tri-oval (blue) implants. (**P**) Lateral stability testing of round and tri-oval implants (arrows) in the mouse maxillae; a stepper motor laterally displaces the implant a known amount while the force to do so is measured by a transducer. (**Q**) Tri-oval implants are significantly more stable than round implants at the time of insertion. Abbreviations: M1, maxillary first molar; M2, maxillary second molar; M3, maxillary third molar; hES, healed extraction site; PED, post-extraction day; imp, implant; IT, insertion torque. Scale bars = 500 µm.

Finite element (FE) modeling provided insight into the relationship between the experimentally-measured lateral stiffness and the elastic properties of the surrounding peri-implant bone [28]. Based on stiffness values from lateral stability testing at post-implant day 3 (PID3), a FE model was used to estimate the elastic modulus of peri-implant tissue. A computer-aided design (CAD) file of each implant was obtained from the manufacturer (Nobel Biocare AB, Göteborg, Sweden) and imported into COMSOL Multiphysics 5.3 when formulating models of the lateral stiffness testing (LST). Each implant was installed to full depth (i.e., eight threads) into a 0.45 mm drill hole made completely through a cylinder (2 mm diameter, 1.45 mm height) of uniform bone having a Young's elastic modulus and Poisson's ratio selected so that the lateral stiffness computed from the FE model matched the experimentally-measured lateral stiffness. A no-slip boundary condition was applied between implant and bone, and the side and bottom surfaces of the bone cylinder were fixed in space. In the FE model simulating LST, a 0.2N lateral load was applied on the side of the implant's top portion, at a height of 0.58 mm above the surface of the bone. The direction of the applied force was perpendicular to the long axis of the implant. The resulting displacement of the implant in the same direction of the lateral force was measured from the displacement output. The ratio of the applied lateral force to the measured lateral displacement at 0.58 mm above the surface of the bone was defined as the lateral stiffness. A typical FE model formulated as described above involved about 238,000 degrees of freedom. To match the results from a given experimental stiffness test of a round or tri-oval implant, the Young's elastic modulus of the bone in the model was parametrically changed until there was a match in lateral stiffness between the FE model and the actual experiment. These FE models demonstrated that the lateral stiffness strongly depended on the Young's elastic modulus of the peri-implant bone.

2.6. Calculating Elastic Modulus of Peri-Implant Bone as a Function of Lateral Stability

Implant insertion caused dynamic tissue remodeling, which could potentially change the tissue elastic modulus in the peri-implant region. Although the changes in peri-implant elastic modulus could not be measured directly on mice, we used FE modeling to generate estimates basing on stiffness values from lateral stability testing at PID3. In the round implant cases, the mean lateral stiffness was 0.00198 N/μm, which corresponded to a modulus of ~2.6 MPa for the peri-implant bone. In the tri-oval implant cases, the mean lateral stiffness was 0.00689 N/μm, which corresponded to a modulus of ~9.2 MPa, a 3.5 times stiffer peri-implant bone than in the case of the round implants.

2.7. Sample Preparation, Tissue Processing, and Histology

Mice were euthanized on PID 3, 7, 10, 14, and 20. For those animals whose implants were to be subjected to mechanical testing, maxillae were harvested with skin and superficial muscles removed, fixed in 100% ethanol, and then subjected to lateral stiffness testing. In cases where implants were evaluated by histology/histomorphometry, tissues were fixed in 4% paraformaldehyde overnight at 4 °C then decalcified in 19% EDTA.

After complete demineralization, specimens were dehydrated through an ascending ethanol series and underwent clearing in xylene prior to paraffin embedding. Before immersion in xylene, implants were gently removed from the samples. Eight-micron-thick longitudinal sections were cut and collected on Superfrost-plus slides [27]. Tissue sections prepared for histology, immunohistochemistry, and immunofluorescence were prepared by one individual then quantified by a blinded individual.

Aniline blue staining was performed to detect osteoid matrix. Tissues sections were also stained with the acidic dye, picrosirius red, to discriminate tightly packed and aligned collagen molecules. Viewed under polarized light, well-aligned fibrillary collagen molecules present polarization colors of longer wavelengths (red) as compared to less organized collagen fibrils that show colors of shorter (green-yellow) wavelengths [27].

2.8. Histomorphometry

Maxillae were embedded in paraffin and sectioned in the transverse planes. The space occupied by the 0.5mm implant was represented across ~60 tissue sections, each of which were 8 μm thick. Of those 60 sections, a minimum of four Aniline blue-stained tissue sections were used for the quantification of new peri-implant bone formation. Each section was photographed using a Leica digital imaging system at 5× and 10× magnification. The digital images were analyzed using ImageJ software 1.4 (National Institute of Mental Health, Bethesda, MD, USA). The percentage of aniline blue-positive new bone (%NB) was calculated using the area occupied by aniline-blue-positive pixels divided by the total number of pixels in the defined region of interest (ROI). Pixel counts from these individual tissue sections were performed in triplicate then averaged for each sample.

2.9. TUNEL Staining, Alkaline Phosphatase Activity, and Tartrate Resistant Acid Phosphatase Activity

TUNEL staining was performed as described by the manufacturer. Briefly, sections were incubated in proteinase K buffer (20 μg/mL in 10 mM Tris pH 7.5), applied to a TUNEL reaction mixture (In Situ Cell Death Detection Kit, Roche, Mannheim, Germany), and mounted with DAPI mounting medium (Vector Laboratories, Burlingame, CA, USA). Slides were viewed under an epifluorescence microscope.

Alkaline phosphatase (ALP) activity was detected by incubation in nitro blue tetrazolium chloride (NBT; Roche, Mannheim, Germany), 5-bromo-4-chloro-3-indolyl phosphate (BCIP; Roche, Mannheim, Germany), and NTM buffer (100 mM NaCl, 100 mM Tris pH 9.5, 5 mM MgCl). After its development, the slides were dehydrated in a series of ethanol and xylene and subsequently cover-slipped with Permount mounting media (Thermo Fisher Scientific, Waltham, MA, USA).

Tartrate-resistant acid phosphatase (TRAP) activity was observed using a leukocyte acid phosphatase staining kit (Sigma, St. Louis, MO, USA). After its development, the slides were dehydrated in a series of ethanol and xylene and subsequently cover-slipped with Permount mounting media (Thermo Fisher Scientific, Waltham, MA, USA).

2.10. Micro-CT Imaging

Scanning and analyses followed published guidelines [29]. Ex vivo high-resolution acquisitions (VivaCT 40, Scanco, Brüttisellen, Switzerland) at 10.5 µm voxel size (55 kV, 145 µA, 347 ms integration time), were performed on post-extraction days 28 and immediately after drill preparation. Multiplanar reconstruction and volume rendering were carried out using OsiriX software (version 5.8, Pixmeo, Bernex, Switzerland).

2.11. Statistical Analyses

For lateral stiffness tests, results are presented as the mean $\pm$ 95% confidence interval. In testing for differences among five means in the stiffness tests for the round or the tri-oval implants at PID 0 through 20, we used one-way ANOVA with PID time as the factor. In comparing the stiffness of round vs. tri-oval implants at any given time point (PID), Student's t-test was used to quantify differences. $p \leq 0.05$ was significant.

3. Results

3.1. Tri-oval Implants Exhibit Higher Primary Stability Compared to Round Implants

Most dental implants are placed into healed sites [30]; to recapitulate this clinical condition, maxillary first molars (mxM1) were extracted from skeletally mature mice (Figure 1A,B). Within seven days, soft tissue healing was complete (Figure 1C). After four weeks, sites were evaluated clinically, by µCT imaging (Figure 1D), and by histology (Figure 1E), which together confirmed complete healing (Figure 1F).

A split-mouth design was then used: osteotomies were produced in healed sites (Figure 1G,H) and two implants were placed, one round (Figure 1I) and the other tri-oval (Figure 1J). All implants were placed ~0.5 mm above the alveolar bone crest and below the plane of occlusion (Figure 1K,L). Insertion torque (IT) was measured using in vitro and in vivo methods. Both analyses indicated that IT values were equivalent between the round and tri-oval implants (Figure 1M,N,O). Primary stability was measured (Figure 1P) and these lateral stability tests demonstrated that tri-oval implants had significantly higher primary stability than round implants (Figure 1Q). How was this greater primary stability achieved?

3.2. The Maxima of a Tri-Oval Implant Provide Higher Stability

Computational models were generated to determine whether a difference in contributed to the higher primary stability of tri-oval implants. These analyses showed that the threads of a round implant penetrated ~25 µm into bone whereas for a tri-oval implant, the maxima penetrated ~45 µm into bone (Figure 2A). Despite the fact that minima regions were not in contact with bone, a tri-oval implant still had a larger calculated BIC (Figure 2B).

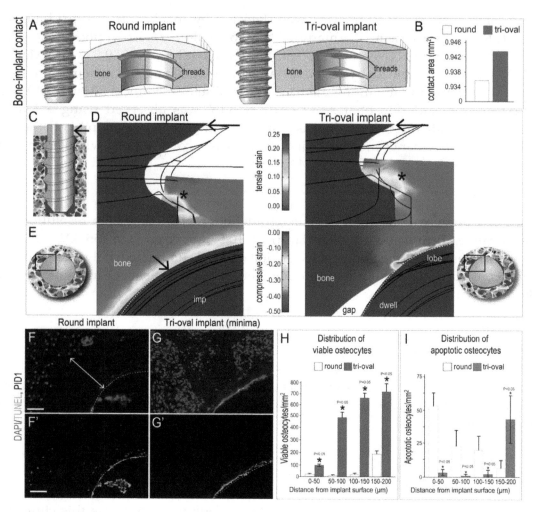

Figure 2. Compared to a round implant, the minima of a tri-oval implant are associated with significantly lower strains and a significantly smaller zone of osteocyte death. (**A**) FE modeling of round (left) and tri-oval (right) implants in bone, using CAD files of the actual implants used in vivo. In a transverse plane, the threads of each type of implant (blue) penetrate the bone, which is modeled as a solid material. (**B**) The calculated bone-implant contact area due to thread penetration. (**C**) Formulation of a FE model of laterally-loaded implant in bone. (**D**) Peri-implant strains surrounding laterally-loaded round and tri-oval implants in the sagittal plane. (**E**) Peri-implant strains arising from initial misfit of the round and tri-oval implants as seen in the transverse plane; only the maxima of the tri-oval implant penetrate the bone. (**F**) DAPI staining of interfacial bone surrounding a representative round implant and (**G**) a representative tri-oval implant; white arrow denotes a circumferential osteocyte-free zone and dotted white line demarcates the osteotomy edge. (**F'**, **G'**) TUNEL staining on adjacent tissue sections. Quantification of the distribution of (**H**) viable and (**I**) apoptotic osteocytes as a function of distance from implant. Abbreviations: imp, implant; PID, post-implant day. Scale bars = 50 μm.

We used FE modeling to understand how the difference in BIC affected peri-implant strains and, in turn, lateral stiffness of the implants. Lateral loading was simulated in the FE model (arrow, Figure 2C) and in both cases the resulting strains concentrated at sites of BIC (Asterix, Figure 2D). The magnitude of these strains, however, was higher in the round implant case (Figure 2D). This meant that when exposed to the same lateral force, the stability of the tri-oval implant was greater than that for the round implant.

The distribution of the peri-implant strains was different, depending on the implant geometry. For example, the round implants had a circumferential zone of high strain whereas the tri-oval implants had strains concentrated only at the maxima; the minima (gaps) had no strain (Figure 2E).

We correlated these strain distributions with biological sequelae. Surrounding round implants was a ~150 μm circumferential zone in which no viable DAPI^{+ve} osteocytes were detectable (white arrow, Figure 2F). Most dying TUNEL^{+ve} osteocytes were found within this same zone (Figure 2F'. Around tri-oval implants, the tri-oval maxima had a similar distribution of dead and dying cells, but in the minima, viable osteocytes were abundant (Figure 2G; quantified in 2H). Dying osteocytes were significantly lower (Figure 2G'; quantified in I). The distribution of DAPI^{+ve} versus dead and TUNEL^{+ve} osteocytes was calculated (Figure 2H, I and Supplemental Figure S1); these data demonstrated that bone viability in the tri-oval minima—which comprised approximately 50% of the circumference of the implant—was significantly higher around the round implants.

3.3. Tri-oval Implants Exhibit Less Bone Resorption, which Allows them to Maintain their Stability Over Time

Peri-implant TRAP activity was more abundant around the round implants (Figure 3A) compared to the tri-oval implants (Figure 3B; quantified in Figure 3C). Resorption removes mineralized matrix, which reduces the elastic modulus of bone and leads to implant instability (white bars, Figure 3D). The tri-oval implants showed no significant loss in stability (blue bars, Figure 3D). Therefore, minimal TRAP activity observed around the tri-oval implants correlated with their greater stability after 3 days.

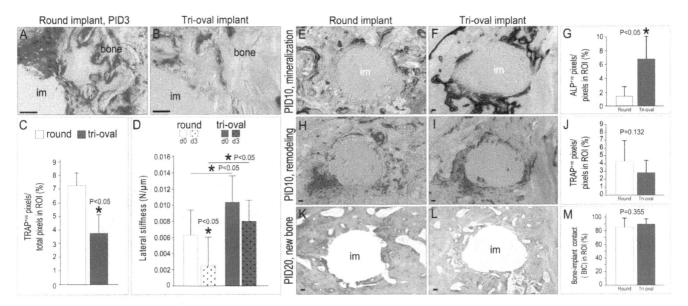

Figure 3. Tri-oval implants exhibits less bone resorption but more robust mineralization. (**A**) TRAP staining of interfacial tissues surrounding a representative round implant on PID3. (**B**) TRAP staining of the minima region around a tri-oval implant on PID3. (**C**) TRAP staining was quantified around the entire circumference of round and tri-oval implants. (**D**) Lateral stiffness test of round and tri-oval implants on PID0 and 3. (**E**) ALP staining of interfacial tissues surrounding a representative round and (**F**) a tri-oval implant on PID10, quantified in (**G**). (**H**) TRAP staining of interfacial tissues surrounding a representative round and (**I**) a tri-oval implant on PID10, quantified in (**J**). (**K**) Aniline blue staining of interfacial tissues surrounding a representative round and (**L**) a tri-oval implant on PID20; quantified in (**M**). Abbreviations as previously stated. Scale bars = 50 μm.

Eventually, both round and tri-oval implants showed evidence of new peri-implant bone mineralization (Figure 3E,F), although the amount of ALP activity was significantly greater around the tri-oval implants (quantified in Figure 3G). This new bone underwent normal remodeling (Figure 3H,I; quantified in Figure 3J). By PID20, both the round and tri-oval implants were fully surrounded by bone (Figure 3K,L; quantified in Figure 3M).

3.4. Tri-Oval Implants Exhibit Superior Osseointegration Compared to Conventional Round Implants

In the experiments conducted thus far, tri-oval implants exhibited better primary stability than round implants, yet both eventually were surrounded by bone. This result was not unexpected because in both cases, implants were placed sub-occlusally, and in previous studies we have shown that sub-occlusal round implants osseointegrate efficiently and effectively [31,32]. Moreover, no differences in quantity of bone or in lateral stability were detected at PID14 (Figure 4B).

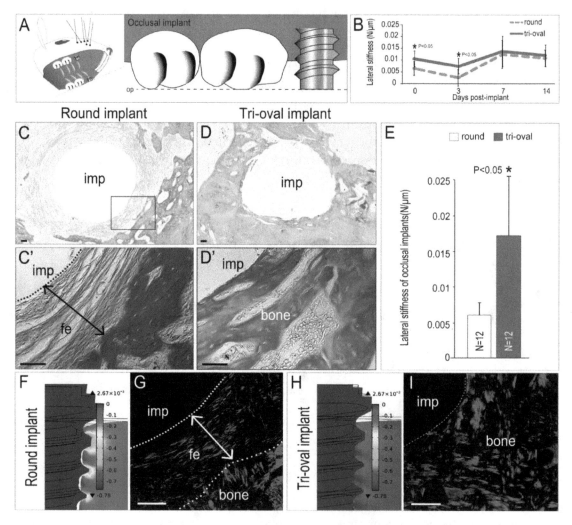

Figure 4. Stability over time as the function of implant geometry. (**A**) Schematic of an occlusal, or functional implant. (**B**) Quantification of lateral stability of sub-occlusal round and tri-oval implants at different timepoints. Aniline blue-stained tissue sections from PID20 through an (**C,C′**) occlusal round implant and (**D,D′**) an occlusal tri-oval implant. (**E**) Quantification of lateral stability of occlusal round and tri-oval implants on PID20. (**F**) In round occlusal implants, FE modeling of peri-implant strain on PID3 and (**G**) picrosirius-red stained tissues from PID20. (**H**) In tri-oval occlusal implants, FE modeling of peri-implant strain on PID3 and (**I**) picrosirius red-stained tissues from PID20. Abbreviations: op, occlusal plane; imp, implant; fe, fibrous encapsulation. Scale bars = 50 μm.

We wondered if the fact that significantly better primary stability exhibited by the tri-oval implant would have a long-term benefit if the implants were immediately loaded. Both the round and tri-oval implants were subjected to functional loading, immediately after placement, which was achieved by positioning the very top of the implant at the same height as the adjacent molar (Figure 4A). The difference in outcome was dramatic: whereas the round implants underwent fibrous encapsulation (Figure 4C,C′), these tri-oval implants osseointegrated (Figure 4D,D′).

Lateral stability results were consistent with histologic/histomorphometric analyses: the soft interfacial tissues surrounding the round implant cases offered little support and consequently, the round implants exhibited poor secondary stability (i.e., small values of lateral stiffness). In comparison, the stiffer interfacial tissues around the tri-oval implants translated into larger lateral stiffness and thus higher secondary stability (Figure 4E).

3.5. The Magnitude of Interfacial Strain is a Key Influence on Whether an Implant will Undergo Fibrous Encapsulation or Osseointegration

Why did these round occlusal implants fail? The key to answering this question lies in the observation that the same round implants can osseointegrate, provided they are placed sub-occlusally to reduce loading (Figure 3). Thus, the round implants failed because they lacked sufficient primary stability (Figure 1Q). We sought to link this observation about stiffness at PID0 with the fates of the implants on PID20, and to do so, we turned again to FE modeling.

Implant stability is a function of the elastic modulus of peri-implant tissue; in other words, the stiffer the tissue, the less the implant will move under loading. FE modeling was used to back-calculate the peri-implant bone modulus that corresponded to the experimentally-measured lateral stability (see Materials and methods). At PID0 and PID3, the peri-implant tissues surrounding trioval implants were 3.5 times stiffer than those surrounding round implants. Using these modulus values, FE models demonstrated that peri-implant strains at PID0 and PID3 were significantly higher around the round occlusal implant (Figure 4F). For example, at the crestal thread tips of an occlusally-loaded round implant, principal compressive strain magnitudes reached >50% (Figure 4F). On the other hand, identically-loaded tri-oval implants were surrounded by stiffer peri-implant tissue and the resulting strains at PID0 and PID3 were less than 10% (Figure 4H). Collectively, these data provide critical insights as to why a round implant with significantly less primary stability underwent fibrous encapsulation when subjected to immediate loading (Figure 4G), whereas a tri-oval implant, with statistically higher primary stability, underwent osseointegration when subjected to the same immediate loading conditions (Figure 4I).

4. Discussion

We coupled mechanical testing with computational studies and histologic/immunohistologic analyses to assess how altering an implant's geometry affected its ability to osseointegrate. We tested implants that were placed below the level of the occlusal plane, and those placed in function. In both scenarios, the tri-oval implants out-performed the round implants. Evidence supporting this conclusion came from mechanical, computational, and biological analyses.

4.1. The Maxima of a Tri-Oval Implant aid in Mechanical Stability

Compared to round implants, the tri-oval implants exhibited better primary stability, which was achieved without using a higher IT (Figure 1). The larger stability was achieved because the maxima of the tri-oval implant penetrated a greater distance into bone than did the threads of the round implant (Figure 2). Based on our data, one might legitimately ask if the novel tri-oval implant design would be negated simply by undersizing the osteotomy for the round implant. In this thought experiment, the threads of the round implant would penetrate deeper into bone and as a result the implant would presumably demonstrate better initial stability. But just as reliably, this scenario would also increase IT [8], peri-implant strain [11], and its associated micro-damage [8,15,33]. In turn, this micro-damage would increase the spatial extent of peri-implant bone resorption (Figure 3) during the early post-operative stages of bone remodeling, which would lower the net modulus of the peri-implant bone and result in a transient decrease of initial stability–as seen for example at PID 3 (Figure 4B).

Clinical observations are consistent with this line of reasoning: in multiple studies, sub-occlusal implants showed a decline in mean ISQ values between weeks 1-4 [34–36]. Friberg also reported a decrease in stability for a majority of sub-occlusal implants [37,38]. Our preclinical study appears to be the first to provide direct molecular, cellular, histologic, and mechanical data to explain how this transient "dip" in implant stability actually occurs.

4.2. The Minima of a Tri-Oval Implant Create a Pro-Osteogenic Environment

Fifty percent of the peri-tri-oval implant environment had very low/no strain (Figure 2E), where damage to the mineralized matrix is minimized, osteocyte death is minimal, and bone resorption is reduced [8,15,33]. Together these events culminated in significantly more new bone around the tri-oval implants (Figures 2 and 3). A similar finding has been reported using a canine implant model, where investigators demonstrated that new woven bone forms first in regions where there is a gap in the bone-implant contact [12]. We find that areas of low/no strain strongly support osteoblast differentiation and new mineralized matrix deposition, provided the osteogenic potential of the bone is good [22].

4.3. Clinical Implications of this Study

Round-shaped implants can osseointegrate, even when subjected to loading immediately after placement. Why, then, did we observe that round implants failed to undergo osseointegration? The answer is straightforward: in those cases where round implants became encapsulated in fibrous tissue it was because loading was allowed on an implant that lacked sufficient primary stability (Figure 1). If the same implant—with the same degree of instability—was buried, then by PID20 it was surrounded by new bone (Figure 3). These data indicate the importance of an "unloaded" healing period proposed by Branemark [39]. What if the healing period is eliminated? Our data predict that healing periods between implant placement and loading could be shortened- or eliminated—without jeopardizing long-term implant success if osteocyte death was minimized during site preparation, and the implant had a geometry that provided both mechanical stability and a pro-osteogenic environment.

5. Conclusions

These multiscale biomechanical analyses demonstrated that the novel tri-oval implant design provided mechanically and biologically favorable environment for peri-implant bone formation and promoted osseointegration.

Author Contributions: Conceptualization: X.Y. and J.A.H.; methodology: X.Y. and J.A.H.; validation: X.Y., J.L., and J.A.H.; data curation: X.Y., J.L., and J.A.H.; formal analysis: X.Y., J.L., W.H., A.G., and J.B.B.; investigation: X.Y. and J.L.; writing—original draft preparation: X.Y. and J.A.H; writing—review and editing: X.Y., J.L., W.H., A.G., J.B.B., and J.A.H.; funding acquisition: X.Y., J.B.B., and J.A.H. All authors gave final approval and agree to be accountable for all aspects of the work.

References

1.   Wennerberg, A.; Albrektsson, T.; Chrcanovic, B. Long-term clinical outcome of implants with different surface modifications. *Eur. J. Oral Implantol.* **2018**, *11* (Suppl. 1), S123–S136.

2.   Gurzawska, K.; Dirscherl, K.; Jorgensen, B.; Berglundh, T.; Jorgensen, N.R.; Gotfredsen, K. Pectin nanocoating of titanium implant surfaces—An experimental study in rabbits. *Clin. Oral Implants Res.* **2017**, *28*, 298–307. [CrossRef] [PubMed]

3.   Cardoso, M.V.; de Rycker, J.; Chaudhari, A.; Coutinho, E.; Yoshida, Y.; Van Meerbeek, B.; Mesquita, M.F.; da Silva, W.J.; Yoshihara, K.; Vandamme, K.; et al. Titanium implant functionalization with phosphate-containing polymers may favour in vivo osseointegration. *J. Clin. Periodontol.* **2017**, *44*, 950–960. [CrossRef] [PubMed]

4.   Cardoso, M.V.; Chaudhari, A.; Yoshihara, K.; Mesquita, M.F.; Yoshida, Y.; Van Meerbeek, B.; Vandamme, K.; Duyck, J. Phosphorylated Pullulan Coating Enhances Titanium Implant Osseointegration in a Pig Model. *Int. J. Oral Maxillofac. Implants* **2017**, *32*, 282–290. [CrossRef]

5. Becker, W.; Hujoel, P.; Becker, B.E.; Wohrle, P. Survival rates and bone level changes around porous oxide-coated implants (TiUnite). *Clin. Implants Dent. Relat. Res.* **2013**, *15*, 654–660. [CrossRef] [PubMed]

6. Branemark, P.I.; Adell, R.; Breine, U.; Hansson, B.O.; Lindstrom, J.; Ohlsson, A. Intra-osseous anchorage of dental prostheses. I. Experimental studies. *Scand. J. Plast. Reconstr. Surg.* **1969**, *3*, 81–100. [CrossRef]

7. Buser, D.; Sennerby, L.; De Bruyn, H. Modern implant dentistry based on osseointegration: 50 years of progress, current trends and open questions. *Periodontology 2000* **2017**, *73*, 7–21. [CrossRef] [PubMed]

8. Cha, J.Y.; Pereira, M.D.; Smith, A.A.; Houschyar, K.S.; Yin, X.; Mouraret, S.; Brunski, J.B.; Helms, J.A. Multiscale analyses of the bone-implant interface. *J. Dent. Res.* **2015**, *94*, 482–490. [CrossRef] [PubMed]

9. Degidi, M.; Perrotti, V.; Strocchi, R.; Piattelli, A.; Iezzi, G. Is insertion torque correlated to bone-implant contact percentage in the early healing period? A histological and histomorphometrical evaluation of 17 human-retrieved dental implants. *Clin. Oral Implants Res.* **2009**, *20*, 778–781. [CrossRef] [PubMed]

10. Meredith, N.; Book, K.; Friberg, B.; Jemt, T.; Sennerby, L. Resonance frequency measurements of implant stability in vivo. A cross-sectional and longitudinal study of resonance frequency measurements on implants in the edentulous and partially dentate maxilla. *Clin. Oral Implants Res.* **1997**, *8*, 226–233. [CrossRef]

11. Wazen, R.M.; Currey, J.A.; Guo, H.; Brunski, J.B.; Helms, J.A.; Nanci, A. Micromotion-induced strain fields influence early stages of repair at bone-implant interfaces. *Acta Biomater.* **2013**, *9*, 6663–6674. [CrossRef] [PubMed]

12. Berglundh, T.; Abrahamsson, I.; Lang, N.P.; Lindhe, J. De novo alveolar bone formation adjacent to endosseous implants. *Clin. Oral Implants Res.* **2003**, *14*, 251–262. [CrossRef] [PubMed]

13. Futami, T.; Fujii, N.; Ohnishi, H.; Taguchi, N.; Kusakari, H.; Ohshima, H.; Maeda, T. Tissue response to titanium implants in the rat maxilla: Ultrastructural and histochemical observations of the bone-titanium interface. *J. Periodontol.* **2000**, *71*, 287–298. [CrossRef] [PubMed]

14. Sandborn, P.M.; Cook, S.D.; Spires, W.P.; Kester, M.A. Tissue response to porous-coated implants lacking initial bone apposition. *J. Arthroplast.* **1988**, *3*, 337–346. [CrossRef]

15. Wang, L.; Wu, Y.; Perez, K.C.; Hyman, S.; Brunski, J.B.; Tulu, U.; Bao, C.; Salmon, B.; Helms, J.A. Effects of Condensation on Peri-implant Bone Density and Remodeling. *J. Dent. Res.* **2017**, *96*, 413–420. [CrossRef] [PubMed]

16. Suarez, D.R.; Valstar, E.R.; Rozing, P.M.; van Keulen, F. Fracture risk and initial fixation of a cementless glenoid implant: The effect of numbers and types of screws. *Proc. Inst. Mech. Eng. H J. Eng. Med.* **2013**, *227*, 1058–1066. [CrossRef]

17. Carlsson, L.; Engman, F.; Fromell, R.; Jörneus, L. Threaded Implant for Obtaining Reliable Anchoring in Bone. EP 1 030 622 B2, 14 May 2014.

18. Reams, J.W.; Goodman, R.E.; Rogers, D.P. Reduced Friction Screw-Type Dental Implant. US5902109, 11 May 1999.

19. Torcasio, A.; Zhang, X.; Van Oosterwyck, H.; Duyck, J.; van Lenthe, G.H. Use of micro-CT-based finite element analysis to accurately quantify peri-implant bone strains: A validation in rat tibiae. *Biomech. Model. Mechanobiol.* **2012**, *11*, 743–750. [CrossRef]

20. Leucht, P.; Kim, J.B.; Wazen, R.; Currey, J.A.; Nanci, A.; Brunski, J.B.; Helms, J.A. Effect of mechanical stimuli on skeletal regeneration around implants. *Bone* **2007**, *40*, 919–930. [CrossRef]

21. Leucht, P.; Monica, S.D.; Temiyasathit, S.; Lenton, K.; Manu, A.; Longaker, M.T.; Jacobs, C.R.; Spilker, R.L.; Guo, H.; Brunski, J.B.; et al. Primary cilia act as mechanosensors during bone healing around an implant. *Med. Eng. Phys.* **2012**, *35*, 392–402. [CrossRef] [PubMed]

22. Li, J.; Yin, X.; Huang, L.; Mouraret, S.; Brunski, J.B.; Cordova, L.; Salmon, B.; Helms, J.A. Relationships among Bone Quality, Implant Osseointegration, and Wnt Signaling. *J. Dent. Res.* **2017**, *96*, 822–831. [CrossRef] [PubMed]

23. Pei, X.; Wang, L.; Chen, C.; Yuan, X.; Wan, Q.; Helms, J.A. Contribution of the PDL to Osteotomy Repair and Implant Osseointegration. *J. Dent. Res.* **2017**, *96*, 909–916. [CrossRef] [PubMed]

24. Meier, E. The Wood Database 2018-2019. Available online: http://www.wood-database.com/ (accessed on 26 January 2019).

25. Seong, W.J.; Kim, U.K.; Swift, J.Q.; Heo, Y.C.; Hodges, J.S.; Ko, C.C. Elastic properties and apparent density of human edentulous maxilla and mandible. *Int. J. Oral Maxillofac. Surg.* **2009**, *38*, 1088–1093. [CrossRef] [PubMed]

26.   Baldi, D.; Lombardi, T.; Colombo, J.; Cervino, G.; Perinetti, G.; Di Lenarda, R.; Stacchi, C. Correlation between Insertion Torque and Implant Stability Quotient in Tapered Implants with Knife-Edge Thread Design. *BioMed Res. Int.* **2018**, *2018*, 7201093. [CrossRef] [PubMed]

27.   Yin, X.; Li, J.; Salmon, B.; Huang, L.; Lim, W.H.; Liu, B.; Hunter, D.J.; Ransom, R.C.; Singh, G.; Gillette, M.; et al. Wnt Signaling and Its Contribution to Craniofacial Tissue Homeostasis. *J. Dent. Res.* **2015**, *94*, 1487–1494. [CrossRef]

28.   Cicciu, M.; Cervino, G.; Milone, D.; Risitano, G. FEM Investigation of the Stress Distribution over Mandibular Bone Due to Screwed Overdenture Positioned on Dental Implants. *Materials* **2018**, *11*, 1512. [CrossRef]

29.   Bouxsein, M.L.; Boyd, S.K.; Christiansen, B.A.; Guldberg, R.E.; Jepsen, K.J.; Muller, R. Guidelines for assessment of bone microstructure in rodents using micro-computed tomography. *J. Bone Min. Res.* **2010**, *25*, 1468–1486. [CrossRef]

30.   Schropp, L.; Isidor, F. Timing of implant placement relative to tooth extraction. *J. Oral Rehabil.* **2008**, *35* (Suppl. 1), 33–43. [CrossRef] [PubMed]

31.   Mouraret, S.; Hunter, D.J.; Bardet, C.; Brunski, J.B.; Bouchard, P.; Helms, J.A. A pre-clinical murine model of oral implant osseointegration. *Bone* **2014**, *58*, 177–184. [CrossRef]

32.   Yin, X.; Li, J.; Chen, T.; Mouraret, S.; Dhamdhere, G.; Brunski, J.B.; Zou, S.; Helms, J.A. Rescuing failed oral implants via Wnt activation. *J. Clin. Periodontol.* **2016**, *43*, 180–192. [CrossRef] [PubMed]

33.   Yuan, X.; Pei, X.; Zhao, Y.; Li, Z.; Chen, C.H.; Tulu, U.S.; Liu, B.; Van Brunt, L.A.; Brunski, J.B.; Helms, J.A. Biomechanics of Immediate Postextraction Implant Osseointegration. *J. Dent. Res.* **2018**, *97*, 987–994. [CrossRef] [PubMed]

34.   Zhou, W.; Han, C.; Yunming, L.; Li, D.; Song, Y.; Zhao, Y. Is the osseointegration of immediately and delayed loaded implants the same?—Comparison of the implant stability during a 3-month healing period in a prospective study. *Clin. Oral Implants Res.* **2009**, *20*, 1360–1366. [CrossRef] [PubMed]

35.   West, J.D.; Oates, T.W. Identification of stability changes for immediately placed dental implants. *Int. J. Oral Maxillofac. Implants* **2007**, *22*, 623–630. [PubMed]

36.   Barewal, R.M.; Stanford, C.; Weesner, T.C. A randomized controlled clinical trial comparing the effects of three loading protocols on dental implant stability. *Int. J. Oral Maxillofac. Implants* **2012**, *27*, 945–956.

37.   Friberg, B.; Sennerby, L.; Meredith, N.; Lekholm, U. A comparison between cutting torque and resonance frequency measurements of maxillary implants. A 20-month clinical study. *Int. J. Oral Maxillofac. Surg.* **1999**, *28*, 297–303. [CrossRef]

38.   Friberg, B.; Sennerby, L.; Linden, B.; Grondahl, K.; Lekholm, U. Stability measurements of one-stage Branemark implants during healing in mandibles. A clinical resonance frequency analysis study. *Int. J. Oral Maxillofac. Surg.* **1999**, *28*, 266–272. [CrossRef]

39.   Branemark, P.I.; Hansson, B.O.; Adell, R.; Breine, U.; Lindström, J.; Hallén, O.; Ohman, A. Osseointegrated implants in the treatment of the edentulous jaw. Experience from a 10-year period. *Scand. J. Plast. Reconstr. Surg. Suppl.* **1977**, *16*, 1–132.

13

Coupling between Osseointegration and Mechanotransduction to Maintain Foreign Body Equilibrium in the Long-Term

Luis Amengual-Peñafiel [1,*], Manuel Brañes-Aroca [2], Francisco Marchesani-Carrasco [3], María Costanza Jara-Sepúlveda [3], Leopoldo Parada-Pozas [4] and Ricardo Cartes-Velásquez [5,6]

[1] Dental Implantology Unit, Hospital Leonardo Guzmán, Antofagasta 1240835, Chile
[2] Faculty of Sciences, Universidad de Chile, Santiago 7800003, Chile; branesmd.1@vtr.net
[3] Clínica Marchesani, Concepción 4070566, Chile; francisco@marchesani.cl (F.M.-C.); mconstanzajara@gmail.com (M.C.J.-S.)
[4] Regenerative Medicine Center, Hospital Clínico de Viña del Mar, Viña del Mar 2520626, Chile; dr.polo@ejerciciosalud.cl
[5] School of Dentistry, Universidad Andres Bello, Concepción 4300866, Chile; cartesvelasquez@gmail.com
[6] Institute of Biomedical Sciences, Universidad Autónoma de Chile, Temuco 4810101, Chile
* Correspondence: luisamengualp@gmail.com

Abstract: The permanent interaction between bone tissue and the immune system shows us the complex biology of the tissue in which we insert oral implants. At the same time, new knowledge in relation to the interaction of materials and the host, reveals to us the true nature of osseointegration. So, to achieve clinical success or perhaps most importantly, to understand why we sometimes fail, the study of oral implantology should consider the following advice equally important: a correct clinical protocol, the study of the immunomodulatory capacity of the device and the osteoimmunobiology of the host. Although osseointegration may seem adequate from the clinical point of view, a deeper vision shows us that a Foreign Body Equilibrium could be susceptible to environmental conditions. This is why maintaining this cellular balance should become our therapeutic target and, more specifically, the understanding of the main cell involved, the macrophage. The advent of new information, the development of new implant surfaces and the introduction of new therapeutic proposals such as therapeutic mechanotransduction, will allow us to maintain a healthy host-implant relationship long-term.

Keywords: oral implants; osseointegration; marginal bone loss; immunomodulation; mechanotransduction

1. Introduction

Titanium dental implants are inserted directly into the bone tissue, a complex and dynamic tissue. This bone tissue not only participates in calcium homeostasis and functions as a hematopoietic organ, but also plays an important role as a regulator of immunity [1].

Recent evidence on foreign body reactions (FBRs) in relation to implantable devices, such as titanium dental implants, reveals that, to achieve a lasting relationship between the implant and the host, titanium implants must have an optimal surface [2], and there must be an adequate healing capacity of the host [3]. Recently, it has been shown that the presence of a titanium implant during bone healing activates the immune system and displays type 2 inflammation, which seems to guide the relationship between the host and the implant [4]. This appears to indicate that osseointegration is a dynamic process, the result of a complex set of reactions in which several mechanisms and pathways of the host interact [1]. If the osseointegration is not altered, a continuous equilibrium occurs in the form of Foreign Body Equilibrium (FBE), which has been documented for 20 years or more in oral implantology [5]. Despite the high rates of survival achieved with titanium dental implants [6], it is necessary to further improve the implant-host relationship to maintain the integrity of the FBE long term; especially when the mechanisms involved in the breakdown of the osseointegration begin to act [7]. Once this occurs the immune system could be activated changing the delicate balance between the osteoblast and the osteoclast, which results in bone resorption [8].

The role of macrophages in osseointegration is greater than expected [1]. Macrophages respond to all implanted materials, which play an essential role in the fate of an implant [9]. Currently, immunomodulation strategies targeting macrophages are being developed around implants, both dental and orthopedic ones; either through new surface treatments [10], the controlled release of specific ions [11] or through specific cytokines [12]. The immunomodulatory effect of the Mesenchymal stem cell (MSC) has also been explored [13], and in this line, the hypothesis of immunomodulation of osseointegration through therapeutic mechanotransduction has recently been proposed, particularly by extracorporeal shock waves therapy (ESWT) [14].

The field of mechanobiology has allowed us to analyze the effects of mechanical forces on cellular processes [15], which has revealed the complex cellular regulation involved in the transduction of mechanical signals [16]. Mechanical stimuli can stimulate the activity not only of bone cells but also MSC [17]. Mechanical stimuli can also change the cellular form and affect the phenotype and function of immune cells, such as macrophage and dendritic cells [18].

This review begins with (i) a discussion of key concepts related to bone tissue and the immune system; (ii) next, we will discuss the FBR, focusing specifically on osseointegration; (iii) to then explore the current strategies of immunomodulation in osseointegrated implants (iv) Finally, we will conclude with a discussion on a topic that may become clinically relevant, the coupling between osseointegration and mechanotransduction to maintain FBE long-term.

2. Bone Tissue and Immune System

The scientific field of osteoimmunology has revealed the vital role of immune cells in the regulation of bone dynamics [19], this has led to the understanding of the existence of different molecular and cellular mechanisms involved in a permanent interaction between bone tissue and the immune system. For this reason, to understand bone healing in general and osseointegration in particular, it is necessary to understand the biology and immunology of bones [20]. Bone is an organ composed of cortical, trabecular, cartilaginous, hematopoietic and connective tissue [21], which is composed by more than 30 different cell populations which reside in the microenvironment of the bone marrow adjacent to an implant. These cell populations, alone or in combination, have the ability to influence the formation and the bone regeneration of the peri-implant environment [2]. In addition, the presence of multiple anatomical and vascular contacts allow for a permanent interaction between the bone tissue and the immune system [22]. In fact, the bone marrow shows structural and functional characteristics that resemble a secondary lymphoid organ. That is why bone marrow is currently considered an immunoregulatory organ, capable of significantly influencing systemic immunity [21].

The cells of the bone tissue and the cells of the immune system share common origins. Osteoclasts (OC) come from stem cells of the monocyte-macrophage cell lineage [22]. However, certain subclasses of circulating monocytes and dendritic cells (DCs) which reside in the bone marrow also have the capacity to transform into OC if they are subjected to certain specific signals [23]. Perhaps this common origin with cells of the immune system could be related to the ability of OCs to recruit CD8 + FoxP3 + T cells and present antigens to them [24,25]. On the other hand, osteoblast (OBs) play a central role in the differentiation of hematopoietic cells [22]. This common origin between osseous and immune cells facilitates understanding of how molecular pathways are involved in bone remodeling (such as in PTH, BMP and Wnt pathway) which also act in regulating the hematopoiesis [26].

Immune cells regulate osteoclastogenesis by three main cytokines: macrophage colony stimulating factor (M-CSF), receptor activator NF kappaB ligand (RANKL) and osteoprotegerin (OPG) [19]. The main element in osteoclastogenesis, the RANKL, can be expressed by activated T lymphocytes, dendritic cells and neutrophils, indicating the participation of these immune cells during osteoclastogenesis [19,21]. The expression of RANKL by activated T cells has been implicated in osteoclastogenesis induced by inflammation, linking adaptive immunity to skeletal biology [27]. This is related to the role of the immune system in several bone diseases, such as osteoporosis, osteoarthritis and rheumatoid arthritis. Several studies have clearly highlighted the role of developing T lymphocytes and the pathophysiology of osteoporosis, which has given birth to a new field of biology called *"immunoporosis"* [28]. Moreover, as the dendritic cells are responsible for the activation of virgin T cells and act as osteoclast precursors, this could be directly involved in osteoclastogenesis induced by inflammation and bone loss [29]. It has been described that persistent inflammation is characterized by the continuous release of proinflammatory cytokines (TNF-a, IL-1a/be IL-6), which is accompanied by a higher RANKL/OPG ratio and an increased osteoclast activity [30]. On the other hand, it has been shown that B cells are an important source of OPG derived from bone marrow, which implies that B cells are one of the main inhibitors of osteoclastogenesis in normal physiology [19].

Macrophages are precursors of osteoclasts, and under the stimulation of M-CSF and RANKL, they can differentiate into osteoclasts during bone remodeling [19]. Bone and bone marrow contain multiple subpopulations of specialized resident macrophages (bone macrophages or osteomacs), which contribute to bone biology and/or hematopoiesis [31]. Macrophages promote osteoblastogenesis in in vitro matrix deposition and they could have an important role in the promotion of bone anabolism, through the provision of trophic support to the osteoblast lineage [32]. In fact, the depletion of macrophages leads to the complete loss of bone formation mediated by osteoblasts in vivo [33]. In addition, they would be important in the reversion phase of a basic multicellular unit (BMU), which separates bone resorption and bone formation [34]. Macrophages are also abundant within the bone callus during the inflammatory phase of bone healing in humans [35], so the presence and diverse functionality of macrophages could allow an important contribution in bone homeostasis and throughout the course of bone healing [32]. Furthermore, the healing of bone fractures is significantly improved in knockout mice lacking T and B cells, which indicates that they may also have a detrimental function during this process. This observation suggests the dual role of immune cells in osteogenesis, through its expression and secretion of a wide range of regulatory molecules [19].

As we have seen, immune cells play an important role in bone homeostasis. Therefore, the insertion of a foreign body into the bone tissue will inevitably be recognized by the immune system, affecting the biological behavior of the bone cells. This event can determine the in vivo destination of an implant or "biomaterial".

3. Foreign Body Reaction and Osseointegration

The interaction between bone tissue and implants involves at least 3 components: immune cells of the host, bone cells of the host and the material [19]. After implantation, the host will experience a response to tissue injury, which will be conditioned by the material present and the degree of the immune response [36].

In general, after a surgical implantation procedure, the damage of the endothelial cells exposes the underlying vascular basement membrane and initiates the coagulation cascade that leads to the formation of a clot of red blood cells-platelets-fibrin. This vascular damage also facilitates the interaction of the implant with blood proteins and interstitial fluids, such as fibrinogen, vitronectin, complement, fibronectin and albumin, which are adsorbed dynamically on the surface of the implant (Vroman effect) in seconds, forming a superficial transient matrix [1,2,7,19,36,37]. This allows physicochemical interactions between the host proteins and the implant's surface, which leads to a change in the molecular conformation of one or more of these host proteins, exposing previously hidden amino acid sequences, which would act as antigenic epitopes [1,7]. Serum factors called "opsonins" will participate in the recognition of the foreign agent, the main ones being immunoglobulin G (IgG) and the complement activated fragment, C3b, allowing for interactions with macrophages through membrane receptors [38]. Hu et al. showed that adsorbed fibrinogen is the main protein responsible for the accumulation of macrophages on the surfaces of implanted biomaterials [39]. It has also been shown that adsorbed fibrinogen exposes two previously hidden amino acids, functioning as epitopes, which allows for interaction with macrophages through the Mac-1 integrin (CD11b/CD18), leading to a proinflammatory environment, modulating the response of the host to the biomaterial in this way [1]. In this same context, it has been suggested that another protein, fibronectin, could participate in the chronic phase of FBR [40].

The complement system seems to play a key role at this early stage [7]. Arvidsson et al. showed that the interaction between titanium and plasma coagulation factors, such as factor XII, could lead to the activation of the complement through the alternative pathway, producing C3b [41]. As is known, immune cells express inactivated C3b/C3b (iC3b) receptors, so that from the early phase of inflammation, the surface of the implant is recognized by the immune system [7]. Recently it has been demonstrated in titanium implants that there is a positive regulation of the C5a-1 receptor (C5aR1) after the inflammatory period, which demonstrates a prolonged activation of innate immunity through the continuous activation of the complement system [4].

After the initial interaction between the blood and the material, acute inflammation begins, which is initiated by the cytokines and chemokines released by the damaged cells, leading to the influx of neutrophils and mononuclear macrophages [19,36]. Neutrophils normally deplete rapidly, undergo apoptosis and disappear from implantation sites within the first two days [19]. The prolonged presence of neutrophils indicates that we are facing active chronic inflammation [36]. This has been observed around titanium implants, probably due to the role of neutrophils in the promotion of vascularization in tissue hypoxia and the ability of the macrophage to suppress the apoptosis of them [4]. It is important to mention that neutrophils, in an effort to degrade the materials, release proteolytic enzymes and reactive oxygen species (ROS), which can corrode the surface of the implanted material [19].

The influx of mononuclear macrophages occurs between 24 and 48 h, which have a phagocytic function that includes the release of proteolytic enzymes that degrade cellular debris and the extracellular matrix (ECM). Currently, these immune cells have aroused great interest among scientists due to their multiple functions in the process of bone healing and high plasticity [19]. Macrophages have been extensively characterized in phenotypes M1 and M2, reflecting the Th1/Th2 nomenclature described for helper T cells [42]. Traditionally, it has been described that M1 proinflammatory macrophages would dominate the early phase of the reparative response and, on the other hand, M2 macrophages (M2a, M2b and M2c), would play a more prominent role during the middle and later stages of the response repair [19]. However, this classification represents only a simplification of the in vivo scenario, since it is very likely that the macrophage phenotype occupies a continuum between the M1 and M2 designations, with transient macrophages with characteristics of both phenotypes present [43]. Therefore, it seems that both phenotypes of macrophages perform essential functions during the process of bone healing, with the macrophage change pattern determining the osteogenesis instead of a specific macrophage phenotype [44].

It has been described that a prolonged M1 polarization phase leads to an increase in fibrosis-enhancing cytokine release pattern by the M2 macrophages, which results in the formation of a fibrocapsule around the biomaterial [19]. This reaction could be related to the "primary failure", which occurs in 1–2% of all dental implants placed, probably due to a series of risk factors that are predisposed to this total failure in osseointegration, like the following: low primary stability, premature loading, traumatic surgery, infection, as well as patient conditions such as smoking or the consumption of some pharmaceutical products [20].

On the contrary, an efficient and timely switch from M1 to M2 macrophage phenotype results in an osteogenic cytokines release and with it the formation of new bone tissue [19]. This second possible reaction is one that would generate the bone encapsulation that allows the commercial use of titanium implants [20]. In commercially pure (c.p.) titanium implants, the presence of the M2 phenotype of the macrophage (most likely M2a) is significantly high, which has been observed as early as 10 days after surgery [4,45]. This indicates that there is an immunomodulated relationship between the titanium implant and the host, which allows the deposit of bone in the implant, and the isolation of this from the space of the bone marrow, through a type of FBR [4]. Albrektsson and colleagues introduce the concept of FBE to describe this phenomenon, osseointegration being considered a mild chronic inflammatory response that allows implant function with a bone-implant interface that remains in a state of equilibrium, susceptible to changes in the environment [5].

Macrophages can swallow particles up to 5 μm, however, if the size of the material or the residue is greater than 50–100 μm, the material is surrounded by macrophages that fuse to form foreign body giant cells (FBGC) [19,46]. This induction of macrophage fusion probably occurs through the secretion of IL-4 and IL-13 by mast cells, basophils, and helper T cells (Th) [40]. It has even been suggested that FBGCs could express phenotypes of M1 and M2 macrophages, depending on the environment, similar to their mononuclear precursors [47]. Although FBGCs are not normally found in healthy tissues, they are abundant around implanted biomaterials, even years after implantation [48]. This is the reason why the presence of FBGC in the interface of the host-implant is an indication of an FBR to the implanted material or device [19,40,46]. Donath et al. described the presence of FGBC on the surface of titanium implants, which were present in multiple cases of FBR through histological studies [49]. It has been seen that the CD11b marker is extremely upregulated at 28 days, demonstrating how macrophages are highly involved in the reaction to titanium implants since this marker has recently been implicated in the fusion of macrophages [4]. For several years, multinucleated giant cells (MNGC) have been described in relation to biomaterials, especially in the case of bone replacement materials, assuming that MNGCs are osteoclasts. However, many studies indicate that these cells actually belong to the cell line of FBGCs, which are of an "inflammatory origin" [47]. It is a fact that osteoclasts can be formed by the fusion of multiple macrophages, and some authors even suggest that macrophages can perform functions of bone resorption [50]. All of the above suggests that FBGS could play a central role in the pathway of bone loss during the FBR [7].

Macrophages and dendritic cells can initiate an adaptive immune response through the presentation of antigens, which can also be particles or ions. When a T cell recognizes an antigen, the T cell is activated (activated TCD4 +) and may have inflammatory secretory profiles (Th1) or anti-inflammatory secretory profiles (Th2) [51]. Recently a constant regulation of CD4 and the negative regulation of CD8, which indicates a reaction of CD4 lymphocytes around the implant, was observed in titanium implants [45]. However, more research is needed to confirm the continued presence of the immune system over time [4].

As we have seen, an implanted device activates the components of the immune system in bone: complement, neutrophils, macrophages and lymphocytes. However, the role of the macrophage in the host-biomaterial relationship is highlighted [4]. Although most implants will be successful, a rejection mechanism may occur. This may be represented by marginal bone loss around the osseointegrated implant, which could be a product of multiple factors such as the implant, the surgical procedure, prosthetic conditions and factors in relation to the patient [20]. The loss of FBE could be the main cause of this peri-implant bone loss. This leaves the door open for the development of different strategies to face the pathology through a deeper understanding of the biology of osseointegration [1].

4. Current Immunomodulation Strategies in Osseointegrated Implants

Titanium is one of the few materials suitable for implantation requirements in the human body, being widely used in oral surgery, maxillofacial surgery, craniofacial surgery and orthopedics. The greater clinical use and popularity of oral implants have led to a growth in demands, with an increasing need for treatments in places where the quality of bone is less than ideal, and in patients with a compromise of scarring products of systemic affections [2]. Although less than 5% of oral implants show failure under optimal clinical conditions. In some cases, through a triad consisting of poor clinical handling, combined with poor implant systems and the treatment of those who are compromised, treating "poor" patients may lead to problems, probably increasing the number of complications [20]. On the other hand, many orthopedic procedures require implants, however, not all implanted devices last forever: up to 15% of the total joint implants require a surgical revision within 15 years of the initial surgery [52]. Therefore, there is a need to improve the biological function and longevity of the implantable devices [20,52].

Recent studies on osseointegrated titanium oral implants demonstrate the presence of the M2 phenotype of the macrophage from the early stage of healing (days) [4,10,45,53]. However, the presence of other chemical elements on the surface of the titanium implant seems to be relevant for the bone balance of osseointegration [2]. Trindade et al. have demonstrated that the bone resorption markers were significantly down-regulated around titanium in turned titanium grade IV implants. Interestingly, the regulation balance of bone resorption RANKL/OPG is suppressed in its entirety, suggesting that bone resorption has been kept to a minimum around Titanium [4]. However, Biguetti et al., using a machined titanium implant of titanium-6 aluminum-4 vanadium alloy, demonstrated the opposite; there was a remarkable remodeling process, evidenced by peaks corresponding to RANKL and OPG, and also an increased area density of osteoclasts. Furthermore, the presence of ten chemical elements in the surface composition of the implants used was determined through an analysis by Energy Dispersive X-ray (EDX): Titanium [Ti], Aluminum [Al], Vanadium [V], Calcium [Ca], Nitrogen [N], Niobium [Nb], Oxygen [O], Phosphorus [P], Sulfur [S] and Zinc [Zn] [53].

In this context, it is noteworthy that c.p. titanium is often alloyed with aluminum and vanadium (Ti6Al4V). However, in some cases, further surface modification procedures such as sand-blasting and acid etching are likely to remove passive layers from the surface of the metal, exposing less stable elements underneath. This could generate an inflammatory response and possible reduction in osteoblast differentiation [2]. Both of these effects can be detrimental to new bone formation and implant integration. However, in relation to the aforementioned, this material has an acceptable clinical success currently [10]. However, the degree of purity of the surfaces is an important issue to consider since there are important studies of oral implants, which reveal the presence of organic and inorganic contaminants onto some surfaces [54,55].

The above could be clinically relevant since, as we know, macrophages respond to all the implanted materials, being fundamental for the fate of an implant [36]. Macrophages are capable of releasing metal ions from solid surfaces in a matter of minutes by dissolucytosis [2]. The fused macrophages in FBGC can remain in the interface biomaterial-tissue, generating a sealed compartment between its surface and the underlying biomaterial, which allows the secretion of different mediators such as ROS, degradative enzymes and acid. Due to this the "frustrated phagocytosis process" being associated with the failure of some implanted devices [48]. Particles, ions, or degradation products from implanted materials or devices may also be recognized as foreign by macrophages and dendritic cells [9,56]. Dendritic cells may also be drawn to the implant site by the recognition of foreign substances, inducing the expansion of CD4 cells [9,21], so that some dental implant could eventually be able to cause a type IV hypersensitivity reaction [57]. Since the bone marrow contains structures in the form of follicles, similar to that observed in lymph nodes or the spleen, although without an organized T and B zone, but these lymphoid follicles can increase in the bone marrow during infections, inflammations and autoimmunity [21].

It has been demonstrated that titanium leakage due to corrosion inevitably results in substantial contact between the foreign material and the tissues. In fact, there was a gradient in titanium intensity from the implant surface and out up to a distance away from it of about 1000 μm [20]. Titanium ions could cause immune responses due to their ability to bind to proteins, such as albumin or transferrin, creating a bioavailable metalloprotein that could serve as an antigen in immunological reactions. Many studies have shown that proinflammatory cytokines such as IL-1β (interleukin 1beta), TNF-α tumor necrosis alpha factor, and GM-CSF (granulocyte-macrophage colony stimulating factor) are jointly regulated after stimulation of a hapten or particles [58]. However, it is likely that this first corrosion is coupled to the acidic environment that inevitably develops after the placement of an implant, a situation that is present until approximately four weeks after surgery when the partial pressure of oxygen has normalized [20]. In all probability at this stage, the released ionic titanium is stabilized by biomolecules such as citrate, an important metal chelator in cellular fluids, forming relatively stable complexes in solutions close to neutral pH [58]. Thereafter it seems likely that titanium corrosion will be quite minimal, provided that there is no more mechanical interruption of the blood flow. The presence of titanium ions in a stage subsequent to osseointegration could generate a synergistic interaction with other negative factors, such as cement particles, leading to marginal bone loss [20].

This scenario where living tissues face the presence of materials in an immunologically active environment allows for a better understanding of the dynamics of osseointegration, and also reveals that the desired FBE in an oral implant can be threatened by clinical conditions [7]. This is why the methods that control the polarization of the macrophage have emerged as an attractive means to reduce inflammatory signaling [19]. It is known that the increase in bone formation correlates with the resolution of the initial inflammatory response. That is, inflammation and osseointegration are inversely proportional [2]. As osseointegration is an immunomodulated inflammatory process, where the immune system is locally up-or down-regulated [57], the precise modulation of postoperative inflammation and the innate immune reaction provide a promising approach for therapeutic purposes [19].

Several immunomodulation strategies have been proposed, mainly through the implanted device, and more recently, the immunomodulation by means of direct stimulation of Human bone marrow-derived mesenchymal stem cell (HBMMSC). This aims to improve integration, avoid fibrosis, prevent bone loss and so increase the useful life of the devices in the human body [14,19,59].

In relation to these immunomodulation strategies through implanted devices, the topographic modification of the titanium dental implant surface has shown a significant positive effect in the speed and degree of osseointegration. In fact, the use of microscale modified implant surfaces has been one of the key factors in increasing the clinical success rate of implants, especially in areas of compromised bone quality [2]. The surface topography of the implant can be optimized at a micro level and nanoscale, influencing properties such as wettability and surface charge, modifying the kinetics of adsorption, the folding of proteins adsorbed onto implant surface and the consequent presentation of bioactive sites to macrophages [51,60]. The geometry of the material may also be relevant for the phenotypic expression of macrophage. It has been demonstrated that micro- and nanopatterned grooves of 400–500 nm wide can influence macrophage elongation, driving macrophages toward an anti-inflammatory, pro-healing phenotype [61]. This interaction of the macrophage with its mechanical environment, that is, the surface of the titanium, is possible through multiple mechanoreceptors on the cell surface, perhaps through integrins [62]. At present, titanium can be alloyed with Zirconium (TiZr). The combination of high-energy and altered surface chemistry (hydrophilic), seems to generate an immunomodulatory effect towards the activation of M2 macrophages, decreasing the presence of FGBC and increasing osseointegration [10].

A growing number of studies report success based on therapies with metal ions such as magnesium, strontium, calcium, among others. These ions can be incorporated into devices, in order to promote osteogenesis coupled with a pro-regenerative immune response. For example, the production of proinflammatory cytokines such as TNF-α, IL-1b, IL-6 and PEG2 has been shown to be reduced in the presence of high concentrations of magnesium, which highlights its role as an immunomodulatory ion [63].

The incorporation of immunomodulatory molecules to the implant constitutes another strategy to modulate the immune response [12,52]. Inflammation could be controlled by the local release of M2 polarizing cytokines such as IL-4, IL-10, IL-13 [64], or the implant could directly inhibit proinflammatory signals, using anti-TNF-α therapy, which are the most potent proinflammatory cytokines that promote the polarization of M1 macrophages [65]. The transcription factor NF-κB has also been pointed out as a possible target to generate implant-mediated immunomodulation. It has been shown that NF-κB decoy can suppress the production of essential chemokines for the recruitment of monocytes, which could avoid the presence of immune cells at the bone-implant interface [66].

In spite of the above-mentioned issues, the biology is more complex. The determination of the appropriate time frame of immunomodulation is critical for optimizing their application. Acute phase inflammation is crucial for proper bone repair after trauma, so the macrophage polarization status also plays a critical role in bone regeneration. As such, the interplay between M1- and M2-dominated microenvironments and the temporal modulation of the transition M1 to M2 provide an interesting line of investigation to pursue new immune-modulatory therapies and improve bone repair and implant integration [52]. One possible method is to utilize a controlled release system to maintain a short period of M1, followed by a transition to M2 polarization via cytokines in a biphasic manner. However, future investigations are necessary [67].

A new therapeutic approach to achieve modulation of the transition from M1 to M2 in the appropriate timeframe could be the MSC of the host, given their innate immunomodulatory capabilities [68]. More than 400 studies have explored the immunomodulatory effect of MSCs for the treatment of various autoimmune conditions, including graft-versus-host disease, diabetes, multiple sclerosis, Crohn's disease, and organ transplantation [69]. In relation to this, a new hypothesis has recently been proposed, that the HBMMSC residing around the peri-implant bone tissue immunomodulate the osseointegration process through the ESWT bio-activation effect. The mechanical stimuli generated by ESWT trigger the release of exosomes by HBMMSCs, generating tolerogenic dendritic cells (Tol-Dcs) and increasing the presence of the M2 phenotype of the macrophage [14].

5. Coupling between Osseointegration and Mechanotransduction to Maintain FBE Long-Term

At present we know that osteogenesis does not depend only on the bone cells of the skeletal system, in fact, there is a multicellular collaboration. Over years, studies have focused on the interaction between bone cells and the material surface, however, now studies in the field of advanced bone materials should involve co-culture systems with the interaction between materials, bone cells, and immune cells. Only then will we know the real osteoimmunomodulatory capacity of the material [19]. However, the complexity becomes even greater when we consider a fourth factor that can become important to maintain the balance of the material-host relationship, the mechanical stimuli. Physical forces also play important roles in embryonic development, tissue homeostasis, and pathogenesis. However, the importance of mechanical signals to control cellular processes has only been recognized more recently. That is why, as interest grows in the field of mechanobiology, new study models are developed to analyze the influence of mechanical forces on cells and tissues [70,71].

The cells are sensitive to shear, tension and compression forces. These mechanical signals have important effects on tissues, such as the production of ECM components [72]. A mechanical alteration can influence gene expression and cellular behavior through the mechanotransduction signal [73]. These mechanical signals would be transmitted by the filaments of the cytoskeleton, such as actin and microtubules, and finally transduced into biochemical signals [74], being the integrins of the cell surface essential for mechanotransduction [75].

The therapeutic mechanotransduction is part of modern Implantology, in fact, good clinical results obtained through progressive loading protocol [76] and immediate loading protocol [77,78], reveal to us that physiological mechanical stimuli can be beneficial to accompany the osseointegration of a dental implant and allow for successful osseointegration [79]. In this sense Duyck et al. demonstrated through a bone chamber model in an animal model that mechanical stimuli are capable of increasing the bone-implant contact (BIC) [80]. However, we also know that mechanical stimuli are key in bone remodeling, so greater trauma can lead to implant failure [20].

At present, ESWT are widely used in the context of therapeutic mechanotransduction. ESWT are supersonic waves, generated by different types of devices, such as electrohydraulic, piezoelectric, electromechanical or pneumatic, which generate transient pressure changes that propagate through the tissues where they are applied [81,82]. ESWT is applied to treat various medical pathologies.

In orthopedics, it is used mainly in the treatment of tendinopathies, the treatment of nonunion in fractures of long bones, avascular necrosis of the femoral head, chronic diabetics, nondiabetic ulcers and ischemic heart disease [83]. In dentistry, ESWT has been used in extracorporeal lithotripsy of salivary stones [84] and painful mielogelosis of the masseter [85]. Recently, Falkensammer et al. used ESWT as a supplement in Orthodontics [86], finding an absence of deleterious effects in the maxillofacial tissues or for pulpal vitality [87].

It has been proposed that the mechanical stimuli generated by ESWT produce an increase in the permeability of the cell membrane, which triggers the release of cytoplasmic ribonucleic acid (RNA) through an active process dependent on exosomes. This event at the cellular level is the one that would produce the effects observed in the accelerated repair of tissues. However, more studies are needed to completely reveal the underlying mechanism [88].

It seems that the bone is programmed to seal immediately any area affecting its integrity, sealing and protecting the marrow content through the restoration of a cortical bone barrier. Therefore, we can assume that the "raw materials" (phosphate, calcium, etc.) could be more available from a source of cortical bone [4]. In this sense, it has been described that oral implants installed in low-density bone tissue (bone type IV) present a higher risk of failure [89]. On the other hand, in patients with osteoporosis, even though there is no difference described to date in the survival rate of oral implants placed in patients with and without osteoporosis, there is an increase in peri-implant bone loss [90]. In orthopedics, it is a proven fact that the fixation of screws and osteosynthesis plates can be hindered in patients with low bone mass and especially with thin cortices. In fact, in osteoporotic fractures, depending on the location, the type of fracture and the surgery performed, the failure rate can reach up to 30% [91]. In this sense, the anabolic effect on the bone described in several studies with the use of ESWT has become particularly attractive [82,92].

Recent research shows that this anabolic bone response through ESWT can also be generated in relation to titanium devices in bone, which could have great therapeutic potential, especially in patients with bone disease. Koolen et al. demonstrated at the histological level that in bone defects reconstructed with a titanium scaffold as a bone substitute show the de novo bone formation after ESWT in rats [93]. In this same line of investigation, Koolen et al. [91] hypothesized that peri-operative shock wave treatment can improve screw fixation and the osteointegration of cortical and cancellous orthopedic screws, especially in osteoporotic patients. They were able to demonstrate in a healthy rodent bones model, that an ESWT immediately after the implantation of titanium screws (Ti6Al4V grade 5) improved screw fixation of the cortical screw, visualized by improved mechanical strength and osseointegration. Another finding was the formation of a neocortex in some animals after treatment. However, the cancellous screw showed no differences in testing after ESWT [91]. In this context, it has been reported that the ESWT not only achieves complete bone healing, but has also been observed to help in the re-attachment of a loose orthopedic screw. This has been observed in a patient with a typical case of non-union treated with ESWT [94].

It has been suggested that these anabolic effects in the bone are due to the fact that shock waves can cause the conversion of progenitor cells into osteogenic precursor cells. Another possibility could be that ESWT induces osteocytic cell death through a mechanism called cavitation. This death of osteocytes could lead to the stimulation of local bone remodeling, activating the osteoblast to produce more osteoid, which could eventually lead to a neocortex [91]. I Osteocytes are important regulators of cellular homeostasis and can act as mechanosensors. In addition, direct contact between dendrites of the osteocytes and the implant surface has been reported after an 8-week osseointegration period in an in vivo model [1]. However, the presence of HBMMSC and immune cells in the peri-implant environment leads us to think that the ESWT could also have a potent immunomodulatory effect in favor of osseointegration [14].

HBMMSC are not only found in the peri-implant environment, but also adhere to the titanium surface [95]. Current evidence indicates that BMMSCs can modulate the immune response by inhibiting polarization induced to M1 macrophages and promote polarization to M2 macrophages through the release of paracrine factors [96]. In addition, HBMMSCs can modulate the immune response through the generation of Tol-DC [97]. This is why the fact that ESWT can act as an effective bioactivator on HBMMSC, increasing its rate of growth, proliferation, migration and reducing apoptosis of these cells, suggests that ESWT could be an adequate tool to express all the potential therapeutic effects of HBMMSC [98]. This evidence suggests that the findings described in relation to ESWT and titanium [91,93,94] are probably a product of the local immunomodulatory effect of HBMMSC [14].

Mechanical signals play an important role in the regulation of immunological and cellular processes in monocytes, macrophages, and dendritic cells [70]. In this sense, recent studies have investigated the anti-inflammatory effect of ESWT in ischemic lesions in the animal model. Scientists have observed that ESWT would regulate the inflammatory reactions reducing the infiltration of inflammatory cells and promoting the differentiation of the M2 macrophage, that is, through the immunomodulation effect [99]. Apparently, the ESWT also exerts direct modulation on the macrophage. It has been demonstrated that the stimulation of macrophages derived from human monocytes with ESWT causes the significant inhibition of some M1 marker genes (CD80, COX2, CCL5) in M1 macrophages and a significant synergistic effect for some M2 marker genes (ALOX15, MRC1, CCL18) in the M2 macrophages. It has also been observed that ESWT affected the production of cytokines and chemokines, inducing, in particular, a significant increase in IL-10 and a reduction in the production of IL-1β [100].

No doubt, infiltrating immune cells play an important role in determining the variable outcome of wound repair in mammals and amphibians. For example, it has been demonstrated that the systemic depletion of macrophages results in a permanent failure in the regenerative capacity of the axolotl, with extensive fibrosis. However, the regenerative capacity of the axolotl is recovered once the macrophage population is restored [101].

While the use of immunomodulatory implants per se (clean implants) generates adequate osseointegration [55], the FBE can be altered under certain clinical conditions, such as overload [1,5,7]. The possibility that we can guide the transition between the M1 inflammatory phase and the M2 anti-inflammatory phase through mechanotransduction makes ESWT a promising therapeutic alternative to improve clinical success in oral implants, maintaining FBE long-term [14]. This could potentially improve the feedback path to the sensory cortex since, as described, the capacity for tactile perception of osseointegrated implants, "osseoperception", increases over time [102]. Furthermore, it has also been proposed that the topical addition of the nerve growth factor (NGF) in oral implants could help to improve this tactile sensitivity in order to minimize occlusal overload [103], and it has been demonstrated that ESWT is effective in increasing the expression of NGF [104].

6. Concluding Remarks

Mechanotransduction can improve the implant-host relationship. However, it is necessary to perform studies at the cellular and molecular level that would allow us to determine both the medical device and the most effective therapeutic range. All of this is in order to improve, maintain and recover the harmony of this triad of elements, i.e., bone cells, immune cells and implants, which finally determines the fate of FBE.

Author Contributions: Writing-Original Draft Preparation, A-P.L.; Writing-Review & Editing, B.-A.M; M.-C.F.; J.-S.M.C.; P.-P.L.; C.-V.R.

References

1.   Trindade, R.; Albrektsson, T.; Wennerberg, A. Current concepts for the biological basis of dental implants: Foreign body equilibrium and osseointegration dynamics. *Oral Maxillofac. Surg. Clin. N. Am.* **2015**, 27, 175–183. [CrossRef] [PubMed]

2.   Hamlet, S.; Ivanovski, S. Inflammatory Cytokine Response to Titanium Surface Chemistry and Topography. In *The Immune Response to Implanted Materials and Devices*; Corradetti, B., Ed.; Springer: Cham, Switzerland, 2017; pp. 151–167. ISBN 978-3-319-45433-7.

3.   Wennerberg, A.; Albrektsson, T. Current challenges in successful rehabilitation with oral implants. *J. Oral Rehabil.* **2011**, *38*, 286–294. [CrossRef] [PubMed]

4.   Trindade, R.; Albrektsson, T.; Galli, S.; Prgomet, Z.; Tengvall, P.; Wennerberg, A. Osseointegration and foreign body reaction: Titanium implants activate the immune system and suppress bone resorption during the first 4 weeks after implantation. *Clin. Implant Dent. Relat. Res.* **2018**, *20*, 82–91. [CrossRef]

5.   Albrektsson, T.; Dahlin, C.; Jemt, T.; Sennerby, L.; Turri, A.; Wennerberg, A. Is marginal bone loss around oral implants the result of a provoked foreign body reaction? *Clin. Implant Dent. Relat. Res.* **2014**, *16*, 155–165. [CrossRef] [PubMed]

6.   Chrcanovic, B.R.; Kisch, J.; Albrektsson, T.; Wennerberg, A. A retrospective study on clinical and radiological outcomes of oral implants in patients followed up for a minimum of 20 years. *Clin. Implant Dent. Relat. Res.* **2018**, *20*, 199–207. [CrossRef] [PubMed]

7.   Trindade, R.; Albrektsson, T.; Tengvall, P.; Wennerberg, A. Foreign Body Reaction to Biomaterials: On Mechanisms for Buildup and Breakdown of Osseointegration. *Clin. Implant Dent. Relat. Res.* **2016**, *18*, 192–203. [CrossRef] [PubMed]

8.   Albrektsson, T.; Canullo, L.; Cochran, D.; De Bruyn, H. "Peri-Implantitis": A Complication of a Foreign Body or a Man-Made "Disease". Facts and Fiction. *Clin. Implant Dent Relat. Res.* **2016**, *18*, 840–849. [CrossRef] [PubMed]

9.   Scarritt, M.E.; Londono, R.; Badylak, S.F. Host Response to Implanted Materials and Devices: An Overview. In *The Immune Response to Implanted Materials and Devices*; Corradetti, B., Ed.; Springer: Cham, Switzerland, 2017; pp. 1–14. ISBN 978-3-319-45433-7.

10.   Hotchkiss, K.M.; Ayad, N.B.; Hyzy, S.L.; Boyan, B.D.; Olivares-Navarrete, R. Dental implant surface chemistry and energy alter macrophage activation in vitro. *Clin. Oral Implants Res.* **2017**, *28*, 414–423. [CrossRef] [PubMed]

11.   Chen, Z.; Mao, X.; Tan, L.; Friis, T.; Wu, C.; Crawford, R.; Xiao, Y. Osteoimmunomodulatory properties of magnesium scaffolds coated with β-tricalcium phosphate. *Biomaterials* **2014**, *35*, 8553–8565. [CrossRef]

12.   Sato, T.; Pajarinen, J.; Behn, A.; Jiang, X.; Lin, T.H.; Loi, F.; Yao, Z.; Egashira, K.; Yang, F.; Goodman, S.B. The effect of local IL-4 delivery or CCL2 blockade on implant fixation and bone structural properties in a mouse model of wear particle induced osteolysis. *J. Biomed. Mater. Res. A* **2016**, *104*, 2255–2262. [CrossRef]

13.   Nojehdehi, S.; Soudi, S.; Hesampour, A.; Rasouli, S.; Soleimani, M.; Hashemi, S.M. Immunomodulatory effects of mesenchymal stem cell-derived exosomes on experimental type-1 autoimmune diabetes. *J. Cell Biochem.* **2018**, *119*, 9433–9443. [CrossRef] [PubMed]

14.   Amengual-Peñafiel, L.; Jara-Sepúlveda, M.C.; Parada-Pozas, L.; Marchesani-Carrasco, F.; Cartes-Velásquez, R.; Galdames-Gutiérrez, B. Immunomodulation of Osseointegration Through Extracorporeal Shock Wave Therapy. *Dent. Hypotheses* **2018**, *9*, 45–50. [CrossRef]

15.   Van der Meulen, M.C.; Huiskes, R. Why mechanobiology? A survey article. *J. Biomech.* **2002**, *35*, 401–404. [CrossRef]

16.   Yusko, E.C.; Asbury, C.L. Force is a signal that cells cannot ignore. *Mol. Biol. Cell* **2014**, *25*, 3717–3725. [CrossRef] [PubMed]

17.   Zhao, L.; Wu, Z.; Zhang, Y. Low-magnitude mechanical vibration may be applied clinically to promote dental implant osseointegration. *Med. Hypotheses* **2009**, *72*, 451–452. [CrossRef] [PubMed]

18.   Mennens, S.F.B.; van den Dries, K.; Cambi, A. Role for Mechanotransduction in Macrophage and Dendritic Cell Immunobiology. *Results Probl. Cell Differ.* **2017**, *62*, 209–242. [CrossRef] [PubMed]

19.   Zetao, C.; Travis, K.; Rachael, M.; Ross, C.; Jiang, C.; Chengtie, W.; Yin, X. Osteoimmunomodulation for the development of advanced bone biomaterials. *Mater. Today* **2016**, *19*, 304–321. [CrossRef]

20.   Albrektsson, T.; Chrcanovic, B.; Östman, P.O.; Sennerby, L. Initial and long-term crestal bone responses to modern dental implants. *Periodontol. 2000* **2017**, *73*, 41–50. [CrossRef]

21.   Zhao, E.; Xu, H.; Wang, L.; Kryczek, I.; Wu, K.; Hu, Y.; Wang, G.; Zou, W. Bone marrow and the control of immunity. *Cell Mol. Immunol.* **2012**, *9*, 11–19. [CrossRef]

22.   Calvi, L.M.; Adams, G.B.; Weibrecht, K.W.; Weber, J.M.; Olson, D.P.; Knight, M.C.; Martin, R.P.; Schipani, E.; Divieti, P.; Bringhurst, F.R.; et al. Osteoblastic cells regulate the haematopoietic stem cell niche. *Nature* **2003**, *425*, 841–846. [CrossRef] [PubMed]

23. Kikuta, J.; Ishii, M. Osteoclast migration, differentiation and function: Novel therapeutic targets for rheumatic diseases. *Rheumatology* **2013**, *52*, 226–234. [CrossRef] [PubMed]

24. Mazo, I.B.; Honczarenko, M.; Leung, H.; Cavanagh, L.L.; Bonasio, R.; Weninger, W. Bone marrow is a major reservoir and site of recruitment for central memory CD8+ T cells. *Immunity* **2005**, *22*, 259–270. [CrossRef] [PubMed]

25. Arboleya, L.; Castañeda, S. Osteoimmunology. *Reumatol. Clin.* **2013**, *9*, 303–315. [CrossRef] [PubMed]

26. Monroe, D.G.; McGee-Lawrence, M.E.; Oursler, M.J.; Westendorf, J.J. Update on Wnt signaling in bone cell biology and bone disease. *Gene* **2012**, *492*, 1–18. [CrossRef] [PubMed]

27. Theill, L.E.; Boyle, W.J.; Penninger, J.M. RANK-L and RANK: T cell, bone loss and mammalian evolution. *Annu. Rev. Immunol.* **2002**, *20*, 795–823. [CrossRef] [PubMed]

28. Srivastava, R.K.; Dar, H.Y.; Mishra, P.K. Immunoporosis: Immunology of Osteoporosis-Role of T Cells. *Front. Immunol.* **2018**, *9*, 657. [CrossRef] [PubMed]

29. Alnaeeli, M.; Park, J.; Mahamed, D.; Penninger, J.M.; Teng, Y.T. Dendritic cells at the osteo-immune interface: Implications for inflammation-induced bone loss. *J. Bone Miner. Res.* **2007**, *22*, 775–780. [CrossRef] [PubMed]

30. Caetano-Lopes, J.; Canhão, H.; Fonseca, J.E. Osteoimmunology-the hidden immune regulation of bone. *Autoimmun. Rev.* **2009**, *8*, 250–255. [CrossRef]

31. Kaur, S.; Raggatt, L.J.; Batoon, L.; Hume, D.A.; Levesque, J.P.; Pettit, A.R. Role of bone marrow macrophages in controlling homeostasis and repair in bone and bone marrow niches. *Semin. Cell Dev. Biol.* **2017**, *61*, 12–21. [CrossRef]

32. Batoon, L.; Millard, S.M.; Raggatt, L.J.; Pettit, A.R. Osteomacs and Bone Regeneration. *Curr. Osteoporos. Rep.* **2017**, *15*, 385–395. [CrossRef]

33. Chang, M.K.; Raggatt, L.J.; Alexander, K.A.; Kuliwaba, J.S.; Fazzalari, N.L.; Schroder, K.; Maylin, E.R.; Ripoll, V.M.; Hume, D.A.; Pettit, A.R. Osteal tissue macrophages are intercalated throughout human and mouse bone lining tissues and regulate osteoblast function in vitro and in vivo. *J. Immunol.* **2008**, *181*, 1232–1244. [CrossRef] [PubMed]

34. Raggatt, L.J.; Wullschleger, M.E.; Alexander, K.A.; Wu, A.C.; Millard, S.M.; Kaur, S.; Maugham, M.L.; Gregory, L.S.; Steck, R.; Pettit, A.R. Fracture healing via periosteal callus formation requires macrophages for both initiation and progression of early endochondral ossification. *Am. J. Pathol.* **2014**, *184*, 3192–3204. [CrossRef] [PubMed]

35. Andrew, J.G.; Andrew, S.M.; Freemont, A.J.; Marsh, D.R. Inflammatory cells in normal human fracture healing. *Acta Orthop. Scand.* **1994**, *65*, 462–466. [CrossRef] [PubMed]

36. Anderson, J.M.; Cramer, S. Perspectives on the inflammatory, healing, and foreign body responses to biomaterials and medical devices. In *Host Response to Biomaterials. The Impact of Host Response on Biomaterial Selection*; Badylak, S., Ed.; Elsevier: New York, NY, USA, 2015; pp. 13–36. ISBN 9780128001967.

37. Hosgood, G. Wound healing. The role of platelet-derived growth factor and transforming growth factor beta. *Vet. Surg.* **1993**, *22*, 490–495. [CrossRef] [PubMed]

38. Anderson, J.M.; Jiang, S. Implications of the Acute and Chronic Inflammatory Response and the Foreign Body Reaction to the Immune Response of Implanted Biomaterials. In *The Immune Response to Implanted Materials and Devices*; Corradetti, B., Ed.; Springer: Cham, Switzerland, 2017; pp. 15–36. ISBN 978-3-319-45433-7.

39. Hu, W.J.; Eaton, J.W.; Ugarova, T.P.; Tang, L. Molecular basis of biomaterial-mediated foreign body reaction. *Blood* **2001**, *98*, 1231–1238. [CrossRef] [PubMed]

40. Christo, S.N.; Diener, K.R.; Bachhuka, A.; Vasilev, K.; Hayball, J.D. Innate Immunity and Biomaterials at the Nexus: Friends or Foes. *BioMed Res. Int.* **2015**. [CrossRef]

41. Arvidsson, S.; Askendal, A.; Tengvall, P. Blood plasma contact activation on silicon, titanium, and aluminum. *Biomaterials* **2007**, *28*, 1346–1354. [CrossRef]

42. Mills, C.D.; Kincaid, K.; Alt, J.M.; Heilman, M.J.; Hill, A.M. M-1/M-2 macrophages and the Th1/Th2 paradigm. *J. Immunol.* **2000**, *164*, 6166–6173. [CrossRef]

43. Mosser, D.M.; Edwards, J.P. Exploring the full spectrum of macrophage activation. *Nat. Rev. Immunol.* **2008**, *8*, 958–969. [CrossRef]

44. Lucas, T.; Waisman, A.; Ranjan, R.; Roes, J.; Krieg, T.; Müller, W.; Roers, A.; Eming, S.A. Differential roles of macrophages in diverse phases of skin repair. *J. Immunol.* **2010**, *184*, 3964–3977. [CrossRef]

45. Trindade, R.; Albrektsson, T.; Tengvall, P.; Wennerberg, A. Bone immune response to Titanium, PEEK and Copper- Osseointegration and the Immune-inflammatory balance. *Clin. Oral Implants Res.* **2018**, *29*, 138. [CrossRef]

46. Anderson, J.M.; Rodriguez, D.T.; Chang, A. Foreign body reaction to biomaterials. *Semin. Immunol.* **2008**, *20*, 86–100. [CrossRef] [PubMed]

47. Barbeck, M.; Booms, P.; Unger, R.; Hoffmann, V.; Sader, R.; Kirkpatrick, C.J.; Ghanaati, S. Multinucleated giant cells in the implant bed of bone substitutes are foreign body giant cells-New insights into the material-mediated healing process. *J. Biomed. Mater. Res. A* **2017**, *105*, 1105–1111. [CrossRef] [PubMed]

48. Scatena, M.; Eaton, K.V.; Jackson, M.F.; Lund, S.A.; Giachelli, C.M. Macrophages: The Bad, the Ugly, and the Good in the Inflammatory Response to Biomaterials. In *The Immune Response to Implanted Materials and Devices*; Corradetti, B., Ed.; Springer: Cham, Switzerland, 2017; pp. 37–62. ISBN 978-3-319-45433-7.

49. Donath, K.; Laass, M.; Günzl, H.J. The histopathology of different foreign body reactions in oral soft tissue and bone tissue. *Virchows Arch. A Pathol. Anat. Histopathol.* **1992**, *420*, 131–137. [CrossRef] [PubMed]

50. Vigneri, A. Macrophage fusion: Molecular mechanisms. *Methods Mol. Biol.* **2008**, *475*, 149–161. [CrossRef]

51. Romagnani, S. T-cell subsets [Th1 versus Th2]. *Ann. Allergy Asthma Immunol.* **2000**, *85*, 9–18. [CrossRef]

52. Lin, T.; Jämsen, E.; Lu, L.; Nathan, K.; Pajarinen, J.; Goodman, S. Modulating Innate Inflammatory Reactions in the Application of Orthopedic Biomaterials. In *Progress in Biology, Manufacturing, and Industry Perspectives*; Li, B., Webster, T., Eds.; Springer: Cham, Switzerland, 2018; pp. 199–218. ISBN 978-3-319-89542-0.

53. Biguetti, C.C.; Cavalla, F.; Silveira, E.M.; Fonseca, A.C.; Vieira, A.E.; Tabanez, A.P.; Rodrigues, D.C.; Trombone, A.P.F.; Garlet, G.P. Oral implant osseointegration model in C57Bl/6 mice: Microtomographic, histological, histomorphometric and molecular characterization. *J. Appl. Oral Sci.* **2018**, *26*, e20170601. [CrossRef]

54. Dohan Ehrenfest, D.M.; Del Corso, M.; Kang, B.; Leclercq, P.; Mazor, Z.; Horowitz, R.A.; Russe, P.; Oh, H.; Zou, D.; Shibli, J.A.; et al. Identification card and codification of the chemical and morphological characteristics of 62 dental implant surfaces. Part 3: Sand-blasted/acid-etched [SLA type] and related surfaces [Group 2A, main subtractive process]. *POSEIDO* **2014**, *2*, 37–55.

55. Clean Implant. Available online: http://www.cleanimplant.com/ (accessed on 25 November 2018).

56. Konttinen, Y.T.; Pajarinen, J.; Takakubo, Y.; Gallo, J.; Nich, C.; Takagi, M.; Goodman, S.B. Macrophage polarization and activation in response to implant debris: Influence by "particle disease" and "ion disease". *J. Long Term Eff. Med. Implants* **2014**, *24*, 267–281. [CrossRef]

57. Albrektsson, T.; Chrcanovic, B.; Mölne, J.; Wennerberg, A. Foreign body reactions, marginal bone loss and allergies to titanium implants. *Eur. J. Oral Implantol.* **2018**, *11*, S37–S46.

58. Høl, P.J.; Kristoffersen, E.K.; Gjerdet, N.R.; Pellowe, A.S. Novel Nanoparticulate and Ionic Titanium Antigens for Hypersensitivity Testing. *Int. J. Mol. Sci.* **2018**, *19*, 1101. [CrossRef]

59. Goodman, S.B.; Gibon, E.; Pajarinen, J.; Lin, T.H.; Keeney, M.; Ren, P.G.; Nich, C.; Yao, Z.; Egashira, K.; Yang, F.; et al. Novel biological strategies for treatment of wear particle-induced periprosthetic osteolysis of orthopaedic implants for joint replacement. *J. R. Soc. Interface* **2014**, *11*, 20130962. [CrossRef]

60. Xu, L.C.; Siedlecki, C.A. Effects of surface wettability and contact time on protein adhesion to biomaterial surfaces. *Biomaterials* **2007**, *28*, 3273–3283. [CrossRef]

61. Luu, T.U.; Gott, S.C.; Woo, B.W.; Rao, M.P.; Liu, W.F. Micro- and Nanopatterned Topographical Cues for Regulating Macrophage Cell Shape and Phenotype. *ACS Appl. Mater. Interfaces* **2015**, *7*, 28665–28672. [CrossRef] [PubMed]

62. Thompson, W.R.; Rubin, C.T.; Rubin, J. Mechanical regulation of signaling pathways in bone. *Gene* **2012**, *503*, 179–193. [CrossRef] [PubMed]

63. Vasconcelos, D.M.; Santos, S.G.; Lamghari, M.; Barbosa, M.A. The two faces of metal ions: From implants rejection to tissue repair/regeneration. *Biomaterials* **2016**, *84*, 262–275. [CrossRef] [PubMed]

64. Martinez, F.O.; Sica, A.; Mantovani, A.; Locati, M. Macrophage activation and polarization. *Front. Biosci.* **2008**, *13*, 453–461. [CrossRef]

65. Gilbert, L.; He, X.; Farmer, P.; Boden, S.; Kozlowski, M.; Rubin, J.; Nanes, M.S. Inhibition of osteoblast differentiation by tumor necrosis factor-alpha. *Endocrinology* **2000**, *141*, 3956–3964. [CrossRef] [PubMed]

66. Lin, T.H.; Pajarinen, J.; Sato, T.; Loi, F.; Fan, C.; Cordova, L.A.; Nabeshima, A.; Gibon, E.; Zhang, R.; Yao, Z.; et al. NF-kappaB decoy oligodeoxynucleotide mitigates wear particle-associated bone loss in the murine continuous infusion model. *Acta Biomater.* **2016**, *41*, 273–281. [CrossRef]

67. Kumar, V.A.; Taylor, N.L.; Shi, S.; Wickremasinghe, N.C.; D'Souza, R.N.; Hartgerink, J.D. Selfassembling multidomain peptides tailor biological responses through biphasic release. *Biomaterials* **2015**, *52*, 71–78. [CrossRef]

68. Viganò, M.; Sansone, V.; d'Agostino, M.C.; Romeo, P.; Perucca Orfei, C.; de Girolamo, L. Mesenchymal stem cells as therapeutic target of biophysical stimulation for the treatment of musculoskeletal disorders. *J. Orthop. Surg. Res.* **2016**, *11*, 163. [CrossRef] [PubMed]

69. Gao, F.; Chiu, S.M.; Motan, D.A.; Zhang, Z.; Chen, L.; Ji, H.L.; Tse, H.F.; Fu, Q.-L.; Lian, Q. Mesenchymal Stem Cell and Immunomodulation: Current Status and Future Prospects. *Cell Death Dis.* **2016**, *7*, e2062. [CrossRef] [PubMed]

70. Guilak, F.; Cohen, D.M.; Estes, B.T.; Gimble, J.M.; Liedtke, W.; Chen, C.S. Control of stem cell fate by physical interactions with the extracellular matrix. *Cell Stem Cell* **2009**, *5*, 17–26. [CrossRef] [PubMed]

71. Carver, W.; Esch, A.M.; Fowlkes, V.; Goldsmith, E.C. The Biomechanical Environment and Impact on Tissue Fibrosis. In *The Immune Response to Implanted Materials and Devices*; Corradetti, B., Ed.; Springer: Cham, Switzerland, 2017; pp. 169–188. ISBN 978-3-319-45433-7.

72. Leung, D.Y.; Glagov, S.; Mathews, M.B. Cyclic stretching stimulates synthesis of matrix components by arterial smooth muscle cells in vitro. *Science* **1976**, *191*, 475–477. [CrossRef] [PubMed]

73. Dunn, S.L.; Olmedo, M.L. Mechanotransduction: Relevance to physical therapist practice—Understanding our ability to affect genetic expression through mechanical forces. *Phys. Ther.* **2016**, *96*, 712–721. [CrossRef] [PubMed]

74. Ingber, D.E. Tensegrity: The architectural basis of cellular mechanotransduction. *Annu. Rev. Physiol.* **1997**, *59*, 575–599. [CrossRef] [PubMed]

75. MacKenna, D.A.; Dolfi, F.; Vuori, K.; Ruoslahti, E. Extracellular signal-regulated kinase and c-Jun NH2-terminal kinase activation by mechanical stretch is integrin-dependent and matrix specific in rat cardiac fibroblasts. *J. Clin. Investig.* **1998**, *101*, 301–310. [CrossRef] [PubMed]

76. Ghoveizi, R.; Alikhasi, M.; Siadat, M.R.; Siadat, H.; Sorouri, M. A radiographic comparison of progressive and conventional loading on crestal bone loss and density in single dental implants: A randomized controlled trial study. *J. Dent.* **2013**, *10*, 155–163.

77. Piattelli, A.; Corigliano, M.; Scarano, A.; Costigliola, G.; Paolantonio, M. Immediate loading of titanium plasma-sprayed implants: An histologic analysis in monkeys. *J. Periodontol.* **1998**, *69*, 321–327. [CrossRef]

78. Huang, H.; Wismeijer, D.; Shao, X.; Wu, G. Mathematical evaluation of the influence of multiple factors on implant stability quotient values in clinical practice: A retrospective study. *Ther. Clin. Risk Manag.* **2016**, *12*, 1525–1532. [CrossRef]

79. Sennerby, L.; Ericson, L.E.; Thomsen, P.; Lekholm, U.; Astrand, P. Structure of the bone-titanium interface in retrieved clinical oral implants. *Clin. Oral Implants Res.* **1991**, *2*, 103–111. [CrossRef] [PubMed]

80. Duyck, J.; Cooman, M.D.; Puers, R.; van Oosterwyck, H.; Sloten, J.V.; Naert, I. A repeated sampling bone chamber methodology for the evaluation of tissue differentiation and bone adaptation around titanium implants under controlled mechanical conditions. *J. Biomech.* **2004**, *37*, 1819–1822. [CrossRef] [PubMed]

81. Ogden, J.A.; Tóth-Kischkat, A.; Schultheiss, R. Principles of shock wave therapy. *Clin. Orthop. Relat. Res.* **2001**, *387*, 8–17. [CrossRef]

82. Van der Jagt, O.P.; Waarsing, J.H.; Kops, N.; Schaden, W.; Jahr, H.; Verhaar, J.A.; Weinans, H. Unfocused extracorporeal shock waves induce anabolic effects in osteoporotic rats. *JBJS* **2011**, *93*, 38–48. [CrossRef] [PubMed]

83. Wang, C.J. Extracorporeal shockwave therapy in musculoskeletal disorders. *J. Orthop. Surg. Res.* **2012**, *7*, 11. [CrossRef] [PubMed]

84. Iro, H.; Schneider, H.T.; Födra, C.; Waitz, G.; Nitsche, N.; Heinritz, H.H.; Benninger, J.; Ell, C. Shockwave lithotripsy of salivary duct stones. *Lancet* **1992**, *339*, 1333–1336. [CrossRef]

85. Kraus, M.; Reinhart, E.; Krause, H.; Reuther, J. Low energy extracorporeal shockwave therapy [ESWT] for treatment of myogelosis of the masseter muscle. *Mund-Kiefer Gesichtschir.* **1999**, *3*, 20–23. [CrossRef]

86. Falkensammer, F.; Rausch-Fan, X.; Schaden, W.; Kivaranovic, D.; Freudenthaler, J. Impact of extracorporeal shockwave therapy on tooth mobility in adult orthodontic patients: A randomized singlecenter placebo-controlled clinical trial. *J. Clin. Periodontol.* **2015**, *42*, 294–301. [CrossRef]

87. Falkensammer, F.; Schaden, W.; Krall, C.; Freudenthaler, J.; Bantleon, H.P. Effect of extracorporeal shockwave therapy [ESWT] on pulpal blood flow after orthodontic treatment: A randomized clinical trial. *Clin. Oral Investig.* **2016**, *20*, 373–379. [CrossRef]

88. Holfeld, J.; Tepeköylü, C.; Reissig, C.; Lobenwein, D.; Scheller, B.; Kirchmair, E.; Kozaryn, R.; Albrecht-Schgoer, K.; Krapf, C.; Zins, K.; et al. Toll-like receptor 3 signalling mediates angiogenic response upon shock wave treatment of ischaemic muscle. *Cardiovasc. Res.* **2016**, *109*, 331–343. [CrossRef]

89. Goiato, M.C.; dos Santos, D.M.; Santiago, J.F.; Moreno, A.; Pellizzer, E.P. Longevity of dental implants in type IV bone: A systematic review. *Int. J. Oral Maxillofac. Surg.* **2014**, *43*, 1108–1116. [CrossRef] [PubMed]

90. De Medeiros, F.C.F.L.; Kudo, G.A.H.; Leme, B.G.; Saraiva, P.P.; Verri, F.R.; Honório, H.M.; Pellizzer, E.P.; Santiago, J.F. Dental implants in patients with osteoporosis: A systematic review with meta-analysis. *Int. J. Oral Maxillofac. Surg.* **2018**, *47*, 480–491. [CrossRef] [PubMed]

91. Koolen, M.K.E.; Kruyt, M.C.; Zadpoor, A.A.; Öner, F.C.; Weinans, H.; van der Jagt, O.P. Optimization of screw fixation in rat bone with extracorporeal shock waves. *J. Orthop. Res.* **2018**, *36*, 76–84. [CrossRef] [PubMed]

92. Van der Jagt, O.P.; Piscaer, T.M.; Schaden, W.; Li, J.; Kops, N.; Jahr, H.; van der Linden, J.C.; Waarsing, J.H.; Verhaar, J.A.; de Jong, M.; Weinans, H. Unfocused extracorporeal shock waves induce anabolic effects in rat bone. *J. Bone Jt. Surg. Am.* **2011**, *93*, 38–48. [CrossRef] [PubMed]

93. Koolen, M.K.E.; Pouran, B.; Öner, F.C.; Zadpoor, A.A.; van der Jagt, O.P.; Weinans, H. Unfocused shockwaves for osteoinduction in bone substitutes in rat cortical bone defects. *PLoS ONE* **2018**, *13*, e0200020. [CrossRef] [PubMed]

94. Loske, A.M. Extracorporeal Shock Wave Therapy, Shock Wave and High Pressure Phenomena. Bone Healing. In *Medical and Biomedical Applications of Shock Waves*; Loske, A.M., Ed.; Springer International Publishing: New York, NY, USA, 2017; p. 222. ISBN 978-3-319-47570-7.

95. Deb, S.; Chana, S. Biomaterials in Relation to Dentistry. *Front. Oral Biol.* **2015**, *17*, 1–12. [CrossRef] [PubMed]

96. Hou, Y.; Zhou, X.; Cai, W.L.; Guo, C.C.; Han, Y. Regulatory effect of bone marrow mesenchymal stem cells on polarization of macrophages. *Zhonghua Gan Zang Bing Za Zhi* **2017**, *25*, 273–278. [CrossRef]

97. English, K.; French, A.; Wood, K.J. Mesenchymal stromal cells: Facilitators of successful transplantation? *Cell Stem Cell* **2010**, *7*, 431–442. [CrossRef]

98. Suhr, F.; Delhasse, Y.; Bungartz, G.; Schmidt, A.; Pfannkuche, K.; Bloch, W. Cell biological effects of mechanical stimulations generated by focused extracorporeal shock wave applications on cultured human bone marrow stromal cells. *Stem Cell Res.* **2013**, *11*, 951–964. [CrossRef]

99. Leu, S.; Huang, T.H.; Chen, Y.L.; Yip, H.K. Effect of Extracorporeal Shockwave on Angiogenesis and Anti-Inflammation: Molecular-Cellular Signaling Pathways. In *Shockwave Medicine*; Wang, C.J., Schaden, W., Ko, J.Y., Eds.; Karger: Basel, Switzerland, 2018; Volume 6, pp. 109–116. [CrossRef]

100. Sukubo, N.G.; Tibalt, E.; Respizzi, S.; Locati, M.; d'Agostino, M.C. Effect of shock waves on macrophages: A possible role in tissue regeneration and remodeling. *Int. J. Surg.* **2015**, *24*, 124–130. [CrossRef]

101. Godwin, J.W.; Pinto, A.R.; Rosenthal, N.A. Macrophages required for regeneration. *Proc. Natl. Acad. Sci. USA* **2013**, *110*, 9415–9420. [CrossRef] [PubMed]

102. Mishra, S.K.; Chowdhary, R.; Chrcanovic, B.R.; Brånemark, P.I. Osseoperception in Dental Implants: A Systematic Review. *J. Prosthodont.* **2016**, *25*, 185–195. [CrossRef] [PubMed]

103. He, H.; Yao, Y.; Wang, Y.; Wu, Y.; Yang, Y.; Gong, P. A novel bionic design of dental implant for promoting its long-term success using nerve growth factor [NGF]: Utilizing nano-springs to construct a stress-cushioning structure inside the implant. *Med. Sci. Monit.* **2012**, *18*, HY42–HY46. [CrossRef] [PubMed]

104. Lee, J.H.; Sung, Y.B.; Jang, S.H. Nerve growth factor expression in stroke induced rats after shock wave. *J. Phys. Ther. Sci.* **2016**, *28*, 3451–3453. [CrossRef] [PubMed]

14

Understanding Peri-Implantitis as a Plaque-Associated and Site-Specific Entity: On the Local Predisposing Factors

Alberto Monje [1,2,*], Angel Insua [2] and Hom-Lay Wang [3]

[1] Department of Periodontology, Universitat Internacional de Catalunya, 08195 Barcelona, Spain
[2] Division of Periodontics, CICOM Periodoncia, 06011 Badajoz, Badajoz, Spain Santiago de Compostela, Spain; ainsua@umich.edu
[3] Department of Periodontics and Oral Medicine, University of Michigan School of Dentistry, Ann Arbor, MI 48109, USA; homlay@umich.edu
* Correspondence: amonjec@umich.edu

Abstract: The prevalence of implant biological complications has grown enormously over the last decade, in concordance with the impact of biofilm and its byproducts upon disease development. Deleterious habits and systemic conditions have been regarded as risk factors for peri-implantitis. However, little is known about the influence of local confounders upon the onset and progression of the disease. The present narrative review therefore describes the emerging local predisposing factors that place dental implants/patients at risk of developing peri-implantitis. A review is also made of the triggering factors capable of inducing peri-implantitis and of the accelerating factors capable of interfering with the progression of the disease.

Keywords: peri-implantitis; peri-implant endosseous healing; dental implantation; dental implant; alveolar bone loss

1. Introduction

Implant dentistry, as a scientific discipline, has grown rapidly over the last four decades with the aim of facilitating early and effective osseointegration affording successful long-term outcomes. Over these years, the onset of complications has been neglected as representing only isolated events. Nowadays, however, due to the increase in prevalence of such problems, one of the major endeavors in this field is the prevention and efficient management of biological complications referred to as peri-implant diseases [1,2].

According to the bacterial theory, peri-implantitis by definition is a chronic inflammatory condition associated with a microbial challenge [3]. Nevertheless, in some cases there may be immunological reasons behind marginal bone loss [4–6] not primarily related to biofilm-mediated infectious processes [7]. Accordingly, a change from a stable immune system, seen during maintained osteointegration, to an active system may lead to the rejection of foreign bodies [7]. In this regard, implant surfaces types, surface wear, or contaminated particles may enhance these immunological reactions [8].

The conversion process from peri-implant mucositis mirrors the progression from gingivitis to periodontitis, with the constant formation of plaque features in the peri-implant tissues, characterized by erythema, bleeding, exudation, and tumefaction. At histological level, the establishment of B- and T-cell-dominated inflammatory cell infiltrates has been evidenced [9]. However, the clinical and histopathological characteristics during the conversion process are still not fully clear. Following conversion, peri-implantitis progresses in a nonlinear and accelerated manner [10].

The epidemiology of peri-implantitis varies widely depending on the given case definition. There has been important controversy regarding the threshold defining physiological peri-implant bone loss. As such, unspecific ranges have been observed in meta-analyses with heterogeneous case definitions. In 2012, the VIII European Workshop of Periodontology underscored that the diagnosis of peri-implantitis should be given on a longitudinal basis of overt progressive bone loss with clinical signs of inflammation [11]. In this regard, a threshold of ≥ 2 mm of peri-implant bone loss could be accepted for the diagnosis of peri-implantitis. More recently, the American Academy of Periodontology and the European Federation of Periodontology have jointly proposed a case definition based on a threshold of ≥ 3 mm [12]. Recent meta-analytical data have suggested the prevalence of peri-implantitis to be 18.5% at patient level and 12.8% at implant level [13], though the prevalence at patient level ranges widely between 1 and 47% [14]. Regardless of the diagnostic criteria proposed, peri-implantitis has been shown to be a site-specific condition. In contrast to periodontitis, which manifests with generalized loss of support, peri-implantitis commonly progresses conditioned by factors predisposing to biofilm accumulation which, under susceptible conditions, triggers a complex inflammatory response.

Strong evidence suggesting an increased risk of peri-implantitis has been obtained in subjects with poor personal- and professional-administered oral hygiene measures, and in individuals with a history of periodontitis [15,16]. Even though other factors and deleterious habits such as smoking [17] or hyperglycemia [18] have been identified as potential risk factors, there is a need for further and stronger evidence to validate their influence upon the development of peri-implantitis [3].

Moreover, in a site-specific condition, attention should focus on those factors which locally might be predisposing for the onset and progression of the disease [19]. Accordingly, the 2017 World Workshop identified evidence linking peri-implantitis to factors that complicate access to adequate oral hygiene, that is, those local conditions that predispose certain implants to develop disease [12].

2. Significance of Terminology for Reaching Consensus

As mentioned above, peri-implantitis and periodontitis occur more frequently under certain systemic conditions and in the presence of deleterious habits. For instance, it is known that major periodontal disease risk factors such as smoking and diabetes alter the epigenetics by downregulating the genic expression of bone matrix proteins that could influence the pathway from peri-implant mucositis to peri-implantitis by suppressing specific transcription factors for osteogenesis, or by activating certain transcription factors for osteoclastogenesis [20,21]. Hence, these systemic conditions may increase the risk of suffering peri-implant diseases.

On the other hand, emerging data point to the influence which certain local factors might have upon the onset and development of disease, since they induce plaque accumulation. These are the so-called predisposing factors. Terminologically, a predisposing factor is a condition that places the given element (dental implant)/individual (patient) at risk of developing a problem (peri-implantitis). In this regard, it is also of interest to underscore that a triggering factor, if not controlled after diagnosing and arresting (or not arresting) the problem (peri-implantitis), represents a perpetuating element that maintains the problem after it has become established [22]. Accelerating factors are therefore defined as those conditions that do not play a role in the onset of a problem (peri-implantitis) but can influence its progression.

3. Are Dental Implants Predisposed to Develop Biological Complications?

The evolution of dental implants and their incorporation to routine practice to restore function and aesthetics of lost or failing dentition have been described as one of the most revolutionary and innovative developments of the twentieth century. In fact, early dental implants were developed with a minimally rough surface microdesign. At that stage in modern implant dentistry, the osseointegration process proved slower and less effective. Long-term findings reported that these implants moreover tended to fail more frequently in the maxilla compared with the mandible. In addition, mean marginal bone loss using primitive implant–abutment connections was shown to be 1.5 mm, with an annual progressive bone loss of 0.1 mm [23,24].

With the development of new technology, the vast majority of commercial implants now have modified (moderately rough) surfaces with the primary aim of securing earlier osseointegration [25]. The incorporation of more biologically acceptable connections may be able to restrict inflammatory infiltration and thus minimize physiological bone loss. Indeed, a clinical study showed that 96% of the implants with a marginal bone loss of >2 mm at 18 months had lost 0.44 mm or more at 6 months postloading [26]. Thus, early healing dictates the long-term life of dental implants and the occurrence of biological complications, as it can be assumed that the establishment of a more anaerobic environment results in greater susceptibility to progressive bone loss.

Advances in the knowledge of bone biology and translational medicine summed to the development of novel armamentaria allow the clinician to minimize physiological bone remodeling. In this regard, excessive physiological bone remodeling (loss) may create a niche for the harboring of periopathogenic microorganisms that can lead to the development of implant biological complications.

4. Peri-Implant Monitoring: Diagnostic Accuracy of Clinical Peri-Implant Parameters

The prompt diagnosis of peri-implant disease is crucial to achieve favorable therapeutic outcomes. While the nonsurgical treatment of peri-implant mucositis is effective, the management of peri-implantitis proves more challenging [27]. Along these lines, it is worth mentioning that the severity and extensiveness of the lesion are crucial factors for successful and maintainable outcomes.

Peri-implantitis develops with progressive bone loss and signs of inflammation. As such, in order to secure an accurate diagnosis, the classical signs of inflammation (i.e., warmth, reddening, tumefaction) and an increased probing depth compared to baseline (assuming a measurement error) must be present [12] (Figure 1; Figure 2), as evidenced by clinical (Table 1) and preclinical studies. Interestingly, during the progression of ligature-induced experimental peri-implantitis, all the clinical parameters are worse due to the degree of inflammation present [28–31].

In this sense, it should be mentioned that disagreement persists concerning the sensitivity of bleeding on probing (BOP) and suppuration as diagnostic criteria. For instance, a human study showed the probability of positive BOP at a peri-implant site with a probing depth of 4 mm to be 27% [32]. The odds for positive BOP was seen to increase 1.6-fold per 1 mm of further probing depth. It has been further evidenced that BOP might be influenced by patient-related factors such as smoking [32]. In fact, understanding of the morphological differences of the periodontal apparatus compared with the peri-implant tissues supports the possibility that the former responds differently to mechanical stimulation. This might explain the poorer sensitivity in the detection of peri-implant diseases compared with periodontal diseases. Likewise, suppuration has been reported in about 10–20% of all peri-implant sites [28,33–36]. Hence, suppuration does not seem to exhibit high sensitivity in the diagnosis of peri-implantitis.

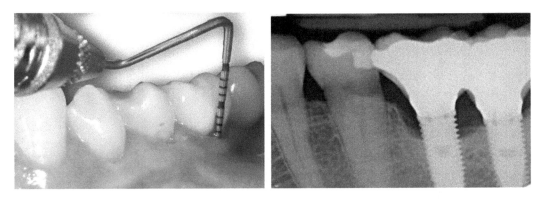

Figure 1. Bleeding on probing and increased probing pocket depth are clinical signs of peri-implantitis. The final diagnosis should be based on the correlation of the clinical data to the radiographic findings.

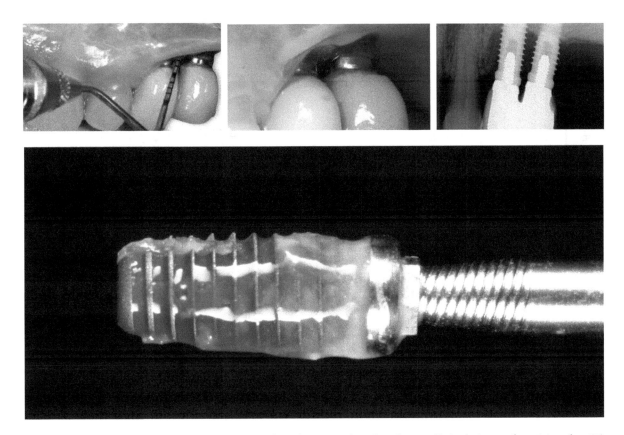

Figure 2. Bleeding on probing and increased probing pocket depth are clinical signs of peri-implantitis. The final diagnosis should be based on the correlation of the clinical data to the radiographic findings. When bone loss is advanced, implant removal is often the most predictable option for dealing with peri-implantitis.

In sum, clinical monitoring of peri-implantitis using a periodontal probe is indicated at each maintenance visit, with the purpose of preventing major biological complications. Nevertheless, the definite diagnosis should be based on the radiographic findings compared to baseline.

Table 1. Clinical characteristics of progressive peri-implant bone loss (peri-implantitis) based on the clinical findings.

Study	Study Design	Follow-Up (Mean)	Methods	Clinical Characteristics of Peri-Implantitis
Fransson et al. 2005, 2008 [37,38]	Cross-sectional	9.4 years	82 patients (197 implants with progressive bone loss/285 implants with stable bone)	• BOP, SUP, recession, and PPD ≥ 6 mm were greater at implants with than without 'progressive' bone loss • The proportion of affected implants that exhibited pus and PPD ≥ 6 mm was higher in smokers than in nonsmokers • SUP, recession, and PPD ≥ 6 mm at an implant in a smoking subject had a 69% accuracy in identifying progressive bone loss
Schwarz et al. 2017 [39]	Cross-sectional	-	60 patients (36 healthy implants/26 with mucositis/167 with peri-implantitis)	• Median PPD was 3 mm at healthy implant sites • Median PPD was 4 mm at peri-implant mucositis sites • Median PPD was 5 mm at peri-implantitis sites • PPD (i.e., by tactile sensation) revealed that 135 of 167 implant sites were associated with a missing buccal bone plate
Schwarz et al. 2017 [40]	Cross-sectional	2.2 years	238 patients (216 implants with mucositis/46 implants diagnosed with peri-implantitis)	• At mucositis sites, the BOP scores ranged between 33% and 50%, while the peak at peri-implantitis sites was 67% • Diseased implant sites were associated with higher frequencies of 4–6 mm PPD versus healthy sites • PPD values of ≥7 mm were only observed in one implant diagnosed with peri-implantitis
Monje et al. 2018 [35]	Case-control	3.17 years	141 patients (90 healthy implants/76 mucositis implants/96 peri-implantitis implants)	• Sites with peri-implant mucositis showed significant levels of BOP (OR = 3.56), redness (OR = 7.66), and PPD (OR = 1.48) compared to healthy sites • Sites exhibiting peri-implantitis showed significant levels of BOP (OR = 2.32), redness (OR = 7.21), PD (OR = 2.43), and SUP (OR = 6.81) compared to healthy sites • PPD was the only diagnostic marker displaying significance comparing peri-implant mucositis and peri-implantitis sites (OR = 1.76) • Tissue-level compared to bone-level implants were less associated with positive SUP (OR = 0.20) and PI (OR = 0.36)
Ramanauskaite et al. 2018 [36]	Cross-sectional	-	269 implants (77 healthy/77 mucositis/115 peri-implantitis)	• In patients diagnosed with peri-implant mucositis, the mean BOP values amounted to 20.83% (43% at implant level) • In patients diagnosed with peri-implantitis, the mean BOP values amounted to 71.33% (86% at implant level) • In patients diagnosed with peri-implantitis, the mean SUP values amounted to 30.16% (17.39% at implant level) • The mean PPD values at implant level were found to be 2.95 mm at healthy implant sites • The mean PPD values at implant level were found to be 3.10 mm at peri-implant mucositis • The mean PPD values at implant level were found to be 4.91 mm at peri-implantitis sites

BOP: bleeding on probing; SUP: suppuration; PPD: probing pocket depth; OR: odds ratio

5. Local Predisposing Factors

5.1. Significance of Soft Tissue Characteristics

The characteristics of the periodontal soft tissues and their association to periodontal conditions have been the subject of debate [41–45]. Based on the existing literature, it seems that attached keratinized gingiva is beneficial in patients with deficient oral hygiene. In contrast, patients with adequate personal- and professional-administered oral hygiene measures do not benefit from attached keratinized gingiva. In fact, movable mucosa facilitates the penetration of biofilm into the crevice, which would trigger the activation of neutrophils and lymphocytes [43]. Hence, in patients not adhering to adequate hygiene, the presence of keratinized attached gingiva might play a pivotal role in the prevention of the disease, in particular in the presence of subgingival restorations.

The influence of keratinized mucosa around dental implants has not been without controversy (Table 2). Early findings indicated that a lack of keratinized mucosa was not associated with less favorable peri-implant conditions [46]. More recent data have shown a wide band of keratinized mucosa to favor improved scores referred to as plaque index, modified gingival index, mucosal recession, and attachment loss [47]. Likewise, it has been demonstrated that the presence of keratinized mucosa around dental implants has a positive impact upon the immunological features, with a negative correlation to prostaglandin E2 levels [48]. This is due in part to a reduced inflammatory condition as a consequence of less discomfort during personal-administered oral hygiene. In fact, two recent clinical studies have shown the presence of ≥2 mm of keratinized mucosa to be crucial for the prevention of peri-implant diseases in erratic maintenance compliers [49] (Figure 3; Figure 4).

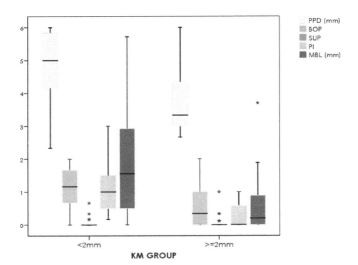

Figure 3. Comparative plot showing the clinical and radiographic differences between <2 mm versus ≥2 mm of peri-implant keratinized mucosa in erratic maintenance compliers [49]. Note: * stand for the outliers

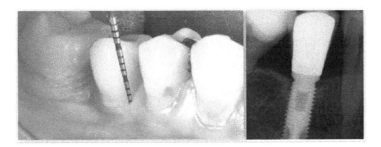

Figure 4. Representative case of an erratic maintenance complier with inadequate personal-administered oral hygiene presenting with healthy clinical and radiographic peri-implant conditions in the presence of 2 mm of keratinized and attached mucosa.

Table 2. Conflicting findings concerning the significance of the presence or lack of keratinized mucosa around dental implants.

Study	Study Design	Implant Function Time (Mean)	Methods	Clinical, Radiographic, and Patient-Reported Outcomes
Wennstrom et al. 1994 [46]	Prospective	5–10 years	39 patients (171 Branemark pure titanium implants)	• 24% of the implants presented with no KM • 13% of the implants presented with <2 mm of KM • 39% of the implants had attached mucosa • Neither attached nor keratinized mucosa were associated to peri-implant conditions
Romanos et al. 2015 [50]	Cross-sectional	9.4 years	118 patients (320 implants) Platform switched dental implants	• A wide band of ≥2 mm of KM was associated with a significantly lower mBI (0.12 ± 0.37; $p < 0.0001$), plaque index (0.45 ± 0.56; $p = 0.001$), and less mucosal recession (0.06 ± 0.23; $p < 0.0001$) than a narrow band of KM (<2 mm) • Considering regular and irregular implant maintenance therapy, a statistically significant difference was found between wide and narrow width of KM • In irregular compliers, the presence of KM is a protective mechanism for better peri-implant conditions
Roccuzzo et al. 2016 [51]	Prospective	10 years	98 patients	• The absence of KM was associated with greater plaque accumulation, greater soft-tissue recession, and a larger number of sites requiring additional surgical and/or antibiotic treatment • Patient-reported outcomes regarding maintenance procedures showed major differences between the groups, favoring the presence of KM
Bonino et al. 2018 [52]	Prospective	6 months	238 patients (216 implants with mucositis/46 implants diagnosed with peri-implantitis)	• Patients without peri-implant KM were less satisfied with the esthetics of the soft tissues around their implants ($p < 0.01$) • Lack of KM was not associated with discomfort during brushing • There was greater recession around implants without KM after 3 months ($p < 0.01$), but not after 6 months
Perussolo et al. 2018 [53]	Prospective	4 years	54 patients (202 implants)	• The values of the clinical parameters were greater in the <2 mm KM band: mean mPI (0.91 ± 0.60), BOP (0.67 ± 0.21), and BD (12.28 ± 17.59) • Marginal bone loss was greater in the KM < 2 mm group (0.26 ± 0.71) than in the KM ≥ 2 mm group (0.06 ± 0.48) • KM width and time in function had a statistically significant effect on marginal bone loss • In the <2 mm KM group, 51.4% presented with discomfort during brushing
Monje et al. 2018 [49]	Cross-sectional	5.73 years	37 patients (66 implants: 26 implants <2 mm/40 implants ≥2 mm) Erratic maintenance compliers (<2×/year)	• On comparing a KM band of <2 mm versus ≥2 mm, and with the exception of suppuration ($p = 0.6$), all the clinical and radiographic parameters were significantly increased when the KM band was <2 mm ($p < 0.001$) • A significant correlation was observed between KM and KT ($r = 0.55$) • A lack of KM did not condition a lack of KT • In the presence of peri-implantitis, only bleeding on probing at the adjacent dentate sites was seen to be increased • Patients had no brushing discomfort with a mean band of KM ≥ 2.5 mm

KM: keratinized mucosa; KT: keratinized gingival tissue; mBI: modified bleeding index; BOP: bleeding on probing; mPI: modified plaque index; BD: brushing discomfort.

Thus, a lack of keratinized mucosa in patients with inadequate oral hygiene could be regarded as a predisposing factor for peri-implant diseases, since it is associated with more recession, less vestibular depth, and more plaque accumulation, which, in turn, may be predisposing to inflammation (i.e., peri-implantitis).

5.2. Surgical Predisposing Factors

5.2.1. Significance of Implant Malpositioning as an Iatrogenic Factor: Critical Bone Dimensions

In the 2017 World Workshop on the classification of Periodontal and Peri-Implant Diseases and Conditions, implant malpositioning was suggested to be a predisposing factor for peri-implantitis due to the limited access for adequate oral hygiene often associated with these implant-supported restorations. If fact, a retrospective study associated implant malpositioning (OR = 48), occlusal overload (OR = 18.7), prosthetic problems (OR = 3.7), and bone grafting procedures (OR = 2.4) with peri-implantitis [54]. An early survey of cases reported in the literature as corresponding to peri-implantitis, following evaluation by a group of independent experts in the field, agreed that >40% of the implants diagnosed with peri-implantitis presented with a too-buccal position, with perfect interexaminer agreement (k = 0.81) [55]. This is in contrast to a four-year clinical study which found implants with residual buccal dehiscence defects to be more prone to develop peri-implantitis [56].

A comprehensive understanding of bone biology is crucial to conceive implant positioning, in particular, too-buccal positioning, as a predisposing factor for peri-implantitis. In a healed ridge, the alveolar process is composed of cortical bone at the outer side, while cancellous bone is featured in the inner structure. The cortical bone receives a blood supply branched from the outside through blood vessels of the periosteal surface, and from the inside from the endosteum [57]. When an implant is inserted with an open-flap procedure, elevation of the periosteum eliminates the periosteal blood supply from the outside. The same process occurs from the inside, since insertion of the implant interrupts the endosteal blood supply. This phenomenon of avascular necrosis is well known in bone biology [58] (Figure 5). A recent study has demonstrated that the critical buccal bone thickness for preventing marked physiological buccal–lingual bone resorption is 1.5 mm. In the absence of this thickness, more pronounced peri-implantitis may occur as a consequence of the microrough surface exposed to the oral cavity-facilitating surface contamination and the chronification of peri-implant infection [59] (Figure 6).

Likewise, apico-coronal implant positioning might dictate the long-term stability of the peri-implant tissues (Figure 7). Based on the hypothesis that too-apical implant positioning may favor the establishment of a microbial anaerobic environment, it is advised that implants be placed within the apico-coronal safety threshold. A recent retrospective analysis has validated this idea. Kumar et al., in nonsplinted single implants in function for at least five years, demonstrated that implant placement at a depth of ≥6 mm from the cementoenamel junction of the adjacent teeth is more commonly associated with peri-implantitis (OR = 8.5) [60]. Similarly, it should be noted that other factors could increase bone loss in these scenarios such as the type of implant–abutment connection (external vs internal vs conical) [61], number of abutment connection/disconnection [62], or the increased difficulty in removing cement remnants in case of cemented restorations [63].

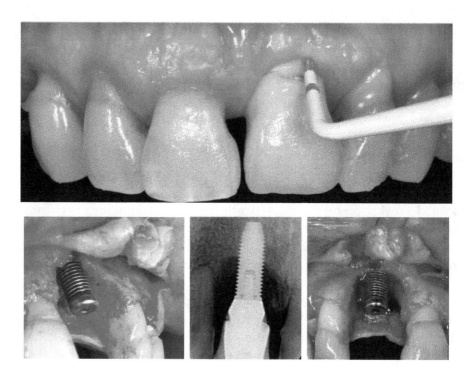

Figure 5. A critical buccal bone thickness of 1.5 mm is essential for preventing excessive physiological and pathological bone loss as a consequence of early avascular necrosis leading to peri-implant bone loss and thus to an increased risk of surface contamination.

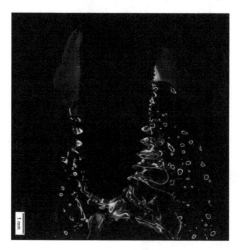

Figure 6. Histological analysis with fluorescent dyes illustrating excessive bone loss as a consequence of ligature-induced peri-implantitis. Note that the lack of fluorescence on the buccal side demonstrates the severe vertical bone resorption that occurs after physiological bone remodeling due to the insufficient critical buccal bone thickness (<1.5 mm).

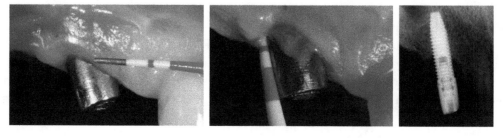

Figure 7. Inadequate apico-coronal implant positioning may favor the establishment of a microbial anaerobic environment that can be predisposing to progressive pathological peri-implant bone loss.

The mesiodistal implant position could be regarded as a predisposing factor for peri-implant bone loss, leading to peri-implantitis due to two main factors: (1) inadequate access for performing correct oral hygiene; and (2) excessive physiological bone remodeling if no safety distance is ensured between two adjacent dental implants or one implant with the adjoining dentition (Figure 8). Classically, the recommendation was to leave 3 mm between dental implants [64]. Even though this is no longer applicable to current implant dentistry due to advances in implant–abutment designs, a safety distance must be observed in order to avoid avascular necrosis of the interimplant cortical bone, with sufficient space to favor adequate personal oral hygiene.

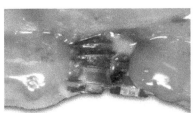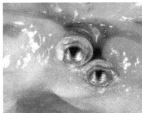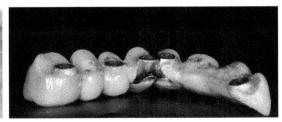

Figure 8. Incorrect implant positioning predisposes dental implants to peri-implant diseases due to the inability to perform correct oral hygiene.

5.2.2. Implant Insertion Torque and Its Interplay with the Hard Tissue Substratum

Implant placement in low-density bone can prove challenging. Thus, in order to ensure adequate primary stability and reduce early osseointegration implant failures, adaptation of the drilling protocol to the bone features has been recommended [65]. In fact, modifications in implant macrodesign, the use of osteotome condenser drills, and underpreparation of the implant socket may increase primary stability and osseointegration [65]. It is important to note that the connections between the trabecular mesh give cancellous bone the capacity to bear loads [66]; atraumatic surgical procedures therefore minimize the risk of bone loss. Thus, the use of drills to condense and densify trabecular bone might disrupt the connectivity of the trabecular network, reduce the capacity of bone to transmit occlusal forces, and result in weak bone that might not guarantee secondary stability due to higher bone turnover [66]. In fact, excessive compression of peri-implant bone by using osteotomes or increased torque may lead to 22–50% more crestal bone loss than conventional implantation [67,68] and also to a 41% reduction in the amount of bone-to-implant contact [69]. Such mechanical devices may damage the canalicular network of the trabecular bone, leading to a change in fluid flow mechanisms, impairment of mechanical stimulation, and delayed new bone formation [69]. Similar undesirable effects may be caused by excessive torque [70], leading to bone compression and delaying bone healing [71] (Figure 9). Areas with minimal bone-to-implant contact and therefore low strain seem to promote faster osteoblast differentiation [66,71,72]. During the first weeks, bone in contact areas around the implant threading is reabsorbed, and bone formation occurs earlier in contact-free areas [73].

The assessment of bone architecture is also relevant for implant drilling [74]. Larger osteocyte necrosis areas were found in trabecular bone versus cortical bone (550 versus 1400 μm, respectively) [65]. A similar increase in osteocyte damaged area was found when drilling speed was raised from 500 to 1500 rpm (600 versus 1400 μm, respectively) [65]. When using a 1.6 mm drill, a distance of 1050 μm of bone damage from the osteotomy center is expected, whereas the distance is about 1400 μm if a 5 mm drill is used [74]. The larger the drill diameter, the greater the tangential speed and centrifugal force, and therefore also the drilling power and energy transmitted to the bone. Lower values of early bone area formation around 5 mm implants versus 3.75 mm implants were found, and the use of large-diameter drills may be one of the underlying reasons [75]. Recently, simplified protocols have been proposed to reduce drilling time. Some authors reported no detrimental effects upon bone formation [75], but less bone formation was found in early stages in other studies [76]. It is important to note that simplified protocols might increase bone compression [76]. Moreover, the drill torque energy applied to the bone increases as the diameters of two consecutive drills increase. This fact might elevate the bone temperature and consequently the area of bone damage [65]. Further, other approaches, such as ultrasonic site preparation, have evidenced better preservation of the bone microarchitecture, resulting in a faster healing response [77].

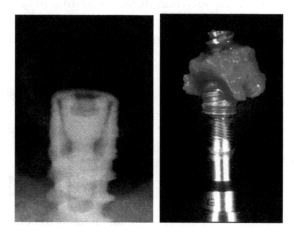

Figure 9. Implant removed four months after placement in the mandible. Note that the implant macrodesign, together with a highly corticalized bone structure, have induced excessive bone loss extending on the coronal portion of the implant and creating bone necrosis on the apical part. The severe bone resorption in the coronal area might have been predisposing to peri-implantitis as a biological complication if the implant had not been removed.

5.3. Significance of Prosthetic Design

Assuming the role of biofilm and its bacterial byproducts in the onset and progression of peri-implantitis, it is conceivable that retentive prosthetic components may promote inflammation (Figure 10). In this regard, Serino and Strom demonstrated that regardless of adequate oral hygiene of the natural dentition in partially edentulous patients, prosthetic design plays a major role in plaque accumulation around implant-supported prostheses. The authors found that adequate oral hygiene could not be performed in 53 out of 58 implants, and that peri-implantitis therefore could be attributed to deficient access for personal oral hygiene [78]. This is a typical scenario in hybrid prostheses, where esthetic requirements are satisfied but long-term implant maintenance is jeopardized owing to poor access for oral hygiene. Similarly, bone-level, implant-supported single crowns with an emergence angle of over 30 degrees and a convex profile have been shown to be factors strongly associated with peri-implantitis. This was not consistent with the findings in tissue-level implants [79]. Hence, convexities and marked emergence profiles should be avoided in the design of single crowns. In any case, patients should be comprehensively instructed to use interproximal brushes to remove food debris or plaque within the implant surroundings [2].

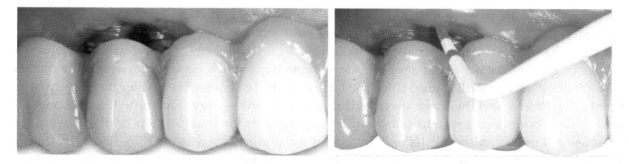

Figure 10. A hybrid prosthesis does not facilitate adequate oral hygiene and favors plaque retention, thereby triggering peri-implantitis.

Into the bargain, conceiving that excessive early bone resorption is often associated with greater late bone loss [26], prosthetic factors associated with minimal physiological bone loss should be noted. In this sense, longer transmucosal abutments (>2 mm) [80] and internal connection (including platform-switching [81] and Morse cone connections [82]) have demonstrated efficient preservation of the peri-implant hard tissue levels.

6. Local Precipitant Factors

The literature describes a few factors (so-called precipitant factors) associated with the triggering of inflammation within the peri-implant sulcus.

6.1. Residual Submucosal Cement

While screw-retained restorations do not necessarily outperform cement-retained prostheses, the presence of residual cement has been shown to have a deleterious effect upon the peri-implant tissues. Wilson et al. demonstrated the triggering role of residual cement, since 81% of the cases developed peri-implantitis, with spontaneous resolution in 74% following mechanical removal of the excess cement [63]. Likewise, Linkevicius et al. demonstrated the effect of residual cement upon peri-implant tissue response. In this scenario, 85% of the cases developed peri-implant disease [83]. Similar findings were obtained by Korsch et al. in a later study affording further insight into the effect of cement type upon the development of pathological complications. It was seen that while methacrylate cement was present in 62% of the suprastructures, zinc oxide eugenol cement could not be detected [84]. As a matter of fact, it was seen that the clinical and radiographic peri-implant conditions were generally unfavorable for implant-retained suprastructures using methacrylate cement, irrespective of cement excess [84]. In view of the significance of the presence of residual cement upon peri-implant tissue stability, it is advisable to use radiopaque cement if needed, with the aim of promptly detecting and removing it.

6.2. Residual Dental Floss

The remnants of floss in the peri-implant sulcus have also been regarded as a triggering factor for peri-implantitis. Van Velzen et al. reported 10 cases with progressive peri-implantitis related to floss remnants. Interestingly, in 90% of the cases, the inflammation resolved spontaneously after mechanical removal of the floss remnants [85]. Thus, caution is required when providing personal oral hygiene instructions involving the use of floss, and patients should be further encouraged to employ interproximal brushes.

7. Local Accelerating Factors: Influence of Surface Topography upon Progressive Bone Loss

In the course of the evolution of implant dentistry, advances in the form of implant surface modifications have led to stronger bone responses and higher implant survival rates [86]. Associations have been reported between significantly greater crestal bone loss and different implant surfaces and topographic features [86]. Furthermore, it has been suggested that surface roughness might have some role in the incidence of peri-implantitis [87] (Figure 11). In contrast, other authors consider that there are no available data confirming an association between implant surface features and the initiation of peri-implantitis or the progression of established peri-implantitis [88]. Ligature animal models have shown an increased risk of peri-implantitis with SLA implants in comparison to machined implants [89], and with TiUnite implants in comparison to machined, SLA, and TiOblast implants [31,90,91]. Similarly, another preclinical study noted significantly greater intrasurgical defect depths, defect widths, probing depths, and radiographic bone loss with TiUnite implants than with Straumann SLA or Biomet T3 implants [92]. Other factors apart from surface features might be relevant in the initial phase; for example, the invaginating grooves and pits on the TiUnite surface might favor bacterial adhesion and protect bacteria from shear forces [92]. Interestingly, a recent systematic review failed to find a long-term association between different surface modifications. Hence, these data in humans suggest that it is possible to achieve very good long-term results with all types of moderately rough implant surfaces [93].

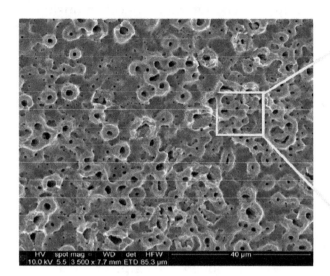 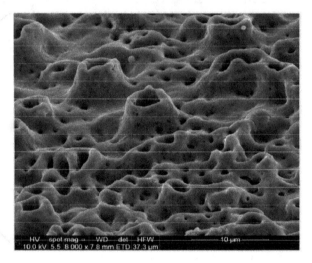

Figure 11. Moderately rough topographic characteristics (RA~1.3 μm) may induce chronification of the inflammatory condition by harboring pathogenic bacteria. This, in turn, may influence the therapeutic outcome. Note the scanning electron microscopic features of the implant surface under high magnification.

Furthermore, the management of established peri-implantitis is possible after surgical treatment, but the therapeutic outcome is also influenced by the implant surface characteristics [90]. In a randomized clinical trial on the effect of adjunctive systemic and local antimicrobial therapy in patients with peri-implantitis, treatment success was reported in 79% of the implants with nonmodified surface features, but in only 34% of the implants with modified surfaces [94]. Similarly, a three-year randomized controlled trial found the surgical treatment of peri-implantitis to be effective, with stable peri-implant marginal bone levels, but here again the nonmodified surfaces yielded significantly better results [95].

Depending on the surface modification methods used, some remnants may persist on the surface and have deleterious effects upon the clinical performance of the implant [87]. These particles and others released from the surface as a result of corrosion and mechanical wear may have cytotoxic effects and stimulate inflammatory reactions [8], leading to osteoclast activation and further peri-implant bone loss. Likewise, it has been recently evidenced that titanium particles derived from implants containing phosphate-enriched titanium oxide, fluoride-modified, and grit-blasted (GB) surface treatments are able to activate CHK2 and trigger the recruitment of BRCA1 in oral epithelial cells. These are markers for detecting activation of the DNA damage response. Accordingly, it can be inferred that titanium particles released into a surgical wound may contribute to the disruption of epithelial homeostasis, and potentially compromise the oral epithelial barrier [96].

8. Other Perspectives to Conceive Peri-Implantitis

Different perspectives to understand peri-implantitis have been further proposed. As such, it has been advocated that peri-implant marginal bone loss might be related to a change in the foreign body equilibrium between the host immune system and the implant device [97]. The biological behavior of the bone cells is mediated by the interaction among immune cells (neutrophils, macrophages, and lymphocytes) and the dental implant (or any kind of foreign body). Briefly, one of the very first interplays around the foreign body is carried out by neutrophils for 24–48 h [98]. The insertion of a dental implant induces a status of hypoxia in the surrounding bone that leads to neutrophil accumulation in order to promote angiogenesis. Also, neutrophil cells may discharge proteolytic enzymes and reactive oxygen species during their function that can erode the implant surface and release metal particles to the tissues [99]. After 48 h, the population of macrophages is higher around the foreign body and these cells may lead the evolution of the immune response. In fact, these cells promote osteoclastogenesis, matrix deposition, and bone anabolism [100], whereas macrophages' absence might impair osteoblast viability and bone formation [101,102]. Neutrophil apoptosis is mediated by macrophages during the shift between inflammatory phase to the healing phase. Also, the polarization between macrophages M1 to M2 and the length of each phase may have clinical effects, thereby an extended M1 phase may lead to a fibrous encapsulation of the fixture and implant failure [103]. On the contrary, higher presence of M2 macrophages has been reported on commercial pure implants [99,104], leading to bone deposition on the surface to isolate the fixture from the surrounding bone.

In addition, macrophages can differentiate into osteoclasts during bone remodeling and have phagocytosis capabilities until 5 μm of particle size [98]. Under presence of larger particles, macrophages tend to fuse to become foreign body giant cells (FBGCs). FBGCs are more frequent around the implant interface [105] than around healthy tissues and this fact might indicate the presence of a foreign body reaction around the dental fixture or the allogenic material.

Hence, under this concept of foreign body reaction, osseointegration is a mild chronic inflammatory and immunologically driven response where the bone–implant interface remains in a state of equilibrium but susceptible to changes in the environment [7,106]. Macrophages, FBGCs, and others approach this new bone barrier and if any disturbing factor occurs, a reactivation of the immuno-inflammatory cells against the foreign body material takes place. The loss of the foreign body equilibrium may thus stand as one of the reasons for this peri-implant bone loss [98].

9. Conclusions

Site-specific diseases are often attributable to local predisposing factors. In the case of plaque-associated peri-implantitis, local contributors, including surgical and prosthetic factors, as well as soft and hard tissue characteristics, may be predisposing factors to biofilm adherence around dental implants, thus leading to inflammation. Moreover, two major precipitant or triggering factors can be identified: residual cement and residual floss. In addition, current evidence seems to suggest that certain surface topographies can further accelerate the process of peri-implantitis.

References

1. Tonetti, M.S.; Chapple, I.L.; Jepsen, S.; Sanz, M. Primary and secondary prevention of periodontal and peri-implant diseases: Introduction to, and objectives of the 11th European Workshop on Periodontology consensus conference. *J. Clin. Periodontol.* **2015**, *42* (Suppl. 16), S1–S4. [CrossRef]
2. Jepsen, S.; Berglundh, T.; Zitzmann, N.U.; Genco, R.; Aass, A.M.; Demirel, K.; Derks, J.; Figuero, E.; Giovannoli, J.L.; Goldstein, M.; et al. Primary prevention of peri-implantitis: Managing peri-implant mucositis. *J. Clin. Periodontol.* **2015**, *42* (Suppl. 16), S152–S157. [CrossRef]
3. Schwarz, F.; Derks, J.; Monje, A.; Wang, H.L. Peri-implantitis. *J. Periodontol.* **2018**, *89* (Suppl. 1), S267–S290. [CrossRef]
4. Albrektsson, T.; Jemt, T.; Mölne, J.; Tengvall, P.; Wennerberg, A. On inflammation-immunological balance theory-A critical apprehension of disease concepts around implants: Mucositis and marginal bone loss may represent normal conditions and not necessarily a state of disease. *Clin. Implant Dent. Relat. Res.* **2019**, *21*, 183–189. [CrossRef] [PubMed]
5. Albrektsson, T.; Chrcanovic, B.; Mölne, J.; Wennerberg, A. Foreign body reactions, marginal bone loss and allergies in relation to titanium implants. *Eur. J. Oral Implantol.* **2018**, *11* (Suppl. 1), S37–S46.
6. Tomas, A.; Luigi, C.; David, C.; Hugo, D.B. "Peri-Implantitis": A Complication of a Foreign Body or a Man-Made "Disease". Facts and Fiction. *Clin. Implant Dent. Relat. Res.* **2016**, *18*, 840–849.
7. Dahlin, C.; Sennerby, L.; Turri, A.; Albrektsson, T.; Jemt, T.; Wennerberg, A. Is Marginal Bone Loss around Oral Implants the Result of a Provoked Foreign Body Reaction? *Clin. Implant Dent. Relat. Res.* **2014**, *16*, 155–165.

8.   Apaza-Bedoya, K.; Tarce, M.; Benfatti, C.A.M.; Henriques, B.; Mathew, M.T.; Teughels, W.; De Souza, J.C.M.;
      Apaza-Bedoya, K. Synergistic interactions between corrosion and wear at titanium-based dental implant
      connections: A scoping review. *J. Periodontal. Res.* **2017**, *52*, 946–954. [CrossRef] [PubMed]

9.   Berglundh, T.; Zitzmann, N.U.; Donati, M. Are peri-implantitis lesions different from periodontitis lesions?
      J. Clin. Periodontol. **2011**, *38* (Suppl. 11), 188–202. [CrossRef]

10.   Derks, J.; Schaller, D.; Håkansson, J.; Wennström, J.L.; Tomasi, C.; Berglundh, T. Peri-implantitis—Onset and
      pattern of progression. *J. Clin. Periodontol.* **2016**, *43*, 383–388. [CrossRef] [PubMed]

11.   Sanz, M.; Chapple, I.L.; Working Group 4 of the VIII European Workshop on Periodontology. Clinical
      research on peri-implant diseases: Consensus report of Working Group 4. *J. Clin. Periodontol.* **2012**, *39* (Suppl.
      12), 202–206. [CrossRef] [PubMed]

12.   Berglundh, T.; Armitage, G.; Araújo, M.G.; Avila-Ortiz, G.; Blanco, J.; Camargo, P.M.; Chen, S.; Cochran, D.;
      Derks, J.; Figuero, E.; et al. Peri-implant diseases and conditions: Consensus report of workgroup 4 of
      the 2017 World Workshop on the Classification of Periodontal and Peri-Implant Diseases and Conditions.
      J. Periodontol. **2018**, *89* (Suppl. 1), S313–S318. [CrossRef]

13.   Rakic, M.; Galindo-Moreno, P.; Monje, A.; Radovanovic, S.; Wang, H.-L.; Cochran, D.; Sculean, A.; Canullo, L.
      How frequent does peri-implantitis occur? A systematic review and meta-analysis. *Clin. Oral Investig.* **2018**,
      22, 1805–1816. [CrossRef] [PubMed]

14.   Derks, J.; Tomasi, C. Peri-implant health and disease. A systematic review of current epidemiology. *J. Clin.
      Periodontol.* **2015**, *42* (Suppl. 16), 158–171. [CrossRef]

15.   Aranda, L.; Diaz, K.; Alarcón, M.; Bagramian, R.; Catena, A.; Wang, H.; Monje, A. Impact of Maintenance
      Therapy for the Prevention of Peri-implant Diseases. A Systematic Review and Meta-analysis. *J. Dent. Res.*
      2015, *95*, 372–379.

16.   Renvert, S.; Persson, G.R. Periodontitis as a potential risk factor for peri-implantitis. *J. Clin. Periodontol.* **2009**,
      36 (Suppl. 10), 9–14. [CrossRef]

17.   Sgolastra, F.; Petrucci, A.; Severino, M.; Gatto, R.; Monaco, A. Smoking and the risk of peri-implantitis.
      A systematic review and meta-analysis. *Clin. Oral Implant Res.* **2015**, *26*, e62–e67. [CrossRef] [PubMed]

18.   Monje, A.; Catena, A.; Borgnakke, W.S. Association between diabetes mellitus/hyperglycaemia and
      peri-implant diseases: Systematic review and meta-analysis. *J. Clin. Periodontol.* **2017**, *44*, 636–648. [CrossRef]
      [PubMed]

19.   Monje, A.; Galindo-Moreno, P.; Canullo, L.; Greenwell, H.; Wang, H.-L. Editorial: From Early Physiological
      Marginal Bone Loss to Peri-Implant Disease: On the Unknown Local Contributing Factors. *Int. J. Periodontics
      Restor. Dent.* **2016**, *35*, 764–765.

20.   Monje, A.; Asa'Ad, F.; Larsson, L.; Giannobile, W.; Wang, H.-L. Editorial Epigenetics: A Missing Link
      Between Periodontitis and Peri-implantitis? *Int. J. Periodontics Restor. Dent.* **2018**, *38*, 476–477. [CrossRef]
      [PubMed]

21.   Larsson, L.; Castilho, R.M.; Giannobile, W.V. Epigenetics and Its Role in Periodontal Diseases: A State-of-the-
      Art Review. *J. Periodontol.* **2015**, *86*, 556–568. [CrossRef] [PubMed]

22.   Racine, N.M.; Riddell, R.R.P.; Khan, M.; Calic, M.; Taddio, A.; Tablon, P. Systematic Review: Predisposing,
      Precipitating, Perpetuating, and Present Factors Predicting Anticipatory Distress to Painful Medical
      Procedures in Children. *J. Pediatr. Psychol.* **2016**, *41*, 159–181. [CrossRef] [PubMed]

23.   Brånemark, P.-I.; Adell, R.; Albrektsson, T.; Lekholm, U.; Lundkvist, S.; Rockler, B. Osseointegrated titanium
      fixtures in the treatment of edentulousness. *Biomaterials* **1983**, *4*, 17–20. [CrossRef]

24.   Adell, R.; Lekholm, U.; Rockler, B.; Brånemark, P.-I. A 15-year study of osseointegrated implants in the
      treatment of the edentulous jaw. *Int. J. Oral Surg.* **1981**, *10*, 387–416. [CrossRef]

25.   Teughels, W.; Van Assche, N.; Sliepen, I.; Quirynen, M. Effect of material characteristics and/or surface
      topography on biofilm development. *Clin. Oral Implants Res.* **2006**, *17* (Suppl. 2), 68–81. [CrossRef]

26.   Galindo-Moreno, P.; León-Cano, A.; Ortega-Oller, I.; Monje, A.; O'valle, F.; Catena, A.; Galindo-Moreno, P.;
      León-Cano, A.; Ortega-Oller, I. Marginal bone loss as success criterion in implant dentistry: Beyond 2 mm.
      Clin. Oral Implants Res. **2015**, *26*, e28–e34. [CrossRef] [PubMed]

27.   Figuero, E.; Graziani, F.; Sanz, I.; Herrera, D.; Sanz, M. Management of peri-implant mucositis and
      peri-implantitis. *Periodontol. 2000* **2014** *66*, 255–273. [CrossRef] [PubMed]

28. Monje, A.; Insua, A.; Rakic, M.; Nart, J.; Moyano-Cuevas, J.L.; Wang, H.-L. Estimation of the diagnostic accuracy of clinical parameters for monitoring peri-implantitis progression: An experimental canine study. *J. Periodontol.* **2018**, *89*, 1442–1451. [CrossRef] [PubMed]

29. Carcuac, O.; Albouy, J.-P.; Linder, E.; Larsson, L.; Abrahamsson, I.; Albouy, J.; Berglundh, T. Experimental periodontitis and peri-implantitis in dogs. *Clin. Oral Implants Res.* **2013**, *24*, 363–371. [CrossRef] [PubMed]

30. Albouy, J.-P.; Abrahamsson, I.; Berglundh, T. Spontaneous progression of experimental peri-implantitis at implants with different surface characteristics: An experimental study in dogs. *J. Clin. Periodontol.* **2012**, *39*, 182–187. [CrossRef] [PubMed]

31. Albouy, J.-P.; Abrahamsson, I.; Persson, L.G.; Berglundh, T. Spontaneous progression of peri-implantitis at different types of implants. An experimental study in dogs. I: Clinical and radiographic observations. *Clin. Oral Implants Res.* **2008**, *19*, 997–1002. [CrossRef] [PubMed]

32. Farina, R.; Filippi, M.; Brazzioli, J.; Tomasi, C.; Trombelli, L. Bleeding on probing around dental implants: A retrospective study of associated factors. *J. Clin. Periodontol.* **2016**, *44*, 115–122. [CrossRef] [PubMed]

33. Fransson, C.; Tomasi, C.; Pikner, S.S.; Gröndahl, K.; Wennström, J.L.; Leyland, A.H.; Berglundh, T. Severity and pattern of peri-implantitis-associated bone loss. *J. Clin. Periodontol.* **2010**, *37*, 442–448. [CrossRef] [PubMed]

34. Fransson, C.; Wennström, J.; Tomasi, C.; Berglundh, T. Extent of peri-implantitis-associated bone loss. *J. Clin. Periodontol.* **2009**, *36*, 357–363. [CrossRef] [PubMed]

35. Monje, A.; Caballe-Serrano, J.; Nart, J.; Penarrocha, D.; Wang, H.-L.; Rakić, M. Diagnostic accuracy of clinical parameters to monitor peri-implant conditions: A matched case-control study. *J. Periodontol.* **2018**, *89*, 407–417. [CrossRef] [PubMed]

36. Ramanauskaite, A.; Becker, K.; Schwarz, F. Clinical characteristics of peri-implant mucositis and peri-implantitis. *Clin. Oral Implants Res.* **2018**, *29*, 551–556. [CrossRef] [PubMed]

37. Fransson, C.; Wennström, J.; Berglundh, T. Clinical characteristics at implants with a history of progressive bone loss. *Clin. Oral Implants Res.* **2008**, *19*, 142–147. [CrossRef] [PubMed]

38. Fransson, C.; Lekholm, U.; Jemt, T.; Berglundh, T. Prevalence of subjects with progressive bone loss at implants. *Clin. Oral Implants Res.* **2005**, *16*, 440–446. [CrossRef] [PubMed]

39. Schwarz, F.; Claus, C.; Becker, K. Correlation between horizontal mucosal thickness and probing depths at healthy and diseased implant sites. *Clin. Oral Implants Res.* **2017**, *28*, 1158–1163. [CrossRef] [PubMed]

40. Schwarz, F.; Becker, K.; Sahm, N.; Horstkemper, T.; Rousi, K.; Becker, J. The prevalence of peri-implant diseases for two-piece implants with an internal tube-in-tube connection: A cross-sectional analysis of 512 implants. *Clin. Oral Implants Res.* **2017**, *28*, 24–28. [CrossRef] [PubMed]

41. Wennström, J.L. Lack of association between width of attached gingiva and development of soft tissue recession. A 5-year longitudinal study. *J. Clin. Periodontol.* **1987**, *14*, 181–184. [CrossRef] [PubMed]

42. Wennström, J.; Lindhe, J. Plaque-induced gingival inflammation in the absence of attached gingiva in dogs. *J. Clin. Periodontol.* **1983**, *10*, 266–276. [CrossRef] [PubMed]

43. Lang, N.P.; Löe, H. The Relationship Between the Width of Keratinized Gingiva and Gingival Health. *J. Periodontol.* **1972**, *43*, 623–627. [CrossRef] [PubMed]

44. Stetler, K.J.; Bissada, N.F. Significance of the Width of Keratinized Gingiva on the Periodontal Status of Teeth with Submarginal Restorations. *J. Periodontol.* **1987**, *58*, 696–700. [CrossRef] [PubMed]

45. Coatoam, G.W.; Behrents, R.G.; Bissada, N.F. The Width of Keratinized Gingiva During Orthodontic Treatment: Its Significance and Impact on Periodontal Status. *J. Periodontol.* **1981**, *52*, 307–313. [CrossRef] [PubMed]

46. Wennström, J.L.; Bengazi, F.; Lekholm, U. The influence of the masticatory mucosa on the peri-implant soft tissue condition. *Implant Dent.* **1994**, *3*, 266. [CrossRef]

47. Lin, G.-H.; Chan, H.-L.; Wang, H.-L. The Significance of Keratinized Mucosa on Implant Health: A Systematic Review. *J. Periodontol.* **2013**, *84*, 1755–1767. [CrossRef] [PubMed]

48. Zigdon, H.; Machtei, E.E. The dimensions of keratinized mucosa around implants affect clinical and immunological parameters. *Clin. Oral Implants Res.* **2008**, *19*, 387–392. [CrossRef] [PubMed]

49. Monje, A.; Blasi, G. Significance of keratinized mucosa/gingiva on peri-implant and adjacent periodontal conditions in erratic maintenance compliers. *J. Periodontol.* **2018**. [CrossRef] [PubMed]

50. Romanos, G.; Grizas, E.; Nentwig, G.H. Association of Keratinized Mucosa and Periimplant Soft Tissue Stability Around Implants with Platform Switching. *Implant Dent.* **2015**, *24*, 422–426. [PubMed]

51. Roccuzzo, M.; Grasso, G.; Dalmasso, P. Keratinized mucosa around implants in partially edentulous posterior mandible: 10-year results of a prospective comparative study. *Clin. Oral Implants Res.* **2016**, *27*, 491–496. [CrossRef] [PubMed]

52. Bonino, F.; Steffensen, B.; Natto, Z.; Hur, Y.; Holtzman, L.P.; Weber, H.-P. Prospective study of the impact of peri-implant soft tissue properties on patient-reported and clinically assessed outcomes. *J. Periodontol.* **2018**, *89*, 1025–1032. [CrossRef] [PubMed]

53. Perussolo, J.; Souza, A.B.; Matarazzo, F.; Oliveira, R.P.; Araújo, M.G. Influence of the keratinized mucosa on the stability of peri-implant tissues and brushing discomfort: A 4-year follow-up study. *Clin. Oral Implants Res.* **2018**, *29*, 1177–1185. [CrossRef] [PubMed]

54. Canullo, L.; Peñarrocha-Oltra, D.; Covani, U.; Botticelli, D.; Serino, G.; Peñarrocha, M.; Peñarrocha-Oltra, D. Clinical and microbiological findings in patients with peri-implantitis: A cross-sectional study. *Clin. Oral Implants Res.* **2016**, *27*, 376–382. [CrossRef] [PubMed]

55. Monje, A.; Galindo-Moreno, P.; Tözüm, T.; Del Amo, F.S.-L.; Wang, H.-L. Into the Paradigm of Local Factors as Contributors for Peri-implant Disease: Short Communication. *Int. J. Oral Maxillofac. Implants* **2016**, *31*, 288–292. [CrossRef] [PubMed]

56. Sahm, N.; Schwarz, F.; Becker, J. Impact of the outcome of guided bone regeneration in dehiscence-type defects on the long-term stability of peri-implant health: Clinical observations at 4 years. *Clin. Oral Implants Res.* **2011**, *23*, 191–196.

57. Roush, J.K.; E Howard, P.; Wilson, J.W. Normal blood supply to the canine mandible and mandibular teeth. *Am. J. Vet. Res.* **1989**, *50*, 904–907. [PubMed]

58. Roux, S.; Orcel, P. Bone loss. Factors that regulate osteoclast differentiation: An update. *Arthritis Res.* **2000**, *2*, 451. [CrossRef] [PubMed]

59. Monje, A.; Insua, A.; Monje, F.; Muñoz, F.; Salvi, G.E.; Buser, D.; Chappuis, V. Diagnostic accuracy of the implant stability quotient in monitoring progressive peri-implant bone loss: An experimental study in dogs. *Clin. Oral Implants Res.* **2018**, *29*, 1016–1024. [CrossRef] [PubMed]

60. Hegde, R.; Ranganathan, N.; Mariotti, A.; Kumar, P.S.; Dabdoub, S.M. Site-level risk predictors of peri-implantitis: A retrospective analysis. *J. Clin. Periodontol.* **2018**, *45*, 597–604.

61. Galindo-Moreno, P.; Fernández-Jiménez, A.; O'Valle, F.; Monje, A.; Silvestre, F.J.; Juodzbalys, G.; Sánchez-Fernández, E.; Catena, A. Influence of the Crown-Implant Connection on the Preservation of Peri-Implant Bone: A Retrospective Multifactorial Analysis. *Int. J. Oral Maxillofac. Implants* **2015**, *30*, 384–390. [CrossRef] [PubMed]

62. Abrahamsson, I.; Berglundh, T.; Lindhe, J. The mucosal barrier following abutment dis/reconnection. An experimental study in dogs. *J. Clin. Periodontol.* **1997**, *24*, 568–572. [CrossRef] [PubMed]

63. Wilson, T.G., Jr. The Positive Relationship Between Excess Cement and Peri-Implant Disease: A Prospective Clinical Endoscopic Study. *J. Periodontol.* **2009**, *80*, 1388–1392. [CrossRef] [PubMed]

64. Tarnow, D.P.; Magner, A.W.; Fletcher, P. The Effect of the Distance from the Contact Point to the Crest of Bone on the Presence or Absence of the Interproximal Dental Papilla. *J. Periodontol.* **1992**, *63*, 995–996. [CrossRef] [PubMed]

65. Aghvami, M.; Brunski, J.B.; Tulu, U.S.; Chen, C.-H.; Helms, J.A. A Thermal and Biological Analysis of Bone Drilling. *J. Biomech. Eng.* **2018**, *140*, 101010. [CrossRef] [PubMed]

66. Wang, L.; Wu, Y.; Perez, K.; Hyman, S.; Brunski, J.; Tulu, U.; Bao, C.; Salmon, B.; Helms, J. Effects of Condensation on Peri-implant Bone Density and Remodeling. *J. Dent. Res.* **2017**, *96*, 413–420. [CrossRef] [PubMed]

67. Buhite, R. Implants in the Posterior Maxilla: A Comparative Clinical and Radiologic Study. *Int. J. Oral Maxillofac. Implants* **2005**, *20*, 231–237. [CrossRef]

68. Anitua, E.; Murias-Freijo, A.; Alkhraisat, M.H. Implant Site Under-Preparation to Compensate the Remodeling of an Autologous Bone Block Graft. *J. Craniofac. Surg.* **2015**, *26*, 374–377. [CrossRef] [PubMed]

69. Büchter, A.; Kleinheinz, J.; Wiesmann, H.P.; Jayaranan, M.; Joos, U.; Meyer, U. Interface reaction at dental implants inserted in condensed bone. *Clin. Oral Implants Res.* **2005**, *16*, 509–517. [CrossRef] [PubMed]

70.   Insua, A.; Monje, A.; Wang, H.-L.; Miron, R.J.; Wang, H. Basis of bone metabolism around dental implants during osseointegration and peri-implant bone loss. *J. Biomed. Mater. Res.* **2017**, *105*, 2075–2089. [CrossRef] [PubMed]

71.   Yin, X.; Mouraret, S.; Cha, J.Y.; Pereira, M.; Smith, A.; Houschyar, K.; Brunski, J.; Helms, J. Multiscale analyses of the bone-implant interface. *J. Dent. Res.* **2015**, *94*, 482–490.

72.   Wang, L.; Aghvami, M.; Brunski, J.; Helms, J. Biophysical regulation of osteotomy healing: An animal study. *Clin. Implant Dent. Relat. Res.* **2017**, *19*, 590–599. [CrossRef] [PubMed]

73.   Berglundh, T.; Abrahamsson, I.; Lang, N.P.; Lindhe, J. De novo alveolar bone formation adjacent to endosseous implants. *Clin. Oral Implants Res.* **2003**, *14*, 251–262. [CrossRef] [PubMed]

74.   Monje, A.; Chan, H.-L.; Galindo-Moreno, P.; Elnayef, B.; Del Amo, F.S.-L.; Wang, F.; Wang, H.-L. Alveolar Bone Architecture: A Systematic Review and Meta-Analysis. *J. Periodontol.* **2015**, *86*, 1231–1248. [CrossRef] [PubMed]

75.   Jimbo, R.; Janal, M.N.; Marin, C.; Giro, G.; Tovar, N.; Coelho, P.G. The effect of implant diameter on osseointegration utilizing simplified drilling protocols. *Clin. Oral Implants Res.* **2014**, *25*, 1295–1300. [CrossRef] [PubMed]

76.   Gil, L.; Sarendranath, A.; Neiva, R.; Marão, H.; Tovar, N.; Bonfante, E.; Janal, M.; Castellano, A.; Coelho, P. Bone Healing Around Dental Implants: Simplified vs Conventional Drilling Protocols at Speed of 400 rpm. *Int. J. Oral Maxillofac. Implants* **2017**, *32*, 329–336. [CrossRef] [PubMed]

77.   Rashad, A.; Sadr-Eshkevari, P.; Weuster, M.; Schmitz, I.; Prochnow, N.; Maurer, P.; Sadr-Eshkevari, P. Material attrition and bone micromorphology after conventional and ultrasonic implant site preparation. *Clin. Oral Implants Res.* **2013**, *24* (Suppl. A100), 110–114. [CrossRef]

78.   Serino, G.; Strom, C. Peri-implantitis in partially edentulous patients: Association with inadequate plaque control. *Clin. Oral Implants Res.* **2009**, *20*, 169–174. [CrossRef] [PubMed]

79.   Katafuchi, M.; Weinstein, B.F.; Leroux, B.G.; Daubert, D.M.; Chen, Y.-W.; Chen, Y. Restoration contour is a risk indicator for peri-implantitis: A cross-sectional radiographic analysis. *J. Clin. Periodontol.* **2018**, *45*, 225–232. [CrossRef] [PubMed]

80.   Ortega-Oller, I.; Monje, A.; Spinato, S.; Catena, A.; León-Cano, A.; Galindo-Moreno, P.; Suárez, F.; Óvalle, F. Prosthetic Abutment Height is a Key Factor in Peri-implant Marginal Bone Loss. *J. Dent. Res.* **2014**, *93* (Suppl. 7), 80–85.

81.   Galindo-Moreno, P.; León-Cano, A.; Monje, A.; Ortega-Oller, I.; O'valle, F.; Catena, A.; Galindo-Moreno, P.; León-Cano, A.; Ortega-Oller, I. Abutment height influences the effect of platform switching on peri-implant marginal bone loss. *Clin. Oral Implants Res.* **2015**, *27*, 167–173. [CrossRef] [PubMed]

82.   Degidi, M.; Daprile, G.; Piattelli, A. Marginal bone loss around implants with platform-switched Morse-cone connection: A radiographic cross-sectional study. *Clin. Oral Implants Res.* **2017**, *28*, 1108–1112. [CrossRef] [PubMed]

83.   Linkevicius, T.; Puisys, A.; Vindasiute, E.; Linkeviciene, L.; Apse, P. Does residual cement around implant-supported restorations cause peri-implant disease? A retrospective case analysis. *Clin. Oral Implants Res.* **2013**, *24*, 1179–1184. [CrossRef] [PubMed]

84.   Korsch, M.; Walther, W. Peri-Implantitis Associated with Type of Cement: A Retrospective Analysis of Different Types of Cement and Their Clinical Correlation to the Peri-Implant Tissue. *Clin. Implant Dent. Relat. Res.* **2015**, *17* (Suppl. 2), 434–443. [CrossRef]

85.   Van Velzen, F.J.J.; Lang, N.P.; Schulten, E.A.J.M.; Bruggenkate, C.M.T. Dental floss as a possible risk for the development of peri-implant disease: An observational study of 10 cases. *Clin. Oral Implants Res.* **2016**, *27*, 618–621. [CrossRef] [PubMed]

86.   Jimbo, R.; Albrektsson, T. Long-term clinical success of minimally and moderately rough oral implants: A review of 71 studies with 5 years or more of follow-up. *Implant Dent.* **2015**, *24*, 62–69. [CrossRef] [PubMed]

87.   De Bruyn, H.; Christiaens, V.; Doornewaard, R.; Jacobsson, M.; Cosyn, J.; Jacquet, W.; Vervaeke, S. Implant surface roughness and patient factors on long-term peri-implant bone loss. *Periodontology 2000* **2017**, *73*, 218–227. [CrossRef] [PubMed]

88.   Renvert, S.; Polyzois, I.; Claffey, N. How do implant surface characteristics influence peri-implant disease? *J. Clin. Periodontol.* **2011**, *38* (Suppl. 11), 214–222. [CrossRef]

89. Berglundh, T.; Abrahamsson, I.; Welander, M.; Lang, N.P.; Lindhe, J. Morphogenesis of the peri-implant mucosa: An experimental study in dogs. *Clin. Oral Implants Res.* **2007**, *18*, 1–8. [CrossRef] [PubMed]

90. Albouy, J.-P.; Abrahamsson, I.; Persson, L.G.; Berglundh, T. Implant surface characteristics influence the outcome of treatment of peri-implantitis: An experimental study in dogs. *J. Clin. Periodontol.* **2010**, *38*, 58–64. [CrossRef] [PubMed]

91. Albouy, J.-P.; Abrahamsson, I.; Persson, L.G.; Berglundh, T. Spontaneous progression of ligatured induced peri-implantitis at implants with different surface characteristics. An experimental study in dogs II: Histological observations. *Clin. Oral Implants Res.* **2009**, *20*, 366–371. [CrossRef] [PubMed]

92. Fickl, S.; Kebschull, M.; Calvo-Guirado, J.L.; Hürzeler, M.; Zuhr, O.; Calvo-Guirado, J.L. Experimental Peri-Implantitis around Different Types of Implants—A Clinical and Radiographic Study in Dogs. *Clin. Implant Dent. Relat. Res.* **2015**, *17* (Suppl. 2), 661–669. [CrossRef]

93. Wennerberg, A.; Albrektsson, T.; Chrcanovic, B. Long-term clinical outcome of implants with different surface modifications. *Eur. J. Oral Implantol.* **2018**, *11* (Suppl. 1), S123–S136. [PubMed]

94. Carcuac, O.; Derks, J.; Charalampakis, G.; Abrahamsson, I.; Berglundh, T.; Wennström, J. Adjunctive Systemic and Local Antimicrobial Therapy in the Surgical Treatment of Peri-implantitis. *J. Dent. Res.* **2016**, *95*, 50–57. [CrossRef] [PubMed]

95. Carcuac, O.; Derks, J.; Abrahamsson, I.; Wennström, J.L.; Petzold, M.; Berglundh, T. Surgical treatment of peri-implantitis: 3-year results from a randomized controlled clinical trial. *J. Clin. Periodontol.* **2017**, *44*, 1294–1303. [CrossRef] [PubMed]

96. Del Amo, F.S.-L.; Rudek, I.; Wagner, V.; Martins, M.; O'Valle, F.; Galindo-Moreno, P.; Giannobile, W.; Wang, H.-L.; Castilho, R. Titanium Activates the DNA Damage Response Pathway in Oral Epithelial Cells: A Pilot Study. *Int. J. Oral Maxillofac. Implants* **2017**, *32*, 1413–1420. [CrossRef] [PubMed]

97. Albrektsson, T.; Buser, D.; Sennerby, L. Crestal Bone Loss and Oral implants. *Clin. Implant Dent. Relat. Res.* **2012**, *14*, 783–791. [CrossRef] [PubMed]

98. Amengual-Peñafiel, L.; Brañes-Aroca, M.; Marchesani-Carrasco, F.; Jara-Sepúlveda, M.C.; Parada-Pozas, L.; Cartes-Velásquez, R. Coupling between Osseointegration and Mechanotransduction to Maintain Foreign Body Equilibrium in the Long-Term: A Comprehensive Overview. *JCM* **2019**, *8*, 139. [CrossRef] [PubMed]

99. Trindade, R.; Albrektsson, T.; Galli, S.; Prgomet, Z.; Tengvall, P.; Wennerberg, A. Osseointegration and foreign body reaction: Titanium implants activate the immune system and suppress bone resorption during the first 4 weeks after implantation. *Clin. Implant Dent. Relat. Res.* **2018**, *20*, 82–91. [CrossRef] [PubMed]

100. Batoon, L.; Millard, S.M.; Raggatt, L.J.; Pettit, A. R Osteomacs and Bone Regeneration. *Curr. Osteoporos. Rep.* **2017**, *15*, 385–395. [CrossRef] [PubMed]

101. Pettit, A.R.; Chang, M.K.; Hume, D.A.; Raggatt, L.-J. Osteal macrophages: A new twist on coupling during bone dynamics. *Bone* **2008**, *43*, 976–982. [CrossRef] [PubMed]

102. Chang, M.K.; Raggatt, L.-J.; Alexander, K.A.; Kuliwaba, J.S.; Fazzalari, N.L.; Schröder, K.; Maylin, E.R.; Ripoll, V.M.; Hume, D.A.; Pettit, A.R.; et al. Osteal Tissue Macrophages Are Intercalated throughout Human and Mouse Bone Lining Tissues and Regulate Osteoblast Function In Vitro and In Vivo. *J. Immunol.* **2008**, *181*, 1232–1244. [CrossRef] [PubMed]

103. Li, B.; Gao, P.; Zhang, H.; Guo, Z.; Zheng, Y.; Han, Y. Osteoimmunomodulation, osseointegration, and in vivo mechanical integrity of pure Mg coated with HA nanorod/pore-sealed MgO bilayer. *Biomater. Sci.* **2018**, *6*, 3202–3218. [CrossRef] [PubMed]

104. Trindade, R.; Albrektsson, T.; Galli, S.; Prgomet, Z.; Tengvall, P.; Wennerberg, A. Bone Immune Response to Materials, Part I: Titanium, PEEK and Copper in Comparison to Sham at 10 Days in Rabbit Tibia. *JCM* **2018**, *7*, 526. [CrossRef] [PubMed]

105. Anderson, J.M.; Rodriguez, A.; Chang, D.T. Foreign body reaction to biomaterials. *Semin. Immunol.* **2008**, *20*, 86–100. [CrossRef] [PubMed]

106. Trindade, R.; Albrektsson, T.; Tengvall, P.; Wennerberg, A. Foreign Body Reaction to Biomaterials: On Mechanisms for Buildup and Breakdown of Osseointegration. *Clin. Implant Dent Relat. Res.* **2016**, *18*, 192–203. [CrossRef] [PubMed]

15

Bone Immune Response to Materials, Part II: Copper and Polyetheretherketone (PEEK) Compared to Titanium at 10 and 28 Days in Rabbit Tibia

Ricardo Trindade [1,*], Tomas Albrektsson [2,3], Silvia Galli [3], Zdenka Prgomet [4], Pentti Tengvall [2] and Ann Wennerberg [1]

[1] Department of Prosthodontics, Institute of Odontology, The Sahlgrenska Academy, University of Gothenburg, 405 30 Gothenburg, Sweden; ann.wennerberg@odontologi.gu.se

[2] Department of Biomaterials, Institute of Clinical Sciences, University of Gothenburg, 405 30 Gothenburg, Sweden; tomas.albrektsson@biomaterials.gu.se (T.A.); pentti.tengvall@gu.se (P.T.)

[3] Department of Prosthodontics, Faculty of Odontology, Malmö University, 205 06 Malmö, Sweden; silvia.galli@mau.se

[4] Department of Oral Pathology, Faculty of Odontology, Malmö University, 205 06 Malmö, Sweden; zdenka.prgomet@mau.se

* Correspondence: ricardo.bretes.trindade@gu.se

Abstract: Osseointegration is likely the result of an immunologically driven bone reaction to materials such as titanium. Osseointegration has resulted in the clinical possibility to anchor oral implants in jaw bone tissue. However, the mechanisms behind bony anchorage are not fully understood and complications over a longer period of time have been reported. The current study aims at exploring possible differences between copper (Cu) and polyetheretherketone (PEEK) materials that do not osseointegrate, with osseointegrating cp titanium as control. The implants were placed in rabbit tibia and selected immune markers were evaluated at 10 and 28 days of follow-up. Cu and PEEK demonstrated at both time points a higher immune activation than cp titanium. Cu demonstrated distance osteogenesis due to a maintained proinflammatory environment over time, and PEEK failed to osseointegrate due to an immunologically defined preferential adipose tissue formation on its surface. The here presented results suggest the description of two different mechanisms for failed osseointegration, both of which are correlated to the immune system.

Keywords: biomaterial; bone; osseointegration; immune; implant; healing; titanium; PEEK; Cu

1. Introduction

Osseointegration [1] is a central event for oral implant function. This specific bone reaction has been described and studied at length for titanium and other materials. Technical innovations have led to improvements of bone reactions, such as material surface topographical changes [2–4] that have been vastly adopted by the oral implant industry, as well as different forms of chemical surface modulations [5,6]. Such surface related innovations have resulted in improved clinical results and widening of clinical indications [7,8]. However, the specific bone related control mechanisms that lead to osseointegration are still in need of scientific analyses, as are the reasons for marginal bone resorption. Generally speaking, the foreign body reaction (FBR) is accepted as the series of host events that follow the introduction of a material into tissues. The host–biomaterial interaction [9] depends on the type of material, clinical handling and on the tissue where the implant is placed (e.g., bone, skin, and blood vessel), as well as the host specific conditions. The immune system has a central role in the FBR [10–12] where the M1/M2-macrophage phenotype balance has been identified as one of the main controlling factors at the cellular level [13]. Macrophages are thus able to shift between an M1-phenotype (proinflammatory) and an M2-phenotype (reparative/anti-inflammatory), with obvious consequences for tissue reaction to biomaterials, and experimental modulation of this balance has been studied to direct a favorable pathway for bone regeneration [14]. The current authors have demonstrated an early M1/M2 shift around titanium, at 10 days of follow-up towards a dominant M2 macrophage phenotype [15], in contrast to other materials such as polyetheretherketone (PEEK) and Copper (Cu) that present mixed M1/M2 phenotypes at the same short term of follow-up. Osseointegration is thus seen as the result of an FBR which in the long run may achieve a foreign body equilibrium allowing for long term loading of implants [16]. However, the basis for the control of bone metabolism around implants in health and disease remains largely unclear [17]. Particularly the events taking place after the inflammatory period of initial healing and a possible immunological regulation of bone metabolism are examples of important fields for further studies. Our group has demonstrated that titanium activates the immune system when compared to a sham site at 10 and 28 days of follow-up [12]. In Part I of this series of studies (where the current work is Part II), the importance of the specific immune response around different materials when compared to a sham site was demonstrated at an early stage of 10 days [15]. The current study aims at comparing materials that do not osseointegrate, i.e., test materials copper (known to induce a pronounced FBR in soft tissues [18]) and PEEK (considered a bioinert material [19]), to a material that osseointegrates, cp titanium (control) at 10 and 28 days, in order to investigate and compare the respective immune modulation reactions between the inflammatory (10 days) and postinflammatory (28 days) stages of bone healing.

2. Materials and Methods

The current study consists of an experiment in the rabbit proximal tibia (metaphysis), comparing bone healing on sites where osteotomies were performed and one of three test materials were placed for comparison: titanium (Ti), copper (Cu), or polyether ether ketone (PEEK), where Ti was a control.

All implants were turned with a threaded 0.6 mm pitch height, 3.75 mm width, and Branemark MkIII design (Figure 1). The Ti implants were made of commercially pure titanium grade IV (98.55% Ti, with specified maximum traces of elements Fe, O, N, H, and C for the remaining 1.45%).

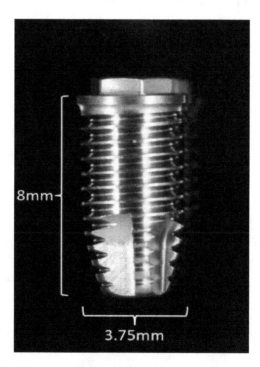

Figure 1. Implant design with 3.75mm width and 8mm length. Representative image of titanium (Ti) implant; copper (Cu) and polyetheretherketone (PEEK) implants with the same design.

2.1. Surgical Procedure

This study was performed on 12 mature, female New Zealand White Rabbits ($n = 6$ for each time point, 10 and 28 days, weight 3 to 4 Kg), with the ethical approval from the Ethics Committee for Animal Research (No. 13-011) of the École Nationale Vétérinaire D'Alfors, Maisons-Alfors, Val-de-Marne, France. The 6 animals at 10 days are the same used for Part I of this series of studies [12]. All care was taken to minimize animal pain or discomfort during and after the surgical procedures. For the surgical procedures, the rabbits were placed under general anesthesia using a mixture of medetomidine (Domitor; Zoetis, Florham Park, NJ, USA), ketamine (Imalgène 1000; Merial, Lyon, France), and diazepam (Valium; Roche, Basel, Switzerland) for induction, then applying subcutaneous buprenorphine (Buprecare; Animalcare, York, UK) and intramuscular meloxicam (Metacam; Boehringer Ingelheim Vetmedica, Inc., Ridgefield, CT, USA). A single incision was performed in the internal knee area on each side and the bone exposed for osteotomies and insertion of implants in the sites mentioned above. The surgical site was sutured with a resorbable suture (Vicryl 3/0; Ethicon, Cincinnati, OH, USA) and hemostasis achieved. Following surgery, Fentanyl patches (Duragesic; Janssen Pharmaceutica, Beerse, Belgium) were applied.

The osteotomies were produced with a sequence of increasing diameter twist drills, from 2 mm to 3.15 mm width, and a final countersink bur prepared the cortical part of the bone. The implants used were 3.75 mm in diameter, placed in an underprepared osteotomy to achieve primary (mechanical) stability.

The rabbits were housed in separate cages and were allowed to move and eat freely.

At 10 and 28 days, the rabbits were sacrificed with a lethal injection of sodium pentobarbital (Euthasol; Virbac, Fort Worth, TX, USA). The 6 animals at each time point had the implants removed through unscrewing. On 4 animals at 10 days and 5 animals at 28 days, bone was collected with a 2 mm twist drill from the periphery of the Ti, Cu, and PEEK sites on the most distal portion, and then processed through quantitative-polymerase chain reaction (qPCR). After this, at each time point, the implant sites were removed en bloc for histological processing on the 6 animals.

2.2. Gene Expression Analysis—qPCR

The bone samples for gene expression analysis at 10 or 28 days were collected from the distal side of the osteotomies of all three groups (following the removal of the implant from the implant sites), with a 2 mm twist drill that removed both cortical and marrow bone in the full length of the osteotomy, to enable the study of the 2 mm peri-implant bone area of each of the Ti, Cu, and PEEK sites. The samples were immediately transferred to separate sterile plastic recipients containing RNAlater medium (AmbionInc, Austin, TX, USA) for preservation. The samples were then refrigerated first at 4 °C and then stored at –20 °C until processing.

2.2.1. mRNA Isolation

Samples were homogenized using an ultrasound homogenizer (Sonoplus HD3100, Brandelin) in 1 ml PureZOL and total RNA was isolated via column fractionalization using the Aurum™ Total RNA Fatty and Fibrous Tissue Kit (Bio-Rad Laboratories Inc.; Hercules, CA, USA) following the manufacturer's instructions. All the samples were DNAse treated using an on-column DNAse I contained in the kit to remove genomic DNA. The RNA quantity for each sample was analyzed in the NanoDrop 2000 Spectrophotometer (Thermo Scientific; Wilmington, DE, USA). BioRad iScript cDNA synthesis kit (Bio-Rad Laboratories Inc.; Hercules, CA, USA) was then used to convert mRNA into cDNA, following the manufacturer's instructions.

qPCR primers (Tataa Biocenter; Gothenburg, Sweden) were designed following the NCBI Sequence database, including the local factors chosen in order to characterize the immune, inflammatory, and bone metabolic pathways (Tables 1 and 2). All primers had efficiency between 90% and 110%.

Table 1. Gene sequences.

Primer	Forward Sequence	Reverse Sequence	Accession No./Transcript ID
NCF-1	TTCATCCGCCACATTGCCC	GTCCTGCCACTTCACCAAGA	NM_001082102.1
CD68	TTTCCCCAGCTCTCCACCTC	CGATGATGAGGGGCACCAAG	ENSOCUT00000010382
CD11b	TTCAACCTGGAGACTGAGAACAC	TCAAACTGGACCACGCTCTG	ENSOCUT00000001589
CD14	TCTGAAAATCCTGGGCTGGG	TTCATTCCCGCGTTCCGTAG	ENSOCUT00000004218
ARG1	GGATCATTGGAGCCCCTTTCTC	TCAAGCAGACCAGCCTTTCTC	NM_001082108.1
IL-4	CTACCTCCACCACAAGGTGTC	CCAGTGTAGTCTGTCTGGCTT	ENSOCUT00000024099
IL-13	GCAGCCTCGTATCCCCAG	GGTTGACGCTCCACACCA	ENSOCUT00000000154
M-CSF	GGAACTCTCGCTCAGGCTC	ACATTCTTGATCTTCTCCAGCAAC	ENSOCUT00000030714
OPG	TGTGTGAATGCGAGGAAGGG	AACTGTATTCCGCTCTGGGG	ENSOCUT00000011149
RANKL	GAAGGTTCATGGTTCGATCTGG	CCAAGAGGACAGGCTCACTTT	ENSOCUT00000024354
TRAP	TTACTTCAGTGGCGTGCAGA	CGATCTGGGCTGAGACGTTG	NM_001081988.1
CathK	GGAACCGGGGCATTGACTCT	TGTACCCTCTGCATTTGGCTG	NM_001082641.1
PPAR-γ	CAAGGCGAGGGCGATCTT	ATGCGGATGGCGACTTCTTT	NM_001082148.1
C3	ACTCTGTCGAGAAGGAACGGG	CCTTGATTTGTTGATGCTGGCTG	NM_001082286.1
C3aR1	CATGTCAGTCAACCCCTGCT	GCGAATGGTTTTGCTCCCTG	ENSOCUT00000007435
CD46	TCCTGCTGTTCACTTTCTCGG	CATGTTCCCATCCTTGTTTACACTT	ENSOCUT00000033915
CD55	TGGTGTTGGGTGGAGTGACC	AGAGTGAAGCCTCTGTTGCATT	ENSOCUT00000031985
CD59	ACCACTGTCTCCTCCCAAGT	GCAATCTTCATACCGCCAACA	NM_001082712.1
C5	TCCAAAACTCTGCAACCTTAACA	AAATGCTTTGACACAACTTCCA	ENSOCUT00000005683
C5aR1	ACGTCAACTGCTGCATCAACC	AGGCTGGGGAGAGACTTGC	ENSOCUT00000029180
CD3	CCTGGGGACAGGAAGATGATGAC	CAGCACCACACGGGTTCCA	NM_001082001.1
CD4	CAACTGGAAACATGCGAACCA	TTGATGACCAGGGGGAAAGA	NM_001082313.2
CD8	GGCGTCTACTTCTGCATGACC	GAACCGGCACACTCTCTTCT	ENSOCUT00000009383
CD19	GGATGTATGTCTGTCGCCGT	AAGCAAAGCCACAACTGGAA	ENSOCUT00000028895
GAPDH	GGTGAAGGTCGGAGTGAACGG	CATGTAGACCATGTAGTGGAGGTCA	NM_001082253.1
ACT-β	TCATTCCAAATATCGTGAGATGCC	TACACAAATGCGATGCTGCC	NM_001101683.1
LDHA	TGCAGACAAGGAACAGTGGA	CCCAGGTAGTGTAGCCCTT	NM_001082277.1

NCF-1 (neutrophil cytosolic factor 1); *CD68* (macrosialin); *CD11b* (*MAC-1*, macrophage marker); *CD14* (monocyte differentiation antigen *CD14*); *ARG1* (Arginase 1); *IL-4* (Interleukin 4); *IL-13* (Interleukin 13); *M-CSF* (colony stimulating factor-macrophage); *OPG* (osteoprotegerin); *RANKL* (Receptor activator of nuclear factor kappa-B ligand); *TRAP* (tartrate resistant acid phosphatase); *CathK* (cathepsin K); *PPAR-γ* (peroxisome proliferator activated receptor gamma); *C3* (complement component 3); *C3aR1* (complement component 3a receptor 1); *CD46* (complement regulatory protein); *CD55* (decay accelerating factor for complement); *CD59* (complement regulatory protein); *C5* (complement component 5); *C5aR1* (complement component 5a receptor 1); *CD3* (T cell surface glycoprotein CD3); *CD4* (T cell surface glycoprotein CD4); *CD8* (T cell transmembrane glycoprotein CD8); *CD19* (B-lymphocyte surface protein CD19); *GAPDH* (glyceraldehyde-3-phosphate dehydrogenase); *ACT-β* (actin beta); *LDHA* (lactate dehydrogenase A).

Table 2. Correspondence between studied gene expression and biological entities.

Biological Entity	Gene
Neutrophil	*NCF-1*
Macrophage	*CD68, CD11b, CD14, ARG1*
Macrophage fusion	*IL-4, IL-13, M-CSF*
Bone resorption	*OPG, RANKL, TRAP, CathK, PPAR-γ*
Complement	Activation: *C3, C3aR1, C5, C5aR1*; Inhibition: *CD46, CD55, CD59*
T lymphocytes	*CD3, CD4, CD8*
B-lymphocytes	*CD19*
Reference genes	*GAPDH, ACT-β, LDHA*

NCF-1 (neutrophil cytosolic factor 1); *CD68* (macrosialin); *CD11b* (*MAC-1*, macrophage marker); *CD14* (monocyte differentiation antigen *CD14*); *ARG1* (Arginase 1); *IL-4* (Interleukin 4); *IL-13* (Interleukin 13); *M-CSF* (colony stimulating factor-macrophage); *OPG* (osteoprotegerin); *RANKL* (Receptor activator of nuclear factor kappa-B ligand); *TRAP* (tartrate resistant acid phosphatase); *CathK* (cathepsin K); *PPAR-γ* (peroxisome proliferator activated receptor gamma); *C3* (complement component 3); *C3aR1* (complement component 3a receptor 1); *CD46* (complement regulatory protein); *CD55* (decay accelerating factor for complement); *CD59* (complement regulatory protein); *C5* (complement component 5); *C5aR1* (complement component 5a receptor 1); *CD3* (T cell surface glycoprotein CD3); *CD4* (T cell surface glycoprotein CD4); *CD8* (T cell transmembrane glycoprotein CD8); *CD19* (B-lymphocyte surface protein CD19); *GAPDH* (glyceraldehyde-3-phosphate dehydrogenase); *ACT-β* (actin beta); *LDHA* (lactate dehydrogenase A).

2.2.2. Amplification Process

Five microliters of SsoAdvanced SYBR™ Green Supermix (Bio-Rad Laboratories Inc.; Hercules, CA, USA) and 1 μL of cDNA template together with 0.4 μM of forward and reverse primer were used in the qPCR reaction. Each cDNA sample was performed on duplicates. The thermal cycles were performed on the CFX Connect Real-Time System (Bio-Rad Laboratories Inc.; Hercules, CA, USA). The CFX Manager Software 3.0 (Bio-Rad, Hercules, CA, USA) was used for the data analysis.

Three genes (*GAPDH, ACT-beta,* and *LDHA*) were selected as reference genes using the geNorm algorithm integrated in the CFX Manager Software. A quantification cycle (Cq) value of the chosen reference genes (Tables 1 and 2) was used as control; hence the mean Cq value of each target gene (Table 1) was normalized against the reference gene's Cq, giving the gene's relative expression. For calculation of fold-change, the $^{\Delta\Delta}$Cq was used, comparing mRNA expressions from the different groups. Significance was set at $p < 0.05$ and the regulation threshold at ×2 fold-change.

2.3. Decalcified Bone Histology

After removal of the implants from the studied Ti, Cu, and PEEK sites on the 6 subjects of each time point, bone was removed en bloc and preserved in 10% formalin (4% buffered formaldehyde; VWR international, Leuven, Belgium) during 48 h for fixation. Samples were decalcified in Ethylene diamine tetra-acetic acid (10% unbuffered EDTA; Milestone srl, BG, Italy) for 4 weeks, with weekly substitution of the EDTA solution, dehydrated and embedded in paraffin (Tissue-Tek TEC; Sakura Finetek Europe BV, Leiden, NL, USA). Samples were sectioned (4-μm-thick) with a microtome (Microm HM355S; Microm International GmbH, Thermo Fischer Scientific, Walldorf, Germany) and stained with Haematoxylin-Eosin (HE) for histological analysis.

2.4. Statistical Analysis

The gene expression statistical analysis was performed using the *t*-test built in the algorithm of the CFX Manager Software 3.0 package (BioRad, Hercules, CA, USA).

3. Results

3.1. Gene Expression Analysis

3.1.1. Days

The gene expression analysis results at 10 days, comparing Cu and PEEK against Ti (control), are displayed in the volcano plots (Figures 2 and 3) and data given in corresponding tables (Tables 3 and 4) with the numerical results expressed in fold-change (regulation, x-axis) and significance (*p* value, y-axis). Data from 10 days have been published in Part I [15] of this study, if with another control.

At 10 days, Cu (vs. Ti, Figure 2 and Table 3) triggered an increased expression of *ARG1* gene (around 14× fold-change). This probably translates to a much higher presence of M2 macrophages (reparative phenotype) around Cu. *NCF1* showed close to a 2× fold upregulation for Cu, and elicited an increased participation of neutrophils at this early stage. Less increased markers, with approximately ×1.5 fold-change were observed for Complement (*C3aR1*), M1-macrophages (*CD14*) [20,21], B-lymphocytes (*CD19*) and Th/Treg-lymphocytes (*CD4*). On the other hand, Cu displayed a downregulation in *TRAP*, *PPAR-gamma* and *OPG*.

At 10 days PEEK (vs. Ti, Figure 3 and Table 4) showed less downregulation of the same bone remodeling markers as Cu, *TRAP, OPG,* and *PPAR-gamma*, as well as the B cell marker *CD19* and macrophage fusion marker *IL-4*. Increased expression of *NCF1* was observed for PEEK, probably translating to an increased presence of neutrophils around this material (as also observed for Cu).

Table 3. Gene expression analysis of Cu compared to Ti (10 days).

Marker	Regulation	*p* Value
PPAR-G	−1.72	0.087477
TRAP	−1.98	0.137344
OPG	−2.03	0.539750

Table 3. *Cont.*

Marker	Regulation	*p* Value
CD3	−1.52	0.411951
IL-4	−1.71	0.185082
ARG1	14.17	0.006031
NCF1	1.96	0.125414
C3aR1	1.66	0.154634
CD14	1.50	0.414019
CD4	1.53	0.431624
CD19	1.64	0.279592

Minus values: downregulation; plus values: upregulation.

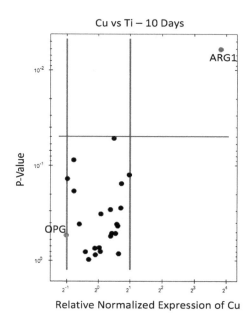

Figure 2. Volcano plot for gene expression of Cu compared to Ti (10 days). Downregulation (vertical green line) and upregulation (vertical red line) set at ×2 regulation. Statistical significance (set at $p < 0.05$) when marker above horizontal blue line.

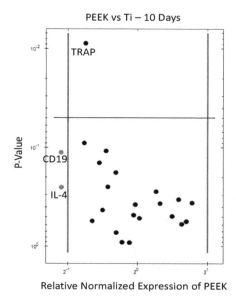

Figure 3. Volcano plot for gene expression of PEEK compared to Ti (10 days). Downregulation (vertical green line) and upregulation (vertical red line) set at ×2 regulation. Statistical significance (set at $p < 0.05$) when marker above horizontal blue line.

Table 4. Gene expression analysis of PEEK compared to Ti (10 days).

Marker	Regulation	p Value
PPAR-G	−1.57	0.550176
TRAP	−1.68	0.008821
OPG	−1.70	0.089695
CD19	−2.14	0.111496
IL-4	−2.14	0.251881
ARG1	1.71	0.361937
NCF1	1.50	0.333874
CD68	1.62	0.556273

Minus values: downregulation; plus values: upregulation.

3.1.2. 28 Days

At 28 days, Cu against Ti (Figure 4 and Table 5), showed upregulation around Cu of *CD68* and *CD14*, as well as *ARG1* (macrophages of both M1-and M2- phenotypes), with M2 far more significant, indicating an overall higher macrophage activation for Cu vs. Ti at 28 days, when compared to 10 days. Complement markers *C3aR1* and *C5aR1* are also upregulated around Cu, as well as *IL-13* (a macrophage fusion marker). On the other hand, there was downregulation of bone remodeling markers *TRAP*, *CATHK*, *PPAR-gamma*, and *RANKL*, as well as *CD3* and *CD4* (T lymphocytes), *C3* complement factor, *CD59* (complement inhibitor), and *IL-4* (the other macrophage fusion marker).

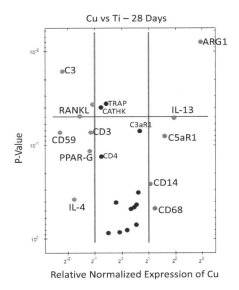

Figure 4. Volcano plot for gene expression analysis of Cu compared to Ti (28 days). Downregulation (vertical green line) and upregulation (vertical red line) set at ×2 regulation. Statistical significance (set at $p < 0.05$) when marker above horizontal blue line.

PEEK vs. Ti at 28 days (Figure 5 and Table 6), showed upregulation of most markers used, with the exception of *TRAP* and *CATHK*, which are effector bone resorption markers that were downregulated. This excessive upregulation indicates a wide and strong immune activation around PEEK compared to Ti at 28 days. However, these results had a limitation in that only two out of the five rabbits used in the study allowed enough mRNA extraction on PEEK samples for gene expression analysis (see Discussion). Nevertheless, both subjects' results were analysed separately for regulation (fold-change) and showed similar responses compatible with that presented in the overall results. However, the significance (p value) should not be taken in consideration here, since the low number of subjects (only 2) renders impossible a statistical analysis.

Table 5. Gene expression analysis of Cu compared to Ti (28 days).

Marker	Regulation	p-Value
C3	−4.64	0.016332
CD59	−4.93	0.073238
RANKL	−2.96	0.049318
PPAR-G	−2.29	0.115578
TRAP	−1.49	0.036164
CATH-K	−1.70	0.039611
CD3	−2.22	0.073334
CD4	−1.69	0.132057
IL-4	−3.43	0.379695
ARG1	7.69	0.007955
CD14	2.09	0.260868
CD68	2.35	0.473322
C5aR1	3.03	0.080240
C3aR1	2.25	0.084210
IL-13	3.84	0.051296

Minus values: downregulation; plus values: upregulation.

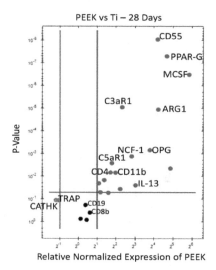

Figure 5. Volcano plot for gene expression analysis of PEEK compared to Ti (28 days). Only 2 subjects to be interpreted with caution. Downregulation (vertical green line) and upregulation (vertical red line) set at ×2 regulation. Statistical significance (set at $p < 0.05$) when marker above horizontal blue line.

Table 6. Gene expression analysis of PEEK compared to Ti (28 days).

Marker	Regulation	p-Value
TRAP	−2.09	0.112708
CATHK	−2.31	0.111423
CD55	18.29	0.000000
C3aR1	8.31	0.000818
C5aR1	3.46	0.002609
CD46	4.68	0.035842
TRAP	−2.09	0.112708
CATHK	−2.31	0.111423
CD55	18.29	0.000000
C3aR1	8.31	0.000818
C5aR1	3.46	0.002609
CD46	4.68	0.035842
CD59	3.03	0.052696
ARG1	18.72	0.000011
CD11b	3.95	0.006903

Table 6. *Cont.*

Marker	Regulation	*p*-Value
CD14	2.14	0.020201
NCF-1	7.04	0.001291
CD3	2.60	0.014589
CD4	3.28	0.006753
CD8b	1.53	0.393394
CD19	1.30	0.182925
MCSF	57.55	0.000000
IL-13	8.11	0.024702
PPAR-G	25.54	0.000000
OPG	13.77	0.000687

Only 2 subjects to be interpreted with caution. Minus values: downregulation; plus values: upregulation.

It is interesting to note that T_{helper}/T_{reg} (*CD4*) was upregulated for Cu at 10 days, but downregulated at 28 days, which could indicate a shift in the presence of T lymphocytes between the two time points and these cells' participation in the biomaterial-associated healing process.

3.2. Comparative Analysis of Gene Expression: 10 vs. 28 Days

The comparison between Cu and PEEK when compared to Ti was divided by respective outcome (Figures 6 and 7): macrophage, complement, neutrophils, lymphocytes, macrophage fusion and bone metabolism. Data from 10 days have been published in Part I [15] of this study, if with another control.

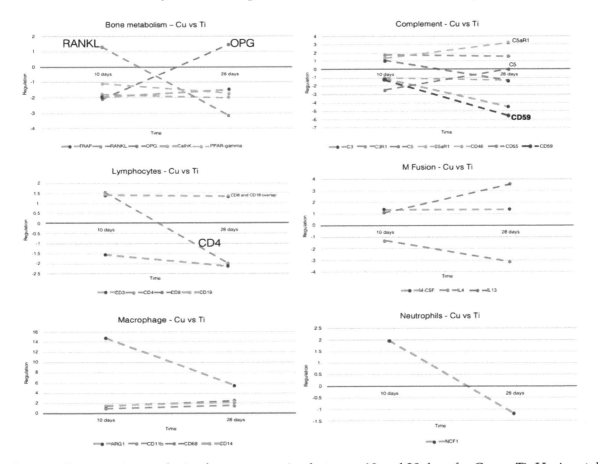

Figure 6. Comparative analysis of gene expression between 10 and 28 days for Cu vs. Ti. Horizontal red line: zero regulation mark; x-axis: time; y-axis: gene marker regulation (10 or 28 days). Intermittent lines do not represent actual results at time points other than 10 or 28 days, but only highlight trend from 10 to 28 days.

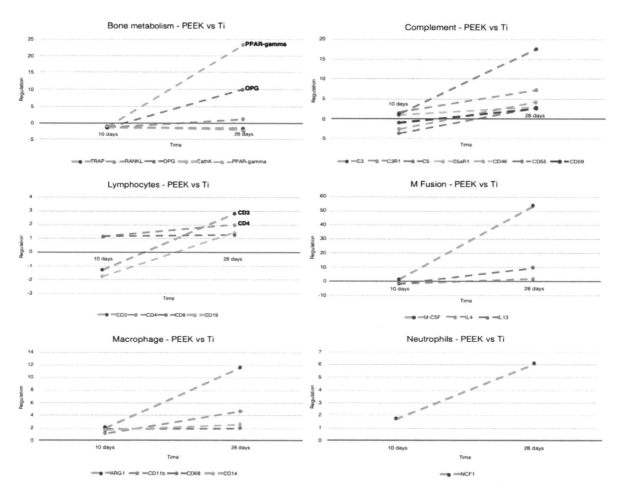

Figure 7. Comparative analysis of gene expression between 10 and 28 days for PEEK vs. Ti. Horizontal red line: zero regulation mark; x-axis: time; y-axis: gene marker regulation (10 or 28 days). Intermittent lines: do not represent actual results at time points other than 10 or 28 days, but only highlight trend from 10 to 28 days.

3.2.1. Cu vs. Ti (Figure 6)

Macrophages: The immune activation was clearly higher around Cu than Ti at both time points. The M2-macrophage phenotype (*ARG1*) was reduced around Cu, but still upregulated when compared to Ti. The M1 markers (combination of *CD68*, *CD11b* and *CD14*) were upregulated slightly around Cu at both 10 and 28 days, i.e., Cu sustained a proinflammatory environment after the acute inflammatory and beginning of the bone remodeling period.

Complement: The results show that *C5* expression increased around Cu from 10 to 28 days, when compared to Ti (both *C5aR1* and *C5* suffered a sharp increase in regulation while the *CD59* (a *C5* inhibitor) was sharply downregulated over time).

Neutrophils: There was a shift observed for *NCF1* from upregulation at 10 days to downregulation at 28 days. This likely indicates a change (reduction) in the presence of neutrophils around Cu.

Lymphocytes: The *CD4* reduction (from up- to downregulated) at 28 days around Cu may indicate a decrease in T_{helper}/T_{reg} function, whereas effector $T_{cytotoxic}$ (*CD8*) and B cells (*CD19*) remain slightly upregulated.

Macrophage fusion: More pronounced *IL4* downregulation and *IL13* upregulation from 10 to 28 days.

Bone metabolism: The *RANKL/OPG* shunt reveals an obvious shift around Cu between 10 and 28 days. *RANKL* changes from upregulated to downregulated and the opposite for *OPG*, which becomes upregulated at 28 days, meaning a suppression of osteoclastogenesis from 10 to 28 days.

3.2.2. PEEK vs. Ti (Figure 7)

It should be noted at 28 days that the results for PEEK should be read with caution since it was only possibility to retrieve mRNA from two of the five samples at 28 days. The possible reasons for this will be discussed below. Data from 10 days have been published in Part I [15] of this study, if with another control.

Macrophages: The macrophage activation around PEEK observed at 10 days and 28 days showed increase in both M1 and M2 markers. This confirms that there was an elevated M1 activation at 28 days, as well as a strong increase in M2-phenotype.

Complement: The results indicate, after 28 days, a continued immune activation around PEEK, especially pronounced for *C3*-related markers (*C3*, *C3aR1*, *CD46*, and *CD55*), and with slight upregulation for *C5*-related markers.

Neutrophils: *NCF1*, the specific neutrophil marker, was at both time points upregulated for PEEK, but showed a sharp increase at 28 days.

Lymphocytes: All lymphocyte markers increased from 10 to 28 days around PEEK. This was especially evident for *CD4+* $T_{h/reg}$ and *CD19+* B cells.

Macrophage fusion: The results indicate a sharp increase in macrophage fusion markers around PEEK, also with a possible contribution to a M2-macrophage phenotype (*IL13*- confirmed by the above mentioned *ARG1* upregulation at 28 days). *M-CSF* also contributes to bone/adipose tissue balance in the osseous tissue, an important finding for PEEK and osseointegration in general, as discussed below.

Bone metabolism: The results suggest formation of adipose-like tissue around PEEK, as expressed by the extreme upregulation of *PPAR-gamma* and by the upregulation of *M-CSF*. Suppression of bone resorption was sustained over time—RANKL still shows at 28 days some upregulation, but was overtaken by a sharp upregulation of *OPG*.

3.3. Histological Analysis

The histological analysis was performed at tissue level. At 10 days (Figures 8–10), Ti presents with initial bone formation within the threads, represented by unorganized collagen proliferation, whereas Cu presents mostly a lytic and cell infiltrate area on the implant surface, followed by a fibrous layer and finally a new bone formation, away from the surface. At 10 days, PEEK demonstrated very little initial bone tissue formation in some threads, but mostly adipose tissue surrounding the implant. Data from 10 days have been published in Part I [15] of this study, if with another control.

At 28 days (Figures 11–13), Ti shows the bone within the threads maturing, while Cu demonstrates a reduction of the cell infiltrate, but still a bone formation away from the implant surface, whereas PEEK presents with mostly adipose tissue around the implant and the little bone tissue formed has not matured (unlike Ti) and shows little calcification.

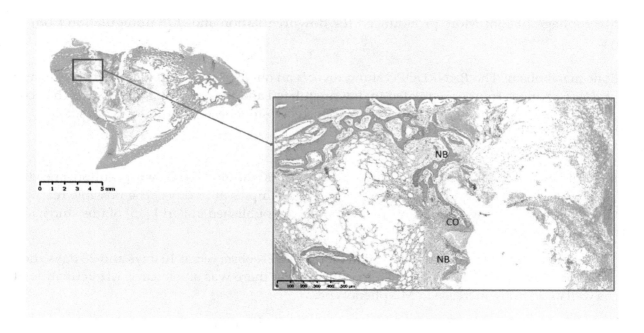

Figure 8. Histological analysis of Ti (10 days). NB: New bone; CO: Contact osteogenesis. Collagen proliferation and some initial calcification to form new bone in the threads. Scale bars: 5 mm and 500 µm.

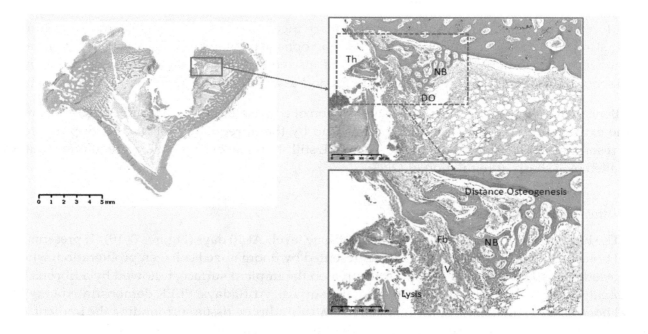

Figure 9. Histological analysis of Cu (10 days). Lytic area next to the implant; Fb: fibroproliferative; NB: New bone; DO: distance osteogenesis; Th: implant thread; V: blood vessel. New bone forming away from the implant surface. Scale bars: 5 mm, 500 µm, and 250 µm clockwise from left.

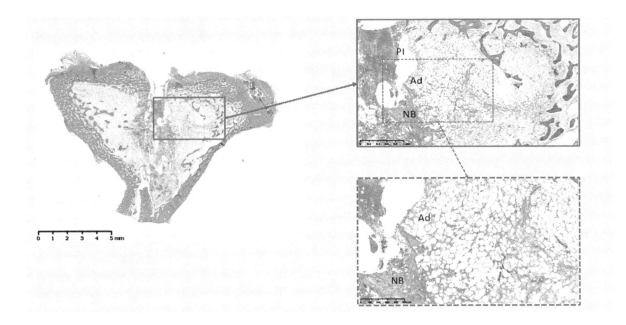

Figure 10. Histological analysis of PEEK (10 days). PI: PEEK implant; NB: New bone; Ad: Adipose tissue. Some collagen proliferation in one thread, adipose tissue also on the implant surface. Scale bars: 5 mm, 1 mm, and 500 μm.

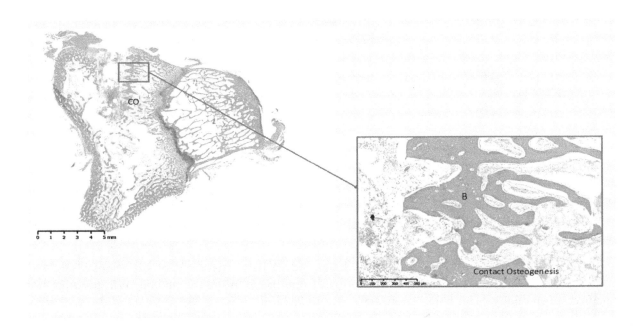

Figure 11. Histological analysis of Ti 28 (days). CO: contact osteogenesis. B: Bone. Formation of mature bone within the implant threads. Scale bars: 5 mm and 500 μm.

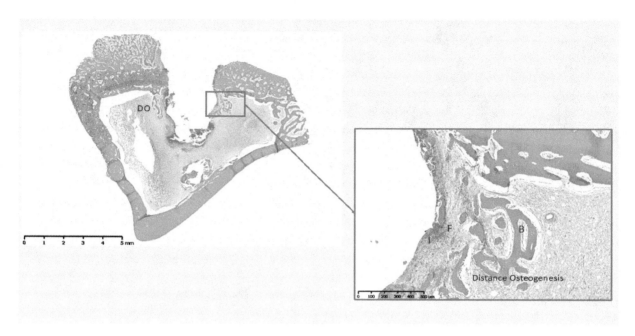

Figure 12. Histological analysis of Cu (28 days). DO: Distance osteogenesis; I: Inflammatory infiltrate; F: fibrous tissue; B: Bone. Formation of bone away from the implant surface, with a reduction of the infiltrate on the implant surface compared to 10 days. Scale bars: 5 mm and 500 μm.

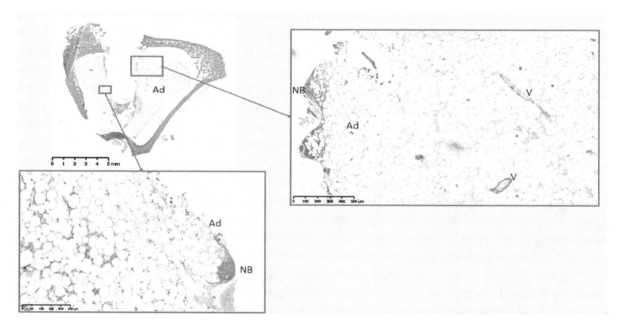

Figure 13. Histological analysis of PEEK (28 days). Ad: Adipose tissue; V: blood vessels; NB: New bone. Mostly adipose tissue proliferation and the bone tissue in the threads has not matured, nor calcified substantially. Scale bars: 5 mm, 500 μm, and 250 μm.

4. Discussion

The osseointegration of materials for biomedical purposes has led to significant advances in patient treatment. Oral implants have become common in clinical practice, and by large base their success on osseointegration of materials such as titanium. Previous studies from the present authors have demonstrated the activation of the immune system around a material placed in bone [12,15], and it was hypothesized that the immune system has a regulatory function on the achievement of osseointegration [11]. In the present experimental study, the bone immune reaction around the materials polyetheretherketone (PEEK) and copper (Cu) was compared to titanium (Ti) as a control, at 10 and 28 days of implantation in rabbit tibia. The current study design aimed at comparing the immune modulation of two materials with poor osseointegration (Cu and PEEK) against a material that osseointegrates (Ti). The comparison between 10 and 28 days is important to understand the evolution of the reaction between the inflammatory period (10 days) and the postinflammatory period (28 days) of healing. Data from 10 days have been published in Part I [15] of this study, but with a Sham (no biomaterial) site as a control.

At 10 days, both PEEK and Cu showed upregulation of markers indicating a higher and different macrophage activity than was found around Ti (confirming the previous study [15]), namely predominantly an M2-phenotype, but also an elevated M1-phenotype. This was more pronounced around Cu than PEEK. At day 10, PEEK did not differ much from Ti, if with higher activation of the immune system (neutrophils and macrophages). This was however observed for Cu, with a higher overall immune activation. Both PEEK and Cu displayed some inhibition of bone resorption when compared to Ti. It is worth noting that PEEK, commonly referred to as a bioinert material [22,23], shows a higher immune activation than Ti at 10 days.

After 28 days of implantation the scenario changes for both PEEK and Cu. Cu shows, as expected, a higher upregulation of the immune markers when compared to Ti, in all its innate components (complement, neutrophils, and macrophages of both M1- and M2-phenotypes). However, the macrophage fusion markers *IL-4* and *IL-13* expressions provide some contradictory indications since *IL-13* was upregulated and *IL-4* downregulated. This could be hypothesized as a stage for initial fusion into foreign body giant cells (FBGCs), but needs confirmation through further studies. Such macrophage fusion is not likely to be guided towards osteoclastogenesis, since bone resorption markers were widely downregulated, hence the macrophage behavior was probably directed towards the formation of FBGCs. However, *IL-13*, also known to induce the M2-phenotype [24] and combined with *ARG1* upregulation, confirms, at 28 days, the elevated M2 phenotype activity around Cu and PEEK compared to Ti, meaning a more pronounced host reparative effort for both materials, even if proinflammatory markers are simultaneously upregulated. The downregulation of bone resorption markers highlights the probable effort around Cu at 28 days, to build bone tissue around the implant for a bony delimitation that, as the histology shows, clearly develops away from the surface of the Cu implant.

PEEK, on the other hand, seems to suffer a vast transformation at 28 days, into a high immune activation in the bone environment surrounding the implant, or rather fails to reduce that immune activation when compared to Ti. Reasons for the high immune upregulation around PEEK at 28 days are not well understood, although the current study results may offer an explanation regarding the bone/adipose tissue balance, as developed below. As mentioned in the results section, the 28 days results for PEEK should be read with caution, since only two subjects out of the five used for gene expression analysis actually enabled collection of enough mRNA to perform the PCR analysis. The difficulty to extract sufficient mRNA from the tissues surrounding PEEK implants was probably due to a low bone tissue formation adjacent to PEEK implants. Furthermore, the reasons behind the classical claim of a supposed bioinertness of PEEK is either that only in vitro studies of it have been presented or that in vivo studies have failed to analyze the immunological response; in contrast, the present results indicate immune activation around PEEK that may persist over extended periods of time.

Regarding the comparison between the two time points of 10 and 28 days, for Cu, the *CD4* expression shifting over time from up- to downregulation, and the maintained upregulation of *CD8* and *CD19* at 28 days, demonstrates a shift in T_{helper}/T_{reg} function whereas effector $T_{cytotoxic}$ and B cells remain slightly upregulated over time. B cells, not only osteoblasts, are known to produce *OPG* in humans [25], which correlates with the increased gene expression of OPG at 28 days and adds another regulatory mechanism of the immune system on bone effector cells, and consequently on the ultimate anabolic/catabolic balance outcome of bone metabolism around implanted materials. It is important to mention that this B cell mechanism is known to be regulated by T cells, and the production of *OPG* by

B/plasma cells can reach 64% of total *OPG* in some mammals [26], thus the present results highlight the immune regulation of bone metabolism around implanted materials.

The notion that Cu starts to enter the remodeling phase and bone production at 28 days, even if at a distance as seen from the histological analysis, is further supported by the results for the above mentioned bone metabolism, with a sharp shift in *RANKL* (upregulated at 10 days and downregulated at 28 days) and in *OPG* (displaying the exact opposite trend) since *RANKL* induces osteoclastogenesis and *OPG* is the decoy molecule that stops this process, the results indicate a shift to a bone reparative environment around Cu at 28 days (through inhibition of the bone resorption inducive mechanisms).

As for the results of the two time point comparisons between PEEK and Ti, the M1-macrophage activation at 28 days may impair bone formation at the PEEK implant surface, with a preferred fatty tissue deposition during repair, as indicated by the upregulation of *PPAR-gamma*, which is produced by differentiated macrophages [27] and in turn triggers the differentiation of adipocytes [28] at 28 days. The upregulation of complement around PEEK, the sharp increase in *NCF1* and the increase in regulation from 10 to 28 days around PEEK for Th/reg and B cells demonstrates that over time a higher immune activity is maintained around PEEK than Ti. This goes beyond the inflammatory period and is most likely proinflammatory.

The upregulation at 28 days of macrophage fusion markers around PEEK indicates also other possible interpretations, such as the M2-phenotype connection of *IL-13* and the fact that *M-CSF*, besides its role in macrophage fusion into either osteoclasts or FBGCs, is intimately related to adipose tissue hyperplasia and growth (through proliferation) [29]. In the present study, the preferential adipose tissue growth observed on PEEK surface is supported at 28 days by the concomitant sharp upregulation of *PPAR-gamma* and *M-CSF*, and downregulation of *TRAP* and *Cathepsin-K* (bone resorption effectors), clearly indicating a sharp imbalance towards adipose tissue formation instead of bone formation around PEEK. It is important to note that in our previous study where Ti was compared to a Sham site at 28 days, no significant differences regarding *PPAR-gamma* or *M-CSF* were observed between the test and control [12], reinforcing the difference observed between PEEK and Ti at 28 days. Fat cell degeneration has previously been described in bone tissue after trauma upon overheating [30]. Such bone/adipose tissue imbalance, tilting towards more adipose tissue formation, has also been demonstrated in osteoporosis studies [31]. The present results after 28 days around PEEK support the description of this new-found mechanism for bone biomaterials. The orchestration of this process by the immune system has also been shown in literature [24], indicating a M1-macrophage chronic inflammation presence in proliferating adipose tissue [32], as well as *CD4+* T$_{helper/reg}$ and *CD19* B cells, as demonstrated in our results with a shift from downregulation at 10 days to upregulation at 28 days. The *PPAR-gamma* and *M-CSF* upregulation reaction likely overrules the OPG upregulation that would suppress bone resorption and increase osteoblast differentiation around PEEK; it is known that bone marrow mesenchymal stem cells (BMMSC) may either differentiate into osteoblasts or adipocytes [33], and PEEK, as demonstrated by the current results, seems to induce immune regulated adipocyte formation and proliferation in its vicinity.

5. Conclusions

Overall, at 10 and 28 days after implantation in rabbit tibia, both Cu and PEEK show a higher immune activation than Ti. This more pronounced and extended immune reaction translates into a prolonged inflammatory phase of the healing period, and may be the cause for the bone tissue failing to form a layer in direct contact with these materials, as shown in the histological sections.

The current results demonstrate that, over time, different materials elicit a different immune regulation of bone metabolism around implanted materials.

From a clinical orofacial perspective, it is fair to state that a fibrous tissue encapsulation or adipose instead of bone tissue formation could also occur around clinically placed titanium implants, should less ideal host conditions be present.

The results from the current study suggest that osseointegration may fail by at least two immunologically regulated mechanisms: (1) soft tissue encapsulation or (2) an imbalance in bone/adipose tissue formation around the implanted material.

Author Contributions: Conceptualization, R.T., T.A., P.T., and A.W.; Methodology, R.T., T.A., P.T., and A.W.; Software, R.T., Z.P., A.W., and S.G.; Validation, R.T. and P.T.; Formal Analysis, R.T. and A.W.; Investigation, R.T. and A.W.; Resources, R.T., P.T., T.A., and A.W.; Data Curation, R.T.; Writing—Original Draft Preparation, R.T. and A.W.; Writing—Review & Editing, P.T., T.A., and A.W.; Visualization, R.T., S.G., and Z.P.; Supervision, A.W., T.A., and P.T.; Project Administration, R.T.; Funding Acquisition, A.W.

References

1. Albrektsson, T.; Brånemark, P.-I.; Hansson, H.-A.; Lindström, J. Osseointegrated titanium implants: Requirements for ensuring a long-lasting, direct bone-to-implant anchorage in man. *Acta Orthop. Scand.* **1981**, *52*, 155–170. [CrossRef] [PubMed]
2. Wennerberg, A.; Albrektsson, T. On implant surfaces: A review of current knowledge and opinions. *Int. J. Oral Maxillofac. Implants* **2010**, *25*, 63–74. [PubMed]
3. Wennerberg, A.; Albrektsson, T.; Andersson, B. Bone tissue response to commercially pure titanium implants blasted with fine and coarse particles of aluminum oxide. *Int. J. Oral Maxillofac. Implants* **1996**, *11*, 38–45. [PubMed]
4. Wennerberg, A.; Albrektsson, T.; Lausmaa, J. Torque and histomorphometric evaluation of c.p. titanium screws blasted with 25- and 75-μm-sized particles of Al2O3. *J. Biomed. Mater. Res.* **1996**, *30*, 251–260. [CrossRef]
5. Buser, D.; Broggini, N.; Wieland, M.; Schenk, R.K.; Denzer, A.J.; Cochran, D.L.; Hoffmann, B.; Lussi, A.; Steinemann, S.G. Enhanced bone apposition to a chemically modified SLA titanium surface. *J. Dent. Res.* **2004**, *83*, 529–533. [CrossRef] [PubMed]
6. Ellingsen, J.E.; Johansson, C.B.; Wennerberg, A.; Holmén, A. Improved retention and bone-to-implant contact with fluoride-modified titanium implants. *Int. J. Oral Maxillofac. Implants* **2004**, *19*, 659–666. [PubMed]
7. Chrcanovic, B.R.; Kisch, J.; Albrektsson, T.; Wennerberg, A. A retrospective study on clinical and radiological outcomes of oral implants in patients followed up for a minimum of 20 years. *Clin. Implant Dent. Relat. Res.* **2018**, *20*, 199–207. [CrossRef] [PubMed]
8. Friberg, B.; Gröndahl, K.; Lekholm, U.; Brånemark, P.-I. Long-term follow-up of severely atrophic edentulous mandibles reconstructed with short brånemark implants. *Clin. Implant Dent. Relat. Res.* **2000**, *2*, 184–189. [CrossRef]
9. Anderson, J.M.; Rodriguez, A.; Chang, D.T. Foreign body reaction to biomaterials. *Semin. Immunol.* **2008**, *20*, 86–100. [CrossRef]
10. Goodman, S.B. Wear particles, periprosthetic osteolysis and the immune system. *Biomaterials* **2007**, *28*, 5044–5048. [CrossRef]
11. Trindade, R.; Albrektsson, T.; Tengvall, P.; Wennerberg, A. Foreign body reaction to biomaterials: On mechanisms for buildup and breakdown of osseointegration. *Clin. Implant Dent. Relat. Res.* **2016**, *18*, 192–203. [CrossRef] [PubMed]
12. Trindade, R.; Albrektsson, T.; Galli, S.; Prgomet, Z.; Tengvall, P.; Wennerberg, A. Osseointegration and foreign body reaction: Titanium implants activate the immune system and suppress bone resorption during the first 4 weeks after implantation. *Clin. Implant Dent. Relat. Res.* **2018**, *20*, 82–91. [CrossRef] [PubMed]
13. Anderson, J.M.; Jones, J.A. Phenotypic dichotomies in the foreign body reaction. *Biomaterials* **2007**, *28*, 5114–5120. [CrossRef] [PubMed]
14. Lin, T.H.; Kohno, Y.; Huang, J.F.; Romero-Lopez, M.; Maruyama, M.; Ueno, M.; Pajarinen, J.; Nathan, K.; Yao, Z.; Yang, F.; et al. Preconditioned or IL4-secreting mesenchymal stem cells enhanced osteogenesis at different stages. *Tissue Eng.* **2019**. [CrossRef] [PubMed]
15. Trindade, R.; Albrektsson, T.; Galli, S.; Prgomet, Z.; Tengvall, P.; Wennerberg, A. Bone immune response to materials, part I: Titanium, PEEK and copper in comparison to sham at 10 days in rabbit tibia. *J. Clin. Med.* **2018**, *7*, 526. [CrossRef] [PubMed]
16. Albrektsson, T.; Dahlin, C.; Jemt, T.; Sennerby, L.; Turri, A.; Wennerberg, A. Is marginal bone loss around oral implants the result of a provoked foreign body reaction? *Clin. Implant Dent. Relat. Res.* **2014**, *16*, 155–165. [CrossRef]

17. Insua, A.; Monje, A.; Wang, H.-L.; Miron, R.J. Basis of bone metabolism around dental implants during osseointegration and peri-implant bone loss. *J. Biomed. Mater. Res.* **2017**, *105*, 2075–2089. [CrossRef]

18. Suska, F.; Emanuelsson, L.; Johansson, A.; Tengvall, P.; Thomsen, P. Fibrous capsule formation around titanium and copper. *J. Biomed. Mater. Res.* **2008**, *85*, 888–896. [CrossRef]

19. Johansson, P.; Jimbo, R.; Kjellin, P.; Currie, F.; Chrcanovic, B.R.; Wennerberg, A. Biomechanical evaluation and surface characterization of a nano-modified surface on PEEK implants: A study in the rabbit tibia. *Int. J. Nanomed.* **2014**, *9*, 3903–3911. [CrossRef]

20. Da Silva, T.A.; Zorzetto-Fernandes, A.L.V.; Cecílio, N.T.; Sardinha-Silva, A.; Fernandes, F.F.; Roque-Barreira, M.C. CD14 is critical for TLR2-mediated M1 macrophage activation triggered by N-glycan recognition. *Sci. Rep.* **2017**, *7*. [CrossRef]

21. McNally, A.K.; Anderson, J.M. Foreign body-type multinucleated giant cells induced by interleukin-4 express select lymphocyte costimulatory molecules and are phenotypically distinct from osteoclasts and dendritic cells. *Exp. Mol. Pathol.* **2011**, *91*, 673–681. [CrossRef] [PubMed]

22. Wenz, L.M.; Merritt, K.; Brown, S.A.; Moet, A.; Steffee, A.D. In vitro biocompatibility of polyetheretherketone and polysulfone composites. *J. Biomed. Mater. Res.* **1990**, *24*, 207–215. [CrossRef] [PubMed]

23. Katzer, A.; Marquardt, H.; Westendorf, J.; Wening, J.V.; von Foerster, G. Polyetheretherketone—Cytotoxicity and mutagenicity in vitro. *Biomaterials* **2002**, *23*, 1749–1759. [CrossRef]

24. Vishwakarma, A.; Bhise, N.S.; Evangelista, M.B.; Rouwkema, J.; Dokmeci, M.R.; Ghaemmaghami, A.M.; Khademhosseini, A. Engineering immunomodulatory biomaterials to tune the inflammatory response. *Trend. Biotechnol.* **2016**, *34*, 470–482. [CrossRef] [PubMed]

25. Yun, T.J.; Chaudhary, P.M.; Shu, G.L.; Kimble Frazer, J.; Ewings, M.K.; Schwartz, S.M.; Pascual, V.; Hood, L.E.; Clark, E.A. OPG/FDCR-1, a TNF receptor family member, is expressed in lymphoid cells and is up-regulated by ligating CD40. *J. Immunol.* **1998**, *161*, 6113–6121.

26. Weitzmann, M.N.; Ofotokun, I. Physiological and pathophysiological bone turnover—Role of the immune system. *Nat. Rev. Endocrinol.* **2016**, *12*, 518–532. [CrossRef]

27. Chinetti, G.; Griglio, S.; Antonucci, M.; Torra, I.P.; Delerive, P.; Majd, Z.; Fruchart, J.-C.; Chapman, J.; Najib, J.; Staels, B. Activation of proliferator-activated receptors α and γ induces apoptosis of human monocyte-derived macrophages. *J. Biol. Chemist.* **1998**, *273*, 25573–25580. [CrossRef]

28. Jiang, C.; Ting, A.T.; Seed, B. PPAR-γ agonists inhibit production of monocyte inflammatory cytokines. *Nature* **1998**, *391*, 82–86. [CrossRef]

29. Levine, J.A.; Jensen, M.D.; Eberhardt, N.L.; O'Brien, T. Adipocyte macrophage colony-stimulating factor is a mediator of adipose tissue growth. *J. Clin. Invest.* **1998**, *101*, 1557–1564. [CrossRef]

30. Eriksson, A.; Albrektsson, T.; Magnusson, B. Assessment of bone viability after heat trauma: A histological, histochemical and vital microscopic study in the rabbit. *Scand. J. Plast. Reconstr. Surg.* **1984**, *18*, 261–268. [CrossRef]

31. Ambrosi, T.H.; Scialdone, A.; Graja, A.; Gohlke, S.; Jank, A.-M.; Bocian, C.; Woelk, L.; Fan, H.; Logan, D.W.; Schurmann, A.; et al. Adipocyte accumulation in the bone marrow during obesity and aging impairs stem cell-based hematopoietic and bone regeneration. *Cell Stem Cell* **2017**, *20*, 771–784. [CrossRef] [PubMed]

32. Kawanashi, N.; Yano, H.; Yokogawa, Y.; Suzuki, K. Exercise training inhibits inflammation in adipose tissue via both suppression of macrophage infiltration and acceleration of phenotypic switching from M1 to M2 macrophages in high-fat-diet-induced obese mice. *Exerc. Immunol. Rev.* **2016**, *16*, 105–118.

33. Bianco, P.; Riminucci, M.; Gronthos, S.; Robey, P.G. Bone marrow stromal stem cells: Nature, biology, and potential applications. *Stem Cells* **2001**, *19*, 180–192. [CrossRef] [PubMed]

16

Osteogenic Cell Behavior on Titanium Surfaces in Hard Tissue

Jung-Yoo Choi [1], Tomas Albrektsson [2,3], Young-Jun Jeon [1] and In-Sung Luke Yeo [4,*]

[1] Dental Research Institute, Seoul National University, Seoul 03080, Korea; jychoi55@snu.ac.kr (J.-Y.C.); yoowjs@snu.ac.kr (Y.-J.J.)

[2] Department of Biomaterials, Sahlgrenska Academy, University of Gothenburg, 40530 Gothenburg, Sweden; tomas.albrektsson@biomaterials.gu.se

[3] Department of Prosthodontics, Faculty of Odontology, Malmö University, 21118 Malmö, Sweden

[4] Department of Prosthodontics, School of Dentistry and Dental Research Institute, Seoul National University, 101 Daehak-ro, Jongro-gu, Seoul 03080, Korea

* Correspondence: pros53@snu.ac.kr

Abstract: It is challenging to remove dental implants once they have been inserted into the bone because it is hard to visualize the actual process of bone formation after implant installation, not to mention the cellular events that occur therein. During bone formation, contact osteogenesis occurs on roughened implant surfaces, while distance osteogenesis occurs on smooth implant surfaces. In the literature, there have been many in vitro model studies of bone formation on simulated dental implants using flattened titanium (Ti) discs; however, the purpose of this study was to identify the in vivo cell responses to the implant surfaces on actual, three-dimensional (3D) dental Ti implants and the surrounding bone in contact with such implants at the electron microscopic level using two different types of implant surfaces. In particular, the different parts of the implant structures were scrutinized. In this study, dental implants were installed in rabbit tibiae. The implants and bone were removed on day 10 and, subsequently, assessed using scanning electron microscopy (SEM), immunofluorescence microscopy (IF), transmission electron microscopy (TEM), focused ion-beam (FIB) system with Cs-corrected TEM (Cs-STEM), and confocal laser scanning microscopy (CLSM)—which were used to determine the implant surface characteristics and to identify the cells according to the different structural parts of the turned and roughened implants. The cell attachment pattern was revealed according to the different structural components of each implant surface and bone. Different cell responses to the implant surfaces and the surrounding bone were attained at an electron microscopic level in an in vivo model. These results shed light on cell behavioral patterns that occur during bone regeneration and could be a guide in the use of electron microscopy for 3D dental implants in an in vivo model.

Keywords: osteogenesis; cell plasticity; dental implants; electron microscopy; scanning transmission electron microscopy; bone-implant interface

1. Introduction

Dental implants are cylindrical prosthetics with screw threads, usually made of titanium (Ti), which are used to replace missing teeth and to support the mastication function of artificial teeth. However, the biological contact with the surface of dental implants is different from that with natural teeth. Osseointegration, the direct contact between bone and implant, is viewed as a hard tissue encapsulation, a foreign body immune reaction that isolates the implant; this bone response is generally accepted as a bio-affinitive reaction to a biocompatible material [1]. To enhance the activity of osteogenic cells in bone integration, the physical and chemical characteristics of the implant surface—including the surface energy, wettability, and topography—are modified, because direct enhancement of the bone surface is much more difficult [2–11]. Such surface treatments can be, in reality, an enhancement to encase the foreign body in hard connective tissue [1,12,13]. Therefore, it is necessary to investigate the in vivo biological response to implant surfaces at the cellular level.

To control the variables, and thereby produce a sound scientific result, in vitro studies using purified cell lines and flat Ti discs with modified surfaces can be performed. However, promising in vitro results in cell responses to such Ti discs do not guarantee obtainment of the desired reactions for Ti implants with the same modified surfaces in in vivo environments. The Ti implants used today to treat patients are screw-shaped, rather than flat disc-shaped. Screw threads have macro- and microstructures—such as roots, flanks, and crests—which the homogeneous Ti disc surfaces for the in vitro experiments are unable to simulate [14]. The cell lines for in vitro tests are usually osteoblast-like cells, rather than human osteogenic cells, and the in vivo environment is very different from an in vitro cell culture medium [5,8,15]. Nonetheless, osteoblastic cell lines in in vitro tests form a simplified system which does not take into account aspects such as immune responses [16]. Therefore, translational evidence is required to create a bridge between the in vitro cell results and the in vivo tissue results—that is, the cellular response to a Ti implant surface in the in vivo environment.

This study aimed to observe Ti implants and the surrounding bone in contact with such implants at the electron microscopic level to identify the in vivo cell responses to the implant surfaces

2. Materials and Methods

2.1. In Vivo Study

This study was approved by the Ethics Committee of the Animal Experimentation of the Institutional Animal Care and Use Committee (CRONEX-IACUC 201702003; Cronex, Hwasung, Korea). All experiments were conducted in accordance with the ARRIVE guidelines for reporting in vivo animal experiments [17]. A total of 8 male New Zealand white rabbits (age: 1–2 years; body weight: 2.6–3.0 kg) with no signs of disease were used. The rabbits were anaesthetized via intramuscular injection of tiletamine/zolazepam (15 mg/kg; Zoletil 50, Virbac Korea Co., Ltd., Seoul, Korea) and xylazine (5 mg/kg; Rompun, Bayer Korea Ltd., Seoul, Korea). Before surgery, the skin over the area of the proximal tibia was shaved and washed with betadine, and an antibiotic (Cefazolin, Yuhan Co., Seoul, Korea) was intramuscularly administered. Lidocaine was locally injected into each surgical site. The skin was incised, and the tibiae were exposed after muscle dissection and periosteal elevation. Drills and profuse sterile saline irrigation were used to prepare the implant sites on the flat tibial surface. The drilling was performed with a final diameter of 4.0 mm at the upper cortical bone, in which the implants were installed in cortical bone and medullary space. Only the V-shaped parts of the threads were engaged (Figure 1A). A total of 5 rabbits received acid-etched (SLA) implants only. Each rabbit received 4 SLA implants, 2 on each side of the rabbit tibia. Three rabbits received turned implants only, each receiving 4 turned implants, 2 on each side of the tibia. The cover screw was covered. The muscle and fascia were sutured with absorbable 4–0 Vicryl sutures, and the outer dermis was closed with a nylon suture. The rabbits were separately housed after surgery. All rabbits were sacrificed via an intravenous overdose of potassium chloride after 10 days of bone healing. After 10 days [1,18,19], the tibiae were exposed, all of the inserted implants were removed through unscrewing, and the surrounding bone was surgically removed en bloc with an adjacent bone collar and immediately placed in Karnovsky's solution for cell fixation in falcon tubes, while the specimens for fluorescence immunocytochemistry were preserved in Roswell Park Memorial Institute (RPMI) media and fetal bovine serum (Gibco, Thermo Fisher Scientific, Waltham, MA, USA) in cell culture dish.

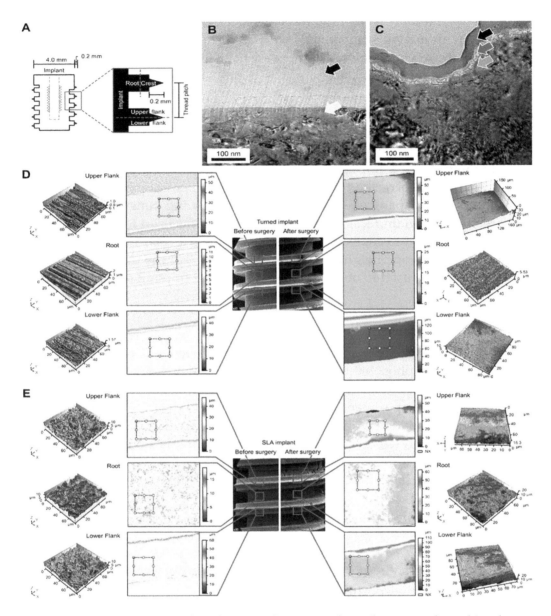

Figure 1. (**A**) Simplified diagram of, and terminology regarding, the screw-shaped implants used in this study. The inner half, close to the minor diameter of the implant, was defined as the root area. The outer half, close to the major diameter of the implant, was called the crest area. The upper half of the thread was defined as the upper flank (UF), and the lower half was the lower flank (LF). (**B**) Cs-corrected transmission electron microscopy (Cs-STEM) analysis retrieved from focused ion beam specimens of the turned and (**C**) acid-etched (SLA) implants on day 10. There were no cells detected on the turned surface (yellow arrow) beneath the Pt-coated layer (black arrow), whereas, cells were detected on SLA surface (red arrow). (**D**) Confocal laser scanning microscopy (CLSM) of the turned and (**E**) SLA surfaces measured in root, UF, and LF. The turned implant revealed a smooth texture, and no cells were seen after in vivo experiment. The SLA implants displayed cell attachment in the root area, depicted as irregular structure of grey color on top of roughened topography in the 3D mapping of the CLSM.

2.2. Sample Preparation and Implant Surface Modification

Herein, 26 Ti sandblasted, large-grit, and SLA implants and 18 turned implants were used (Deep Implant System, Inc., Seongnam, Korea). The implants were made of grade 4 commercially pure Ti by computer numerical control (CNC) machining. The implant surface was called 'turned' when the surface had no further modification after CNC machining. The SLA surface was made by sandblasting the implant surface with 250–500 μm alumina particles and by etching the surface with HCl/H$_2$SO$_4$

acid mixture. All of the implants were 4.0 mm in diameter and 5.0 mm in length. A total of 20 SLA implants were used in an in vivo study, and 6 were used in the surface analysis, while 12 turned implants were used in the in vivo analysis, and 6 were used in the surface analysis.

2.3. Surface Characteristics

Among the 6 SLA implants and 6 turned implants used in the surface analysis, 2 of each type of implant were used for scanning electron microscopy (SEM; Hitachi S-4700, Hitachi, Tokyo, Japan), 2 were used for confocal laser scanning microscopy (CLSM; LSM 800, Carl Zeiss AG, Oberkochen, Germany), and the remaining 2 implants were used for focused ion beam (FIB; Helios 650, FEI, Hillsboro, OR, USA) and Cs-corrected transmission electron microscopy (Cs-STEM; JEM-ARM200F, Cold FEG, FEOL Ltd., Tokyo, Japan), which are capable of producing transmission electron microscopy (TEM) images directly from an undecalcified specimen. SEM was used to observe the topographical features, while CLSM was used to analyze the surface roughness levels. The measured area roughness parameters included the average height deviation value (S_a) and the developed surface area ratio (S_{dr}). FIB and Cs-STEM were used to observe the undecalcified implant surface directly without any resin embedding.

2.4. Scanning Electron Microscopy (SEM) Analysis

The retrieved implant specimens and surrounding bony specimens were fixed with Karnovsky's solution and washed in 0.1 M phosphate buffer saline (PBS) 3 times every 15 min. The specimens were dehydrated through a graded 70–100% ethanol series and then treated with hexamethyldisilazane for 15 min. The surrounding bone specimens were cut in half around the round hole in which the implant had been inserted, after degradation with 80% ethanol using rotary discs within an appropriate amount of time. Prior to the SEM analysis, the implant and bone specimens were sputter coated with a thin film of platinum to protect the implant and bony surfaces. All specimens were handled with Ti forceps and surgical gloves in a clean laboratory environment. Each implant and bone sample was attached using adhesive carbon tape, as well as aluminum tape, on the SEM sample stub. The samples were inserted into a Hitachi S-4700 (Hitachi, Tokyo, Japan), which was operated at 20 kV.

2.5. Immunofluorescence Microscopy (IF) Analysis

Prior to the sacrifice of the rabbit tibiae, the implants were removed from each tibia and, along with the surrounding bone, the specimens were preserved for 3 h in the refrigerator in the RPMI media, which contained penicillin (50 U/mL) and streptomycin (50 µg/mL). The cells underwent immunostaining and were incubated for 15 min with a protein block (DAKO, Agilent, Santa Clara, CA, USA, X0909) to remove non-specific binding protein. The cells were then incubated for 30 min with a diluted osteocalcin primary antibody (1:100 dilution in 3% bovine serum albumin (BSA), #MA120788, Thermo Fisher Scientific, USA). After being rinsed in PBS, these cells were incubated for 1 h with a diluted secondary antibody (1:200 diluted goat anti-mouse IgG-FITC in 3% BSA, #A10530, Thermo Fisher Scientific, Waltham, MA, USA) in a dark room and washed with PBS. Subsequently, nuclear counterstaining was performed using Hoechst 33342 (Thermo Fisher Scientific, Waltham, MA, USA) (1:10,000 dilution) for 5 min. After the counterstaining, the images were obtained by fluorescence microscopy using Axio Observer.A1 (Carl Zeiss, Jena, Germany).

2.6. Transmission Electron Microscopy (TEM) Analysis

Prior to sacrifice, the implants were removed, and the cells were isolated with a cell scraper and fixed in Karnovsky's solution. After sacrifice, the cells from the bony structures around the area where implants had been placed were collected and fixed in Karnovsky's solution. They were washed in 0.1 M PBS 3 times every 15 min. The specimens were dehydrated through a graded 70–100% ethanol series, exchanged with propylene oxide, and embedded in a mixture of Epon 812 and Araldite. Ultrathin sections (70 nm) were cut using a Leica EM UC6 Ultramicrotome (Leica, Vienna, Austria). A ribbon of serial ultrathin sections from each bony specimen and implant were collected on copper grids and stained with uranyl acetate and lead citrate. The serial fields were photographed at ×500 magnification using a JEOL 1400-Flash electron microscope (JEOL, Tokyo, Japan) operated at 120 kV.

2.7. TEM Sample Preparation by Focused Ion Beam (FIB)

The implant specimens were fixed with Karnovsky's solution and washed in 0.1 M PBS 3 times every 15 min. The specimens were dehydrated through a graded 70–100% ethanol series and finally treated with hexamethyldisilazane for 15 min. A Helios 650 (FEI, Hillsboro, OR, USA) dual-beam FIB system was used for the TEM sample preparation. The specimens were deposited with a platinum layer to protect the implant and bony surfaces prior to milling. A Ga^+ ion beam accelerated voltage of 30 kV was used for milling. The TEM sample (under 100 nm) was attached to a Cu TEM grid. The TEM analysis at Cs-STEM was observed using a JEM-AFM200F (Cold FEG, JEOL, Tokyo, Japan).

3. Results

3.1. Parts of the Implant

The distribution of the main locations of cells was classified into three major structures within the implant: The root, the lower flank (LF), and the upper flank (UF). The implants used in this study were specially designed: The sharp V-shape parts for the firm engagement of bone, and the square area between the threads for the biologic response with no physical intervention such as stress (Figure 1A).

3.2. TEM Sample Preparation by Focused Ion Beam (FIB)

Surface characteristics along with cell attachment were probed using Cs-TEM from the FIB system. The cells were detected directly from an undecalcified specimen without the need to undergo cell isolation. The cells on the turned surface were unseen (Figure 1B), while on the SLA surface, organic matter was detected under the Pt-coated layer (Figure 1C).

3.3. Confocal Laser Scanning Microscopy (CLSM) Analysis of the Implant

The different topographical features [10,20,21] of the implants may affect cell attachment. Therefore, CLSM was used to measure the height parameters (S_a), as well as the hybrid parameters (S_{dr}), for the root, UF, and LF areas. The S_a values for the turned surface were 0.163 μm, 0.086 μm, and 0.098 μm, and the S_{dr} values were 10.3%, 8.2%, and 12.1% in the root, UF, and LF, respectively (Figure 1D). On the SLA surfaces, the S_a values were 1.14 μm, 1.17 μm, and 1.09 μm, and the S_{dr} values were 237%, 235%, and 239% for the root, UF, and LF, respectively. The S_a and S_{dr} values differed in terms of surface characteristics, with the SLA being higher; however, based on the different structural components, no differences were found in either the S_a or S_{dr}. After the cells were fixed, the 3D topographical mapping of the cells also showed higher cell quantities in the root area of the SLA implants (Figure 1E). To see the correlation of the surrounding bone and the retrieved implant, the topographical parameters of the bone were also tested, but unfortunately, due to the sputtering of the Pt, the parameters could not be calculated in the bone area.

3.4. Scanning Electron Microscopy (SEM) Analysis of the Implant

In our research, the cell attachment and spreading varied depending on the structural differences in the implant thread. Cells were not attached in turned surfaces in all parts of the implants (Figure 2A). In the root area of SLA implants, an active cellular event took place. The cells were aggregated and spread out effectively, with their cellular processes extended. The fibrin of the cell could be detected. In the crest area, osteocytes and their processes were observed on both the UF and LF. However, they were not as active as the cells in the root area, in which the cells maintained a round shape, insufficiently spreading, and were in a static form (Figure 2B).

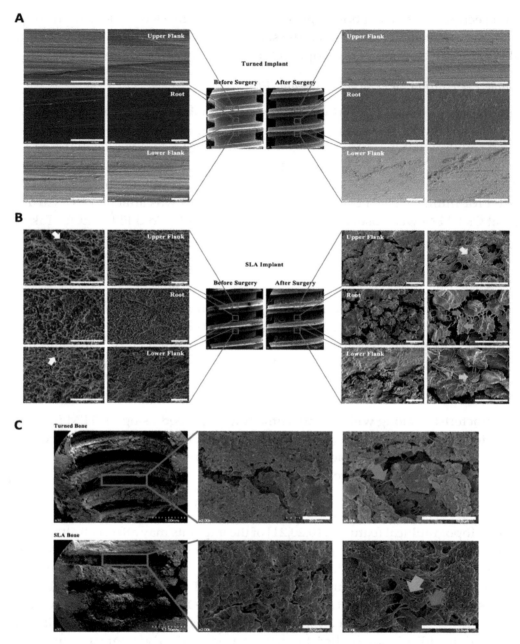

Figure 2. (**A**) Scanning Electron Microscopy (SEM) analysis of the turned implants. The smooth surface is displayed with many turned grooves. No cells were attached after 10 days. (**B**) SEM analysis of sandblasted, large-grit, and SLA implants. The surface characteristics of the SLA implants, which are typically porous, with honeycomb shapes (white arrow); the rather sharp peaks (left top white arrow) are definite, and the texture of the surface is rough. On the right-hand-side, the cells (green arrow) are shown to be mainly attached and actively spread out in the root area, with their filopodia extended (blue arrow). The fibrin can be seen on the cells (red arrow). In the UF, osteocytes and their processes are seen (yellow arrow). In the LF, the cell process is being extended, getting ready to migrate. The round cells are in static status (orange arrow). (**C**) SEM analysis of the surrounding bone of the removed turned and SLA implants at day 10. In the upper row, the overall image reveals traces of the smooth implant surface; thus, the bone texture is rather regular. The formation of the fibrin network is shown beneath some active cells (blue arrow). The lower row demonstrates the surrounding bone of the removed SLA implant. The texture of the bone is rather rough compared with that of the turned implant. The red blood cells can be seen underneath the cells. The mineralization grains (green arrow) are shown, and collagen (red arrow) is depicted well with striped bands. Scale bars = 10 μm.

3.5. Scanning Electron Microscopy (SEM) Analysis of the Surrounding Bone of the Retrieved Implant

The SEM analysis of the surrounding bone of the retrieved turned implants revealed a fibrin network among the cells, whereas a striped pattern of supposed collagen bands was elucidated in the SLA implants. In the area where the bone was in contact with the UF and LF, a bone matrix was formed, while the crest area of the thread showed a fibrin network and an active cellular response. In the surrounding bone of the SLA-retrieved implants, the texture of the bone surface was rougher compared to that of the turned implants. Red blood cells were embedded, and a mineralization process had occurred in the crest area where the collagen bands were visible; cell folding could be observed with granules (Figure 2C).

3.6. Immunofluorescence Microscopy (IF) Analysis

Among the cells attached on the SLA surfaces, osteogenic cells needed to be identified because they are the key cells in bone formation. Accordingly, the attachment of osteogenic cells to the implant surface was confirmed through the use of osteocalcin—antibody targeted for rabbits in vivo. Immunofluorescence microscopy enabled the development of images of osteogenic cells on the SLA implants and the surrounding bone after 10 days, and consequently, confirmed the existence of osteogenic cells on the implant surface. While osteogenic cells were detected on the implant surface, the surrounding bone showed few osteogenic cells (Figure 3A).

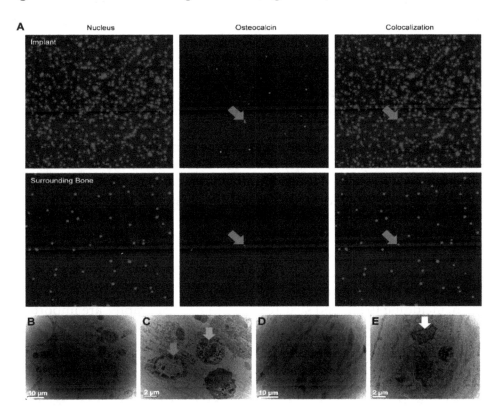

Figure 3. (**A**) Immunofluorescence microscopy (IF) of the SLA implants and surrounding bone on day 10, including nucleus, marker, and colocalization. Osteogenic cells (red arrow) are attached to the SLA implant surface rather than to the surrounding bone, which showed few osteogenic cells. The magnification of the photographs is ×200. (**B**) Transmission electron microscopy (TEM) analysis of retrieved SLA implant at day 10. (**C**) Macrophages (blue arrow) and osteogenic cell (red arrow) can be seen in the SLA implants. (**D**) TEM analysis of surrounding bone on day 10. (**E**) In the surrounding bone, osteocytes (white arrow) were detected.

3.7. Transmission Electron Microscopy (TEM) Analysis

The samples were also scrutinized by TEM. The TEM images of the SLA implants revealed macrophages and osteogenic cells (Figure 3B,C), while in the surrounding bone, osteocytes were detected (Figure 3D,E).

4. Discussion

In the present study, we aimed to determine the cell activity that occurs during the bone-forming process. We targeted the challenges concerning the lack of actual visualization of bone formation, and put much effort into presenting data on the active process in a bony environment with an actual 3D implant structure rather than the flat Ti discs used in in vitro studies. Our experimental data showed that a positive cell reaction occurred on the SLA surfaces, whereas the turned surfaces lacked cell adhesion. Meanwhile, the surrounding bone of the turned surface implants exhibited active cellular events. This may be confirmation of contact osteogenesis on the SLA surfaces. Whilst distance osteogenesis appears to occur around the smooth turned surfaces, it is well known that rougher turned surfaces (that were not investigated in this paper) also display contact osteogenesis [19,22–24].

According to the IF results seen, confirmation of osteogenic cells on the roughened implant surfaces might be further evidence of contact osteogenesis. However, further investigation is required to determine why only few osteogenic cells were detected on the bone surface—which is considered to be the place for distance osteogenesis. In addition, although limitations exist, in that cell classification is difficult in FIB specimens, the results reveal further evidence of contact osteogenesis on the SLA surface. Investigations are needed to better understand the link between such a phenomenon and the higher clinical long-term survival rate of implants with the SLA surfaces (over 95%), compared to that of turned implants (81–91%) [25,26].

The cells on the Ti implant surfaces seemed to be able to read the configuration of the structural parts of the implant. Considering the fact that implant geometry is a major factor in the initial stability of an implant inserted into bone and that osseointegration contributes to the subsequent stability, such SEM results imply that the initial, or primary, stability is associated with the shape of the crest area and that the secondary, or biological, stability is mainly connected to the cellular behavior at the root area [27,28].

Under the circumstances of immobility, exogenous foreign material such as Ti implants, exhibit bone demarcation instead of implant rejection; hence, the stability-enhancing structures of an implant may be of particular importance [29]. Cylindrical implants without threads have uniform but weak attachment to the bone, which is especially weak to shear stress. This weakness may have been one reason why the cylindrical implants displayed a lot of bone resorption in situ [30]. With regards to the electron microscopic images captured in the in vivo environment of this study, all the implant components shown, including the thread structure and microtopography, are important in the cellular response during the osseointegration process. Altering the surface roughness of a material may affect the biological processes regulating the behavioral mechanisms (e.g., cell activity, adhesion) of osteoblastic/immune cells, such extracellular protein deposition at the moment of implantation has an influence on the cellular behavior which later leads to differences in in vivo outcomes [31,32]. This study was qualitative. Quantitative investigations are necessary for various modified surfaces. Recently, implants made of other materials—including ceramic and polyetheretherketone (PEEK)—have been developed, the surfaces of which need to be further investigated with respect to this in vivo cellular response [33,34].

This study successfully presented direct evidence of the behavior of osteogenic cells on the implant surface in an in vivo environment at the electron microscopic level. According to the interpreted data herein, in the bone surrounding dental implants, cell behavior is determined by the treated surface of the implant, whereas cells attached to the SLA implants seem to be able to read the configuration of different implant structures and develop an attachment pattern that conforms to those structures.

Author Contributions: Conceptualization, J.-Y.C. and Y.-J.J.; Methodology, J.-Y.C., Y.-J.J., and T.A.; Software, J.-Y.C.; Validation, J.-Y.C., T.A., and I.-S.L.Y.; Formal Analysis, J.-Y.C. and Y.-J.J.; Investigation, J.-Y.C.; Resources, J.-Y.C., T.A., Y.-J.J., and I.-S.L.Y.; Data Curation, J.-Y.C., T.A., Y.-J.J., and I.-S.L.Y.; Writing—Original Draft Preparation, J.-Y.C.; Writing—Review & Editing, J.-Y.C., T.A., and I.-S.L.Y.; Visualization, J.-Y.C., T.A., Y.-J.J., and I.-S.L.Y.; Supervision, I.-S.L.Y.; Project Administration, J.-Y.C. and I.-S.L.Y.; Funding Acquisition, I.-S.L.Y.

References

1. Trindade, R.; Albrektsson, T.; Galli, S.; Prgomet, Z.; Tengvall, P.; Wennerberg, A. Osseointegration and foreign body reaction: Titanium implants activate the immune system and suppress bone resorption during the first 4 weeks after implantation. *Clin. Implant Dent. Relat. Res.* **2018**, *20*, 82–91. [CrossRef] [PubMed]
2. Kohles, S.S.; Clark, M.B.; Brown, C.A.; Kenealy, J.N. Direct assessment of profilometric roughness variability from typical implant surface types. *Int. J. Oral Maxillofac. Implants* **2004**, *19*, 510–516.
3. Yeo, I.S.; Han, J.S.; Yang, J.H. Biomechanical and histomorphometric study of dental implants with different surface characteristics. *J. Biomed. Mater. Res. B Appl. Biomater.* **2008**, *87*, 303–311. [CrossRef] [PubMed]
4. Choi, J.Y.; Lee, H.J.; Jang, J.U.; Yeo, I.S. Comparison between bioactive fluoride modified and bioinert anodically oxidized implant surfaces in early bone response using rabbit tibia model. *Implant Dent.* **2012**, *21*, 124–128. [CrossRef]
5. Kang, H.K.; Kim, O.B.; Min, S.K.; Jung, S.Y.; Jang, D.H.; Kwon, T.K.; Min, B.M.; Yeo, I.S. The effect of the dltiddsywyri motif of the human laminin alpha2 chain on implant osseointegration. *Biomaterials* **2013**, *34*, 4027–4037. [CrossRef]
6. Koh, J.W.; Kim, Y.S.; Yang, J.H.; Yeo, I.S. Effects of a calcium phosphate-coated and anodized titanium surface on early bone response. *Int. J. Oral Maxillofac. Implants* **2013**, *28*, 790–797. [CrossRef] [PubMed]
7. Kwon, T.K.; Lee, H.J.; Min, S.K.; Yeo, I.S. Evaluation of early bone response to fluoride-modified and anodically oxidized titanium implants through continuous removal torque analysis. *Implant Dent.* **2012**, *21*, 427–432. [CrossRef]
8. Yeo, I.S.; Min, S.K.; Kang, H.K.; Kwon, T.K.; Jung, S.Y.; Min, B.M. Identification of a bioactive core sequence from human laminin and its applicability to tissue engineering. *Biomaterials* **2015**, *73*, 96–109. [CrossRef] [PubMed]
9. Wennerberg, A.; Albrektsson, T.; Chrcanovic, B. Long-term clinical outcome of implants with different surface modifications. *Eur. J. Oral Implantol.* **2018**, *11* (Suppl. 1), S123–S136. [PubMed]
10. Wennerberg, A.; Albrektsson, T. On implant surfaces: A review of current knowledge and opinions. *Int. J. Oral Maxillofac. Implants* **2010**, *25*, 63–74. [PubMed]
11. Choi, J.Y.; Jung, U.W.; Kim, C.S.; Jung, S.M.; Lee, I.S.; Choi, S.H. Influence of nanocoated calcium phosphate on two different types of implant surfaces in different bone environment: An animal study. *Clin. Oral Implants Res.* **2013**, *24*, 1018–1022. [CrossRef] [PubMed]
12. Albrektsson, T.; Chrcanovic, B.; Molne, J.; Wennerberg, A. Foreign body reactions, marginal bone loss and allergies in relation to titanium implants. *Eur. J. Oral Implantol.* **2018**, *11* (Suppl. 1), S37–S46.
13. Albrektsson, T. On implant prosthodontics: One narrative, twelve voices-1. *Int. J. Prosthodont.* **2018**, *31*, s11–s14.
14. Choi, J.Y.; Kang, S.H.; Kim, H.Y.; Yeo, I.L. Control variable implants improve interpretation of surface modification and implant design effects on early bone responses: An in vivo study. *Int. J. Oral Maxillofac. Implants* **2018**, *33*, 1033–1040. [CrossRef] [PubMed]
15. Min, S.K.; Kang, H.K.; Jang, D.H.; Jung, S.Y.; Kim, O.B.; Min, B.M.; Yeo, I.S. Titanium surface coating with a laminin-derived functional peptide promotes bone cell adhesion. *Biomed. Res. Int.* **2013**, *2013*, 638348. [CrossRef]
16. Araújo-Gomes, N.; Romero-Gavilán, F.; Sánchez-Pérez, A.M.; Gurruchaga, M.; Azkargorta, M.; Elortza, F.; Martinez-Ibañez, M.; Iloro, I.; Suay, J.; Goñi, I. Characterization of serum proteins attached to distinct sol-gel hybrid surfaces. *J. Biomed. Mater. Res. B Appl. Biomater.* **2018**, *106*, 1477–1485. [CrossRef]
17. Kilkenny, C.; Browne, W.J.; Cuthi, I.; Emerson, M.; Altman, D.G. Improving bioscience research reporting: The arrive guidelines for reporting animal research. *Vet. Clin. Pathol.* **2012**, *41*, 27–31. [CrossRef]
18. Trindade, R.; Albrektsson, T.; Galli, S.; Prgomet, Z.; Tengvall, P.; Wennerberg, A. Bone immune response to materials, part i: Titanium, peek and copper in comparison to sham at 10 days in rabbit tibia. *J. Clin. Med.* **2018**, *7*, 526. [CrossRef]

19. Choi, J.Y.; Sim, J.H.; Yeo, I.L. Characteristics of contact and distance osteogenesis around modified implant surfaces in rabbit tibiae. *J. Periodontal Implant Sci.* **2017**, *47*, 182–192. [CrossRef] [PubMed]

20. Wennerberg, A.; Albrektsson, T. Effects of titanium surface topography on bone integration: A systematic review. *Clin. Oral Implants Res.* **2009**, *20* (Suppl. 4), 172–184. [CrossRef]

21. Yeo, I.S. Reality of dental implant surface modification: A short literature review. *Open Biomed. Eng. J.* **2014**, *8*, 114–119. [CrossRef] [PubMed]

22. Albrektsson, T.; Brånemark, P.I.; Hansson, H.A.; Lindström, J. Osseointegrated titanium implants. Requirements for ensuring a long-lasting, direct bone-to-implant anchorage in man. *Acta Orthop. Scand.* **1981**, *52*, 155–170. [CrossRef]

23. Davies, J.; Turner, S.; Sandy, J.R. Distraction osteogenesis—A review. *Br. Dent. J.* **1998**, *185*, 462–467. [CrossRef] [PubMed]

24. Davies, J.E. Mechanisms of endosseous integration. *Int. J. Prosthodont.* **1998**, *11*, 391–401.

25. Buser, D.; Janner, S.F.; Wittneben, J.G.; Brägger, U.; Ramseier, C.A.; Salvi, G.E. 10-year survival and success rates of 511 titanium implants with a sandblasted and acid-etched surface: A retrospective study in 303 partially edentulous patients. *Clin. Implant Dent. Relat. Res.* **2012**, *14*, 839–851. [CrossRef]

26. Adell, R.; Lekholm, U.; Rockler, B.; Brånemark, P.I. A 15-year study of osseointegrated implants in the treatment of the edentulous jaw. *Int. J. Oral Surg.* **1981**, *10*, 387–416. [CrossRef]

27. Kwon, T.K.; Kim, H.Y.; Yang, J.H.; Wikesjö, U.M.; Lee, J.; Koo, K.T.; Yeo, I.S. First-order mathematical correlation between damping and resonance frequency evaluating the bone-implant interface. *Int. J. Oral Maxillofac. Implants* **2016**, *31*, 1008–1015. [CrossRef]

28. Meredith, N. Assessment of implant stability as a prognostic determinant. *Int. J. Prosthodont.* **1998**, *11*, 491–501.

29. Donath, K.; Laass, M.; Günzl, H.J. The histopathology of different foreign-body reactions in oral soft tissue and bone tissue. *Virchows Arch. A Pathol. Anat. Histopathol.* **1992**, *420*, 131–137. [CrossRef]

30. Chrcanovic, B.R.; Albrektsson, T.; Wennerberg, A. Reasons for failures of oral implants. *J. Oral Rehabil.* **2014**, *41*, 443–476. [CrossRef]

31. Romero-Gavilán, F.; Gomes, N.C.; Ródenas, J.; Sánchez, A.; Azkargorta, M.; Iloro, I.; Elortza, F.; García Arnáez, I.; Gurruchaga, M.; Goñi, I.; et al. Proteome analysis of human serum proteins adsorbed onto different titanium surfaces used in dental implants. *Biofouling* **2017**, *33*, 98–111. [CrossRef] [PubMed]

32. Dodo, C.G.; Senna, P.M.; Custodio, W.; Paes Leme, A.F.; Del Bel Cury, A.A. Proteome analysis of the plasma protein layer adsorbed to a rough titanium surface. *Biofouling* **2013**, *29*, 549–557. [CrossRef]

33. Bormann, K.H.; Gellrich, N.C.; Kniha, H.; Schild, S.; Weingart, D.; Gahlert, M. A prospective clinical study to evaluate the performance of zirconium dioxide dental implants in single-tooth edentulous area: 3-year follow-up. *BMC Oral Health* **2018**, *18*, 181. [CrossRef] [PubMed]

34. Najeeb, S.; Zafar, M.S.; Khurshid, Z.; Siddiqui, F. Applications of polyetheretherketone (peek) in oral implantology and prosthodontics. *J. Prosthodont. Res.* **2016**, *60*, 12–19. [CrossRef] [PubMed]

Permissions

All chapters in this book were first published by MDPI; hereby published with permission under the Creative Commons Attribution License or equivalent. Every chapter published in this book has been scrutinized by our experts. Their significance has been extensively debated. The topics covered herein carry significant findings which will fuel the growth of the discipline. They may even be implemented as practical applications or may be referred to as a beginning point for another development.

The contributors of this book come from diverse backgrounds, making this book a truly international effort. This book will bring forth new frontiers with its revolutionizing research information and detailed analysis of the nascent developments around the world.

We would like to thank all the contributing authors for lending their expertise to make the book truly unique. They have played a crucial role in the development of this book. Without their invaluable contributions this book wouldn't have been possible. They have made vital efforts to compile up to date information on the varied aspects of this subject to make this book a valuable addition to the collection of many professionals and students.

This book was conceptualized with the vision of imparting up-to-date information and advanced data in this field. To ensure the same, a matchless editorial board was set up. Every individual on the board went through rigorous rounds of assessment to prove their worth. After which they invested a large part of their time researching and compiling the most relevant data for our readers.

The editorial board has been involved in producing this book since its inception. They have spent rigorous hours researching and exploring the diverse topics which have resulted in the successful publishing of this book. They have passed on their knowledge of decades through this book. To expedite this challenging task, the publisher supported the team at every step. A small team of assistant editors was also appointed to further simplify the editing procedure and attain best results for the readers.

Apart from the editorial board, the designing team has also invested a significant amount of their time in understanding the subject and creating the most relevant covers. They scrutinized every image to scout for the most suitable representation of the subject and create an appropriate cover for the book.

The publishing team has been an ardent support to the editorial, designing and production team. Their endless efforts to recruit the best for this project, has resulted in the accomplishment of this book. They are a veteran in the field of academics and their pool of knowledge is as vast as their experience in printing. Their expertise and guidance has proved useful at every step. Their uncompromising quality standards have made this book an exceptional effort. Their encouragement from time to time has been an inspiration for everyone.

The publisher and the editorial board hope that this book will prove to be a valuable piece of knowledge for researchers, students, practitioners and scholars across the globe.

List of Contributors

Ling Li, Heithem Ben Amara, Jun-Beom Lee, Yong-Moo Lee and Ki-Tae Koo
Department of Periodontology and Dental Research Institute, School of Dentistry, Seoul National University, Seoul 03080, Korea

Jungwon Lee
One-Stop Specialty Center, Seoul National University Dental Hospital & Department of Periodontology, School of Dentistry, Seoul National University, Seoul 03080, Korea

Ki-Sun Lee
Department of Prosthodontics, Korea University Ansan Hospital, Ansan 15355, Gyeonggi-do, Korea

Sang-Wan Shin
Department of Advanced Prosthodontics, Graduate School of Clinical Dentistry, Korea University, Seoul 02841, Korea

Byoungkook Kim and Pangyu Kim
3D Printer R&D Team, Dentium Co., Ltd., Suwon 16229, Gyeonggi-do, Korea

Ji-Youn Hong
Department of Periodontology, Periodontal-Implant Clinical Research Institute, School of Dentistry, Kyung Hee University, 26, Kyungheedae-ro, Dongdaemun-gu, Seoul 02447, Korea

Seok-Yeong Ko
Department of Periodontology, College of Dentistry and Institute of Oral Bioscience, Jeonbuk National University, 567, Baekje-daero, Deokjin-gu, Jeonju-si, Jeollabuk-do 54896, Korea

Luca Comuzzi
Private practice, via Raffaello 36/a, 31020 San Vendemiano (TV), Italy

Yun-Young Chan
Department of Dentistry, Inha International Medical Center, 424, Gonghang-ro, 84-gil, Unseo-dong, Jung-gu, Incheon 22382, Korea

Su-Hwan Kim
Department of Periodontics, Asan Medical Center, 88, Olympic-ro 43-gil, Songpa-gu, Seoul 05505, Korea
Department of Dentistry, University of Ulsan College of Medicine, 88, Olympic-ro 43-gil, Songpa-gu, Seoul 05505, Korea

Jeong-Ho Yun
Department of Periodontology, College of Dentistry and Institute of Oral Bioscience, Jeonbuk National University, 567, Baekje-daero, Deokjin-gu, Jeonju-si, Jeollabuk-do 54896, Korea
Research Institute of Clinical Medicine of Jeonbuk National University-Biomedical Research Institute of Jeonbuk National University Hospital, 20, Geonjiro, Deokjin-gu, Jeonju-si, Jeollabuk-do 54907, Korea

Saverio Cosola
Oral Surgery Unit, Department of Stomatology, Faculty of Medicine and Dentistry, University of Valencia, 13, 46010 Valencia, Spain
Tuscan Stomatologic Institute, via Aurelia, 335, 55041 Lido di Camaiore, Italy

Simone Marconcini, Michela Boccuzzi and Ugo Covani
Tuscan Stomatologic Institute, via Aurelia, 335, 55041 Lido di Camaiore, Italy

Giovanni Battista Menchini Fabris
Tuscan Stomatologic Institute, via Aurelia, 335, 55041 Lido di Camaiore, Italy
Department of Stomatology, University of Studies Guglielmo Marconi, 44, 00193 Roma, Italy

Miguel Peñarrocha-Diago and David Peñarrocha-Oltra
Oral Surgery Unit, Department of Stomatology, Faculty of Medicine and Dentistry, University of Valencia, 13, 46010 Valencia, Spain

Wonsik Lee
Advanced Process and Materials R&D Group, Korea Institute of Industrial Technology, 7-47 Songdo-dong, Yeonsu-gu, Incheon 406-840, Korea

Margherita Tumedei and Giovanna Iezzi
Department of Medical, Oral and Biotechnological Sciences, University "G. D'Annunzio" of Chieti-Pescara, 66100 Chieti, Italy

Adriano Piattelli
Department of Medical, Oral and Biotechnological Sciences, University "G. D'Annunzio" of Chieti-Pescara, 66100 Chieti, Italy
Catholic University of San Antonio de Murcia (UCAM), Av. de los Jerónimos, Guadalupe, 135 30107 Murcia, Spain
Villaserena Foundation for Research, 65121 Città Sant'Angelo (Pescara), Italy

Andrés Parrilla-Almansa and Silvia Sánchez-Sánchez
Image Diagnostic Service, Virgen de la Arrixaca University Hospital, El Palmar, 30120 Murcia, Spain

Carlos Alberto González-Bermúdez
Faculty of Medicine, Universidad de Murcia, Instituto Murciano de Investigación Biosanitaria Virgen de la Arrixaca (IMIB-Arrixaca), 30.100 Murcia, Spain

Luis Meseguer-Olmo
Department of Orthopaedic Surgery and Trauma, School of Medicine, Lab of Regeneration and Tissue Repair, UCAM-Universidad Catolica San Antonio de Murcia, Guadalupe, 30107 Murcia, Spain

Carlos Manuel Martínez-Cáceres
Pathology Unit, Biomedical Research Institute of Murcia (IMIB-Arrixaca-UMU), El Palmar, 30120 Murcia, Spain

Francisco Martínez-Martínez
Orthopaedic and Trauma Service, Virgen de la Arrixaca University Hospital, El Palmar, 30120 Murcia, Spain

José Luis Calvo-Guirado
Department of Oral Surgery and Implant Dentistry, Faculty of Health Sciences, UCAM- Universidad Católica San Antonio de Murcia, Guadalupe, 30107 Murcia, Spain

Juan José Piñero de Armas
Cátedra Internacional de Análisis Estadístico y Big Data, Universidad Católica de Murcia, 30107 Murcia, Spain

Juan Manuel Aragoneses
Department of Dental Research in Universidad Federico Henriquez y Carvajal (UFHEC), Santo Domingo 10107, Dominican Republic

Nuria García-Carrillo
Department of Medicina Oral, Facultad de Medicina, Universidad de Murcia, Instituto Murciano de Investigación Biosanitaria Virgen de la Arrixaca (IMIB-Arrixaca), 30.100 Murcia, Spain

Piedad N. De Aza
Instituto de Bioingenieria, Universidad Miguel Hernandez, 03202 Elche, Spain

Lilian C. Anami
Department of Dentistry, Santo Amaro University (UNISA), São Paulo 04743-030, Brazil

Jung-Yoo Choi
Dental Research Institute, Seoul National University, Seoul 03080, Korea

Jae-Il Park
Animal Facility of Aging Science, Korea Basic Science Institute, Gwangju 61186, Korea

Yong-Seok Jang, Min-Ho Lee and Tae-Sung Bae
Department of Dental Biomaterials, Institute of Biodegradable Materials, BK21 plus Program, School of Dentistry, Chonbuk National University, Jeonju 54896, Korea

Sang-Hoon Oh
Haruan Dental Clinic, Department of Dental Biomaterials, Institute of Biodegradable Materials, BK21 plus Program, School of Dentistry, Chonbuk National University, Jeonju 54896, Korea

Won-Suck Oh
Department of Biologic and Materials Sciences Division of Prosthodontics, School of Dentistry, University of Michigan, Ann Arbor, MI 48109, USA

Jung-Jin Lee
Department of Prosthodontics, Institute of Oral Bio-Science, School of Dentistry, Chonbuk National University and Research Institute of Clinical Medicine of Chonbuk National University-Biomedical Research Institute of Chonbuk National University Hospital, Jeonju 54907, Korea

João P. M. Tribst, Amanda M. O. Dal Piva, Alexandre L. S. Borges and Marco A. Bottino
Department of Dental Materials and Prosthodontics, São Paulo State University (Unesp/SJC), Institute of Science and Technology, São José dos Campos 12245-000, Brazil

Taek-Ka Kwon
Division of Prosthodontics, Department of Dentistry, St. Catholic Hospital, Catholic University of Korea, Suwon 16247, Korea

Cornelis J. Kleverlaan
Department of Dental Materials Science, Academic Centre for Dentistry Amsterdam (ACTA), Universiteit van Amsterdam and Vrije Universiteit, 1081 LA Amsterdam, The Netherlands

Ki-Seong Kim and Young-Jun Lim
Department of Prosthodontics and Dental Research Institute, School of Dentistry, Seoul National University, Seoul 03080, Korea

Ricardo Trindade and Ann Wennerberg
Department of Prosthodontics, Faculty of Odontology, The Sahlgrenska Academy, University of Gothenburg, 405 30 Gothenburg, Sweden

Xing Yin and Jingtao Li
State Key Laboratory of Oral Diseases & National Clinical Research Center for Oral Diseases, West China Hospital of Stomatology, Sichuan University, Chengdu 610041, China
Division of Plastic and Reconstructive Surgery, Department of Surgery, Stanford School of Medicine, Stanford, CA 94305, USA

Waldemar Hoffmann and Angelines Gasser
Nobel Biocare Services AG, Zurich-Airport, 8058 Zurich, Switzerland

John B. Brunski and Jill A. Helms
Division of Plastic and Reconstructive Surgery, Department of Surgery, Stanford School of Medicine, Stanford, CA 94305, USA

Luis Amengual-Peñafiel
Dental Implantology Unit, Hospital Leonardo Guzmán, Antofagasta 1240835, Chile

Pentti Tengvall
Department of Biomaterials, Institute of Clinical Sciences, University of Gothenburg, 405 30 Gothenburg, Sweden

Francisco Marchesani-Carrasco and María Costanza Jara-Sepúlveda
Clínica Marchesani, Concepción 4070566, Chile

Leopoldo Parada-Pozas
Regenerative Medicine Center, Hospital Clínico de Viña del Mar, Viña del Mar 2520626, Chile

Ricardo Cartes-Velásquez
School of Dentistry, Universidad Andres Bello, Concepción 4300866, Chile
Institute of Biomedical Sciences, Universidad Autónoma de Chile, Temuco 4810101, Chile

Alberto Monjesz
Department of Periodontology, Universitat Internacional de Catalunya, 08195 Barcelona, Spain
Division of Periodontics, CICOM Periodoncia, 06011 Badajoz, Badajoz, Spain Santiago de Compostela, Spain

Angel Insua
Division of Periodontics, CICOM Periodoncia, 06011 Badajoz, Badajoz, Spain Santiago de Compostela, Spain

Hom-Lay Wang
Department of Periodontics and Oral Medicine, University of Michigan School of Dentistry, Ann Arbor, MI 48109, USA

Ricardo Trindade and Ann Wennerberg
Department of Prosthodontics, Institute of Odontology, The Sahlgrenska Academy, University of Gothenburg, 405 30 Gothenburg, Sweden

Silvia Galli
Department of Prosthodontics, Faculty of Odontology, Malmö University, 205 06 Malmö, Sweden

Zdenka Prgomet
Department of Oral Pathology, Faculty of Odontology, Malmö University, 205 06 Malmö, Sweden

Manuel Brañes-Aroca
Faculty of Sciences, Universidad de Chile, Santiago 7800003, Chile

Jung-Yoo Choi and Young-Jun Jeon
Dental Research Institute, Seoul National University, Seoul 03080, Korea

Tomas Albrektsson
Department of Biomaterials, Sahlgrenska Academy, University of Gothenburg, 40530 Gothenburg, Sweden
Department of Prosthodontics, Faculty of Odontology, Malmö University, 21118 Malmö, Sweden
Department of Biomaterials, Institute of Clinical Sciences, University of Gothenburg, 405 30 Gothenburg, Sweden
Department of Prosthodontics, Faculty of Odontology, Malmö University, 205 06 Malmö, Sweden

In-Sung Luke Yeo
Department of Prosthodontics, School of Dentistry and Dental Research Institute, Seoul National University, 101 Daehak-ro, Jongro-gu, Seoul 03080, Korea

Index

Printed in the USA
CPSIA information can be obtained
at www.ICGtesting.com
JSHW051358091023
49903JS00006B/192